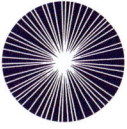

AMERICAN ACADEMY
OF OPHTHALMOLOGY®

13

Refractive Surgery

Last major revision 2017–2018

2018-2019
BCSC

Basic and Clinical Science Course™

Protecting Sight. Empowering Lives.®

The American Academy of Ophthalmology is accredited by the Accreditation Council for Continuing Medical Education (ACCME) to provide continuing medical education for physicians.

The American Academy of Ophthalmology designates this enduring material for a maximum of 10 *AMA PRA Category 1 Credits*™. Physicians should claim only the credit commensurate with the extent of their participation in the activity.

CME expiration date: June 1, 2020. *AMA PRA Category 1 Credits*™ may be claimed only once between June 1, 2017, and the expiration date.

BCSC® volumes are designed to increase the physician's ophthalmic knowledge through study and review. Users of this activity are encouraged to read the text and then answer the study questions provided at the back of the book.

To claim *AMA PRA Category 1 Credits*™ upon completion of this activity, learners must demonstrate appropriate knowledge and participation in the activity by taking the posttest for Section 13 and achieving a score of 80% or higher. For further details, please see the instructions for requesting CME credit at the back of the book.

The Academy provides this material for educational purposes only. It is not intended to represent the only or best method or procedure in every case, nor to replace a physician's own judgment or give specific advice for case management. Including all indications, contraindications, side effects, and alternative agents for each drug or treatment is beyond the scope of this material. All information and recommendations should be verified, prior to use, with current information included in the manufacturers' package inserts or other independent sources, and considered in light of the patient's condition and history. Reference to certain drugs, instruments, and other products in this course is made for illustrative purposes only and is not intended to constitute an endorsement of such. Some material may include information on applications that are not considered community standard, that reflect indications not included in approved FDA labeling, or that are approved for use only in restricted research settings. **The FDA has stated that it is the responsibility of the physician to determine the FDA status of each drug or device he or she wishes to use, and to use them with appropriate, informed patient consent in compliance with applicable law.** The Academy specifically disclaims any and all liability for injury or other damages of any kind, from negligence or otherwise, for any and all claims that may arise from the use of any recommendations or other information contained herein.

AAO, AAOE, American Academy of Ophthalmology, Basic and Clinical Science Course, BCSC, EyeCare America, EyeNet, EyeSmart, EyeWiki, Femtocenter, Focal Points, IRIS, ISRS, OKAP, ONE, Ophthalmic Technology Assessments, *Ophthalmology, Ophthalmology Retina,* Preferred Practice Pattern, ProVision, The Ophthalmic News & Education Network, and the AAO logo (shown on cover) and tagline (Protecting Sight. Empowering Lives.) are, among other marks, the registered trademarks and trademarks of the American Academy of Ophthalmology.

Cover image: From BCSC Section 12, *Retina and Vitreous.* End-stage chorioretinal atrophy in pathologic myopia. *(Courtesy of Richard F. Spaide, MD.)*

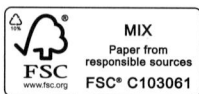

MIX
Paper from
responsible sources
FSC
www.fsc.org   FSC® C103061

Printed in the United States of America.

Basic and Clinical Science Course

Louis B. Cantor, MD, Indianapolis, Indiana, *Senior Secretary for Clinical Education*

Christopher J. Rapuano, MD, Philadelphia, Pennsylvania, *Secretary for Lifelong Learning and Assessment*

George A. Cioffi, MD, New York, New York, *BCSC Course Chair*

Section 13

Faculty

M. Bowes Hamill, MD, *Chair,* Houston, Texas

Renato Ambrósio Jr, MD, PhD, Rio de Janeiro, Brazil

Gregg J. Berdy, MD, St Louis, Missouri

Richard S. Davidson, MD, Denver, Colorado

Parag A. Majmudar, MD, Chicago, Illinois

Sherman W. Reeves, MD, MPH, Minnetonka, Minnesota

Neda Shamie, MD, Century City, California

George O. Waring IV, MD, Charleston, South Carolina

The Academy wishes to acknowledge the *American Society of Cataract and Refractive Surgeons (ASCRS)* for recommending faculty members to the BCSC Section 13 committee.

The Academy also wishes to acknowledge the following committees for review of this edition:

Committee on Aging: Jean R. Hausheer, MD, Lawton, Oklahoma; Sumitra S. Khandelwal, MD, Houston, Texas

Vision Rehabilitation Committee: Deepthi M. Reddy, MD, Houston, Texas

Practicing Ophthalmologists Advisory Committee for Education: Bradley D. Fouraker, MD, *Primary Reviewer,* Tampa, Florida; Edward K. Isbey III, *Chair,* Asheville, North Carolina; Alice L. Bashinsky, MD, Asheville, North Carolina; David J. Browning, MD, PhD, Charlotte, North Carolina; Steven J. Grosser, MD, Golden Valley, Minnesota; Stephen R. Klapper, MD, Carmel, Indiana; James A. Savage, MD, Memphis, Tennessee; Michelle S. Ying, MD, Ladson, South Carolina

EB

European Board of Ophthalmology: Jesper Hjortdal, MD, PhD, *EBO Chair,* Aarhus, Denmark; Marie-José Tassignon, MD, PhD, FEBO, *EBO Liaison,* Antwerp, Belgium; Roberto Bellucci, MD, Verona, Italy; Daniel Epstein, MD, PhD, Bern, Switzerland; José L. Güell, MD, FEBO, Barcelona, Spain; Markus Kohlhaas, MD, Dortmund, Germany; Rudy M.M.A. Nuijts, MD, PhD, Maastricht, the Netherlands

Financial Disclosures

Omega Ophthalmics (C), Perfect Lens (C), Refocus Group (C), RevitalVision (C), Strathspey Crown (O), Visiometrics (C)

The other authors and reviewers state that within the past 12 months prior to their contributions to this CME activity and for the duration of development, they have had no financial interest in or other relationship with any entity discussed in this course that produces, markets, resells, or distributes ophthalmic health care goods or services consumed by or used in patients, or with any competing commercial product or service.

*C = consultant fees, paid advisory boards, or fees for attending a meeting; L = lecture fees (honoraria), travel fees, or reimbursements when speaking at the invitation of a commercial sponsor; O = equity ownership/stock options of publicly or privately traded firms (excluding mutual funds) with manufacturers of commercial ophthalmic products or commercial ophthalmic services; P = patents and/or royalties that might be viewed as creating a potential conflict of interest; S = grant support for the past year (all sources) and all sources used for a specific talk or manuscript with no time limitation

Recent Past Faculty

Elizabeth A. Davis, MD
Eric D. Donnenfeld, MD
J. Bradley Randleman, MD
Christopher J. Rapuano, MD
Steven I. Rosenfeld, MD
Donald T.H. Tan, MD
Brian S. Boxer Wachler, MD

In addition, the Academy gratefully acknowledges the contributions of numerous past faculty and advisory committee members who have played an important role in the development of previous editions of the Basic and Clinical Science Course.

American Academy of Ophthalmology Staff

Dale E. Fajardo, EdD, MBA, *Vice President, Education*
Beth Wilson, *Director, Continuing Professional Development*
Ann McGuire, *Acquisitions and Development Manager*
Stephanie Tanaka, *Publications Manager*
D. Jean Ray, *Production Manager*
Kimberly Torgerson, *Publications Editor*
Beth Collins, *Medical Editor*
Naomi Ruiz, *Publications Specialist*

American Academy of Ophthalmology
655 Beach Street
Box 7424
San Francisco, CA 94120-7424

Contents

6   Photoablation: Complications and Adverse Effects . . . 101

General Introduction

The Basic and Clinical Science Course (BCSC) is designed to meet the needs of residents and practitioners for a comprehensive yet concise curriculum of the field of ophthalmology. The BCSC has developed from its original brief outline format, which relied heavily on outside readings, to a more convenient and educationally useful self-contained text. The Academy updates and revises the course annually, with the goals of integrating the basic science and clinical practice of ophthalmology and of keeping ophthalmologists current with new developments in the various subspecialties.

The BCSC incorporates the effort and expertise of more than 90 ophthalmologists, organized into 13 Section faculties, working with Academy editorial staff. In addition, the course continues to benefit from many lasting contributions made by the faculties of previous editions. Members of the Academy Practicing Ophthalmologists Advisory Committee for Education, Committee on Aging, and Vision Rehabilitation Committee review every volume before major revisions. Members of the European Board of Ophthalmology, organized into Section faculties, also review each volume before major revisions, focusing primarily on differences between American and European ophthalmology practice.

Organization of the Course

The Basic and Clinical Science Course comprises 13 volumes, incorporating fundamental ophthalmic knowledge, subspecialty areas, and special topics:

1 Update on General Medicine
2 Fundamentals and Principles of Ophthalmology
3 Clinical Optics
4 Ophthalmic Pathology and Intraocular Tumors
5 Neuro-Ophthalmology
6 Pediatric Ophthalmology and Strabismus
7 Orbit, Eyelids, and Lacrimal System
8 External Disease and Cornea
9 Intraocular Inflammation and Uveitis
10 Glaucoma
11 Lens and Cataract
12 Retina and Vitreous
13 Refractive Surgery

In addition, a comprehensive Master Index allows the reader to easily locate subjects throughout the entire series.

References

Readers who wish to explore specific topics in greater detail may consult the references cited within each chapter and listed in the Basic Texts section at the back of the book.

These references are intended to be selective rather than exhaustive, chosen by the BCSC faculty as being important, current, and readily available to residents and practitioners.

Multimedia

This edition of Section 13, *Refractive Surgery,* includes videos related to topics covered in the book. The videos were selected by members of the BCSC faculty and are available to readers of the print and electronic versions of Section 13 (www.aao.org/bcscvideo _section13). Mobile-device users can scan the QR code below (a QR-code reader must already be installed on the device) to access the video content.

Self-Assessment and CME Credit

Each volume of the BCSC is designed as an independent study activity for ophthalmology residents and practitioners. The learning objectives for this volume are given on page 1. The text, illustrations, and references provide the information necessary to achieve the objectives; the study questions allow readers to test their understanding of the material and their mastery of the objectives. Physicians who wish to claim CME credit for this educational activity may do so by following the instructions given at the end of the book.

Conclusion

The Basic and Clinical Science Course has expanded greatly over the years, with the addition of much new text, numerous illustrations, and video content. Recent editions have sought to place a greater emphasis on clinical applicability while maintaining a solid foundation in basic science. As with any educational program, it reflects the experience of its authors. As its faculties change and medicine progresses, new viewpoints emerge on controversial subjects and techniques. Not all alternate approaches can be included in this series; as with any educational endeavor, the learner should seek additional sources, including Academy Preferred Practice Pattern Guidelines.

The BCSC faculty and staff continually strive to improve the educational usefulness of the course; you, the reader, can contribute to this ongoing process. If you have any suggestions or questions about the series, please do not hesitate to contact the faculty or the editors.

The authors, editors, and reviewers hope that your study of the BCSC will be of lasting value and that each Section will serve as a practical resource for quality patient care.

Objectives

Upon completion of BCSC Section 13, *Refractive Surgery,* the reader should be able to

- state the contributions of the cornea's shape and tissue layers to the optics of the eye and how these components are affected biomechanically by different types of keratorefractive procedures

- describe the basic concepts of wavefront analysis and its relationship to different types of optical aberrations

- identify the general types of lasers used in refractive surgeries

- explain the steps—including medical and social history, ocular examination, and ancillary testing—in evaluating whether a patient is an appropriate candidate for refractive surgery

- for incisional keratorefractive surgery (radial keratotomy, transverse keratotomy, arcuate keratotomy, and limbal relaxing incisions), describe the history, patient selection, surgical techniques, outcomes, and complications

- list the various types of corneal onlays and inlays that have been used for refractive correction

- for surface ablation procedures, describe patient selection, epithelial removal, refractive outcomes, and complications

- describe patient selection, surgical techniques, outcomes, and complications for laser in situ keratomileusis (LASIK)

- describe the different methods for creating a LASIK flap using a microkeratome or a femtosecond laser as well as the instrumentation and possible complications associated with each

- explain recent developments in the application of wavefront technology to surface ablation and LASIK

- for conductive keratoplasty, state a brief overview of history, patient selection, and safety issues

- describe how intraocular surgical procedures, including refractive lens exchange with intraocular lens (IOL) implantation or phakic IOL implantation, can be used in refractive correction, with or without corneal intervention

- describe the different types of IOLs used for refractive correction

- explain the leading theories of accommodation and how they relate to potential treatment of presbyopia

- describe nonaccommodative and accommodative approaches to the treatment of presbyopia

- state considerations for, and possible contraindications to, refractive surgery in patients with preexisting ocular and/or systemic disease

- list some of the effects of prior refractive procedures on later IOL calculations, contact lens wear, and ocular surgery

Introduction

Of all the subspecialties within ophthalmology, refractive surgery may be the most rapidly evolving. However, the language associated with the recording of visual acuity is also changing. For this edition, the BCSC Section 13 Committee uses the following conventions with respect to the recording of corrected and uncorrected visual acuity. Where the Section used the term *corrected distance visual acuity (CDVA)* in the previous edition, it now uses *best-corrected visual acuity (BCVA),* followed by the newer term on first mention within a chapter. Similarly, *uncorrected distance visual acuity (UDVA)* will be replaced by *uncorrected visual acuity (UCVA).* A visual acuity conversion chart is available on the inside front cover.

Refractive surgeons, as in all medical specialties, also use numerous abbreviations and acronyms in discussing and describing their field, especially for the continually emerging and changing refractive procedures. The following list of frequently used terms is included as an aid to readers while reading this text as well as the refractive surgery literature in general.

Abbreviations and Acronyms Common to Refractive Surgery

ACS anterior ciliary sclerotomy

AHWP Asian Harmonization Working Party (for device regulation)

AK arcuate keratotomy

ArF argon-fluoride (laser)

ASA advanced surface ablation (synonym for *photorefractive keratectomy,* PRK)

BCVA best-corrected visual acuity (also called *corrected distance visual acuity,* **CDVA**)

CCD charge-coupled device

CCL corneal crosslinking (also CXL)

CDVA corrected distance visual acuity (also called *best-corrected visual acuity,* **BCVA**)

CE mark Conformité Européene mark (product approval used in European countries, similar to US FDA approval)

CK conductive keratoplasty

CXL corneal crosslinking (also CCL)

D diopter

DALK deep anterior lamellar keratoplasty

DLK diffuse lamellar keratitis

DMEK Descemet membrane endothelial keratoplasty

DSEK Descemet stripping endothelial keratoplasty

EDOF extended depth of focus (intraocular lens)

Epi-LASIK epipolis laser in situ keratomileusis

Femto-LASIK femtosecond laser in situ keratomileusis

FLEx femtosecond lenticule extraction

GAT Goldmann applanation tonometry

GHTF Global Harmonization Task Force (international medical device regulation)

HDE Humanitarian Device Exemption

Hex K hexagonal keratotomy

Ho:YAG holmium-yttrium-aluminum-garnet (laser)

ICL implantable collamer lens

ICRS intrastromal corneal ring segments

IOL intraocular lens

IOP intraocular pressure

I–S inferior–superior (value)

KC keratoconus

LASEK laser subepithelial keratomileusis

LASIK laser in situ keratomileusis

logMAR base-10 logarithm of the minimum angle of resolution

LRI limbal relaxing incision

LTK laser thermokeratoplasty

MFIOL multifocal intraocular lens

Nd:YAG neodymium-doped yttrium aluminum garnet (laser)

OCT optical coherence tomography

PCO posterior capsule opacification

PERK Prospective Evaluation of Radial Keratotomy (study)

PIOL phakic intraocular lens

PISK pressure-induced stromal keratopathy

PKP penetrating keratoplasty

PMD pellucid marginal degeneration

PMMA polymethyl methacrylate

PRK photorefractive keratectomy

PTK phototherapeutic keratectomy

ReLEx refractive lenticule extraction

RGP rigid gas-permeable (contact lenses)

RK radial keratotomy

RLE refractive lens exchange

RMS root mean square

RSB residual stromal bed

SIM K corneal power (K) simulation measurements

SMILE small-incision lenticule extraction

UCVA uncorrected visual acuity (also called *uncorrected distance visual acuity*, **UDVA**)

UDVA uncorrected distance visual acuity (also called *uncorrected visual acuity*, **UCVA**)

CHAPTER 1

The Science of Refractive Surgery

The goal of refractive surgery is to reduce dependence on contact lenses or glasses for use in routine daily activities. A wide variety of surgical techniques and technologies are available, and all require an appropriate preoperative evaluation to determine the best technique and ensure the optimal outcome for each patient individually.

Refractive surgical procedures can be categorized broadly as *corneal* or *intraocular* (Table 1-1). Keratorefractive (corneal) procedures include incisional, laser ablation, lamellar implantation, corneal collagen shrinkage, and corneal crosslinking techniques. Intraocular refractive procedures include phakic intraocular lens (PIOL) implantation and cataract surgery or refractive lens exchange (RLE) with implantation of a monofocal, toric, multifocal, accommodative, or extended depth of focus intraocular lens. Each technique has advantages and disadvantages and should be specifically matched to the patient.

This chapter reviews the fundamental corneal properties relevant to refractive surgery (focusing on keratorefractive procedures), corneal imaging for refractive surgery, and the effects of keratorefractive surgery on the cornea. It includes review of the optical principles discussed in BCSC Section 3, *Clinical Optics;* refractive errors (both lower- and higher-order aberrations); corneal biomechanics; corneal topography and tomography; wavefront analysis; laser biophysics and laser–tissue interactions; corneal biomechanical changes after surgery; and corneal wound healing.

Corneal Optics

The air–tear-film interface provides the majority of the optical power of the eye. Although a normal tear film has minimal deleterious effect, an abnormal tear film can have a dramatic impact on vision. For example, either excess tear film (eg, epiphora) or altered tear film (eg, dry eye or blepharitis) can decrease visual quality.

The optical power of the eye derives primarily from the anterior corneal curvature, which produces about two-thirds of the eye's refractive power, approximately +48.00 diopters (D). The overall corneal power is less (approximately +42.00 D) as a result of the negative power (approximately –6.00 D) of the posterior corneal surface. Standard keratometers and Placido-based (ie, based on an analysis of corneal reflections of a concentric ring image) corneal topography instruments measure the anterior corneal radius of curvature and *estimate* total corneal power from these front-surface measurements. These instruments extrapolate the central corneal power *(K)* by measuring the rate of change in curvature from the paracentral 3–4-mm zone; this factor takes on crucial importance

Table 1-1 Overview of Refractive Procedures

Location	Type of Procedure	Specific Procedures	Common Abbreviations	Refractive Error Treated
Corneal	Incisional	Radial keratotomy	RK	Myopia (historical)
		Astigmatic keratotomy		
		Arcuate keratotomy	AK	Astigmatism
		Femtosecond laser-assisted arcuate keratotomy	FLAAK	Astigmatism
		Limbal relaxing incisions	LRI	Astigmatism
		Ruiz procedure		Astigmatism (historical)
		Hexagonal keratotomy	Hex K	Hyperopia (historical)
	Excimer laser	Surface ablation		Myopia, hyperopia, astigmatism
		Photorefractive keratectomy	PRK	+6.00 to −14.00 D
		Laser subepithelial keratomileusis	LASEK	+6.00 to −14.00 D
		Epipolis laser in situ keratomileusis	Epi-LASIK	+6.00 to −14.00 D
		Lamellar		
		Laser in situ keratomileusis	LASIK	+6.00 to −14.00 D
		Femtosecond laser in situ keratomileusis	Femto-LASIK	+6.00 to −14.00 D
		Refractive lenticule	ReLEx FLEx, SMILE	Investigational
	Nonlaser lamellar	Epikeratophakia, epikeratoplasty		Myopia, hyperopia, astigmatism (historical)
		Myopic keratomileusis		Myopia (historical)
		Intrastromal corneal ring segments	ICRS	Myopia, keratoconus
	Collagen shrinkage	Laser thermokeratoplasty	LTK	Hyperopia, astigmatism (historical)
		Conductive keratoplasty	CK	Hyperopia, astigmatism +0.75 to +3.25 D
	Corneal crosslinking		CCL, CXL	Keratoconus
Intraocular	Phakic	Anterior chamber phakic intraocular lens (IOL) implantation		Myopia (in development)
		Iris-fixated phakic IOL implantation		Myopia (−5.00 to −20.00 D)
		Posterior chamber phakic IOL implantation		Myopia (−3.00 to −20.00 D)
	Pseudophakic	Refractive lens exchange (multifocal/accommodating/extended depth of focus IOLs)	RLE	Myopia, hyperopia, presbyopia
		Refractive lens exchange (toric IOL)		Myopia, hyperopia, astigmatism

in the determination of IOL power after keratorefractive surgery (see Chapter 11). The normal cornea flattens from the center to the periphery by up to 4.00 D (this progressive flattening toward the peripheral cornea is referred to as a *prolate* shape) and is flatter nasally than temporally.

The majority of keratorefractive surgical procedures change the refractive state of the eye by altering corneal curvature. The tolerances involved in altering corneal dimensions are relatively small. For instance, changing the refractive status of the eye by 2.00 D may require altering the cornea's thickness by less than 30 μm. Thus, achieving predictable results is sometimes problematic because minuscule changes in the shape of the cornea may produce large changes in refraction.

Refractive Error: Optical Principles and Wavefront Analysis

One of the major applications of the wave theory of light is in wavefront analysis (see also BCSC Section 3, *Clinical Optics*). Currently, wavefront analysis can be performed clinically by 4 methods: Hartmann-Shack, Tscherning, thin-beam single-ray tracing, and optical path difference. Each method generates a detailed report of lower-order aberrations (sphere and cylinder) and higher-order aberrations (spherical aberration, coma, and trefoil, among others). This information is useful both in calculating custom ablations to enhance vision or correct optical problems and in explaining patients' visual symptoms.

Measurement of Wavefront Aberrations and Graphical Representations

Although several techniques are available for measuring wavefront aberrations, the most popular in clinical practice is based on the Hartmann-Shack wavefront sensor. With this device, a low-power laser beam is focused on the retina. A point on the retina acts as a point source, and the reflected light is then propagated back (anteriorly) through the optical elements of the eye to a detector. In an aberration-free eye, all the rays would emerge in parallel, and the reflected wavefront would be a flat plane. In reality, the wavefront is not flat. To determine the shape of the reflected wavefront, an array of lenses samples parts of the wavefront and focuses light on a detector (Fig 1-1A). The extent of the divergence of the lenslet images from their expected focal points determines the wavefront error (Fig 1-1B). Optical aberrations measured by the aberrometer can be resolved into a variety of basic *shapes,* the combination of which represents the total aberration of the patient's ocular system, just as conventional refractive error is a combination of sphere and cylinder.

Currently, wavefront aberrations are most commonly specified by *Zernike polynomials,* which are the mathematical formulas used to describe the surfaces shown in Figures 1-2 through 1-6. Each aberration may be positive or negative in value and induces predictable alterations in the image quality. The magnitude of these aberrations is expressed as a root mean square (RMS) error, which is the deviation of the wavefront averaged over the entire wavefront. The higher the RMS value is, the greater is the overall aberration for a given eye. The majority of patients have total RMS values less than 0.3 μm for a 6-mm pupil. Most higher-order Zernike coefficients have mean values close to zero. The most important Zernike coefficients affecting visual quality are coma, spherical aberration, and trefoil.

A   CCD image   CCD camera   Lenslet array

B

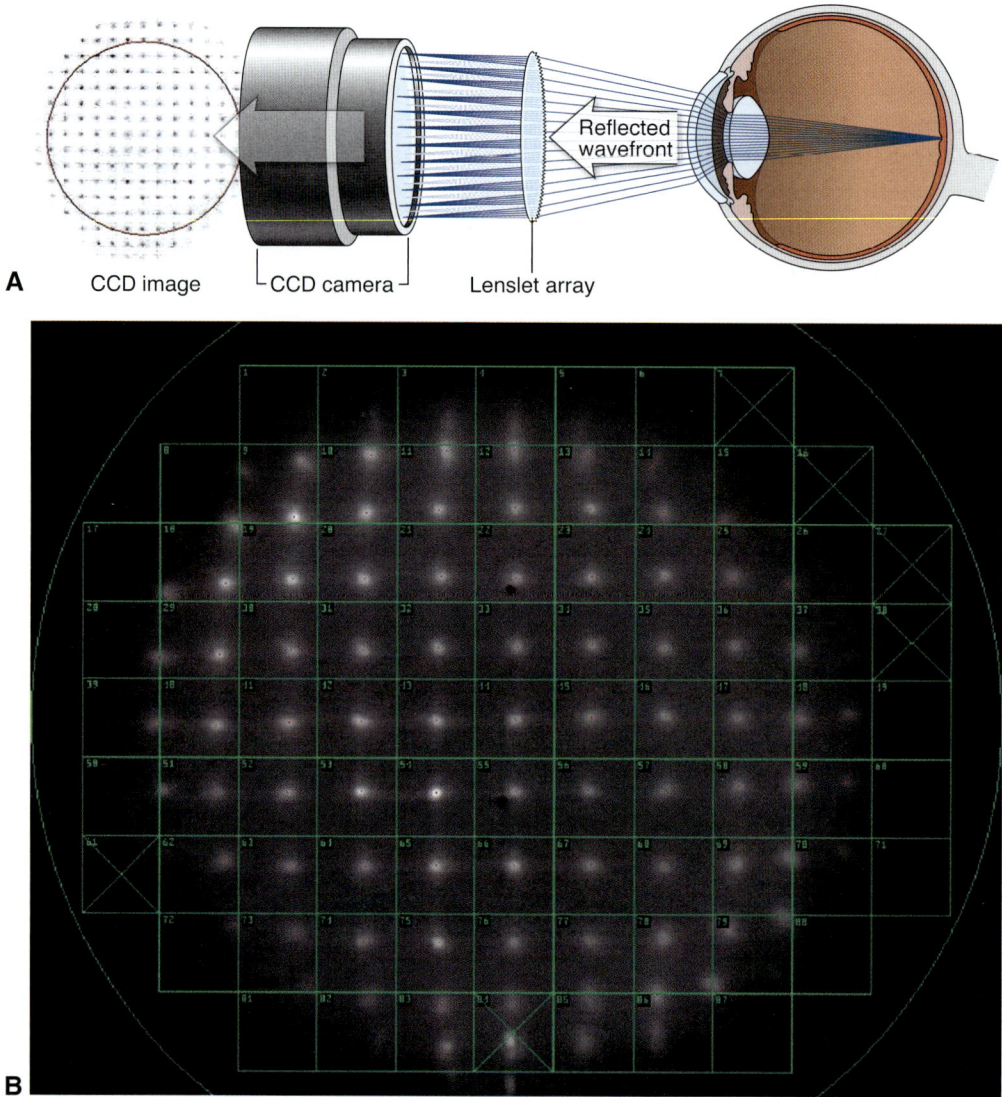

Figure 1-1   **A,** Schematic of a Hartmann-Shack wavefront sensor. As can be seen, the reflected wavefront passes through a grid of small lenses (the *lenslet array*), and the images formed are focused onto a charge-coupled device (CCD) chip. The degree of deviation of the focused images from the expected focal points determines the aberration and thus the wavefront error. **B,** An example of the images formed after the wavefront passes through the lenslet array. The green overlay lattice is registered to correspond to each lenslet in the array. *(Part A redrawn by Mark Miller from a schematic image courtesy of Abbott Medical Optics Inc.; part B reproduced from http://what-when-how.com; https://goo.gl/Asc06o.)*

Fourier analysis is an alternative method of evaluating the output from an aberrometer. Fourier analysis involves a sine wave–derived transformation of a complex shape. Compared with shapes derived from Zernike polynomial analysis, the shapes derived from Fourier analysis are more detailed, theoretically allowing for the measurement and treatment of more highly aberrant corneas.

Lower-Order Aberrations

Myopia, hyperopia, and regular astigmatism are all lower-order (second-order) aberrations that can be expressed as wavefront aberrations. Myopia produces *positive defocus* (Fig 1-2), whereas hyperopia produces *negative defocus.* Regular (cylindrical) astigmatism produces a wavefront aberration that has orthogonal (ie, facing at right angles) and oblique components (Fig 1-3). Other lower-order aberrations are non–visually significant aberrations known as *first-order aberrations,* such as vertical and horizontal prisms and zero-order aberrations (piston).

Higher-Order Aberrations

Wavefront aberration is highly dependent on pupil size, with increased higher-order aberrations apparent as the pupil dilates. Higher-order aberrations also increase with age, although the clinical effect is thought to be balanced by the increasing miosis of the pupil with age. Although lower-order aberrations decrease after laser vision correction, higher-order aberrations, particularly spherical aberration and coma, may increase after conventional surface ablation, laser in situ keratomileusis (LASIK), or radial keratotomy (RK) for myopia. This increase is correlated with the degree of preoperative myopia. After standard hyperopic laser vision correction, higher-order aberrations increase even more than they do in myopic eyes but in the opposite (toward negative values) direction. Compared with conventional treatments, customized excimer laser treatments may decrease the number of induced higher-order aberrations and provide a higher quality of vision, particularly in mesopic conditions.

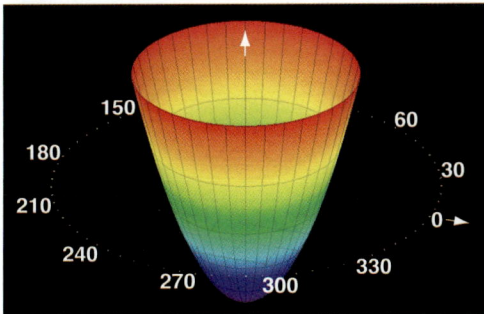

Figure 1-2 Zernike polynomial representation of defocus. *Arrows* indicate z axis (*arrow* emerging from cone) and zero axis. *(Courtesy of Tracey Technologies.)*

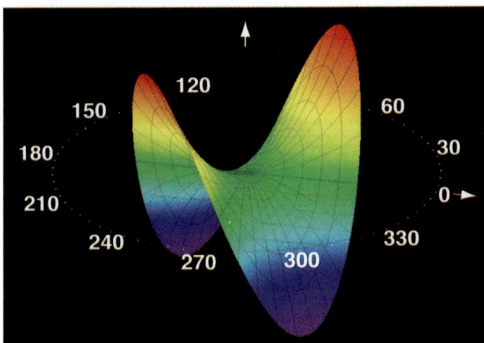

Figure 1-3 Zernike polynomial representation of astigmatism. *(Courtesy of Tracey Technologies.)*

Spherical aberration

When peripheral light rays impacting a lens or the cornea focus in front of more central rays, the effect is called spherical aberration (Fig 1-4). Clinically, this radially symmetric fourth-order aberration is the cause of night myopia and is commonly increased after RK and myopic LASIK and surface ablation. It results in halos around point images. Spherical aberration is the most significant higher-order aberration. It may increase depth of field but decreases contrast sensitivity.

Coma and trefoil

With coma, a third-order aberration, rays at one edge of the pupil come into focus before rays at the opposite edge do (Fig 1-5). As can be seen by examining the illustrations, light rays entering the system do not focus on a plane; rather, one edge of the incoming beam focuses either in front of or behind the opposite edge of the beam. If one were to examine the image generated by an incoming light beam passing through an optical system with a coma aberration, the image would appear "smeared," looking somewhat like a comet with a zone of sharp focus at one edge of the image tailing off to a fuzzy focus at the opposite edge of the beam. Coma is common in patients with decentered corneal grafts, keratoconus, and decentered laser ablations.

Trefoil, also a third-order aberration, can occur after refractive surgery. Trefoil produces less degradation in image quality than does coma of similar RMS magnitude (Fig 1-6).

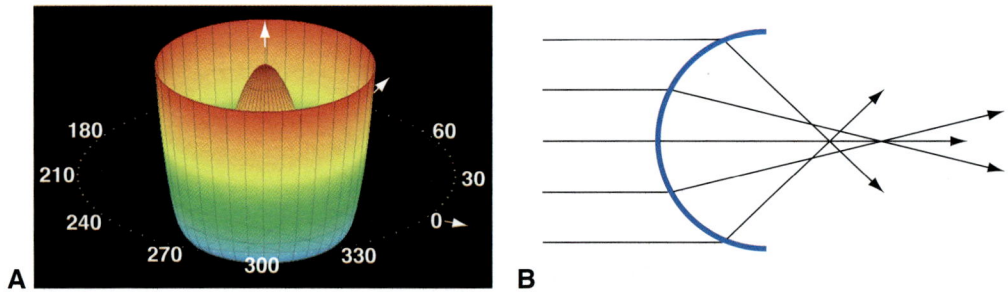

Figure 1-4 **A,** Zernike polynomial representation of spherical aberration. **B,** A schematic diagram of spherical aberration. Parallel rays impacting a spherical lens are refracted more acutely in the periphery than in the center of the lens. *(Part A courtesy of Tracey Technologies; part B developed by M. Bowes Hamill, MD.)*

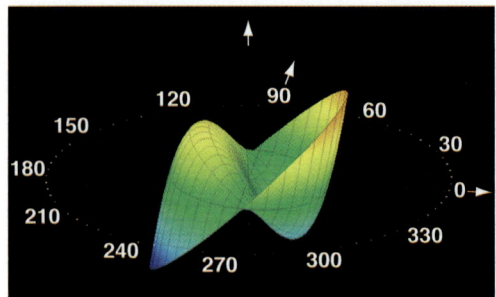

Figure 1-5 Zernike polynomial representation of coma. *(Courtesy of Tracey Technologies.)*

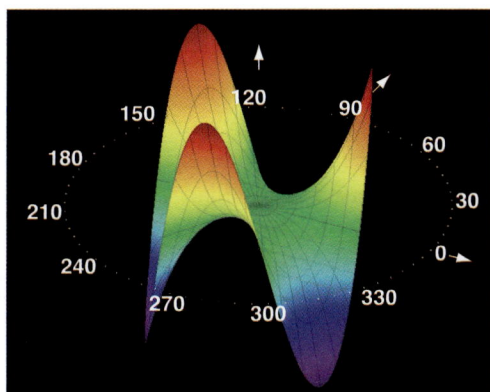

Figure 1-6 Zernike polynomial representation of trefoil. *(Courtesy of Tracey Technologies.)*

Other higher-order aberrations

There are numerous other higher-order aberrations, of which only a small number are of clinical interest. As knowledge of surgically induced aberration increases, more of the basic types of aberrations may become clinically relevant.

Effect of excimer laser ablation on higher-order aberrations

Whereas use of conventional (non–wavefront-guided) excimer laser ablations typically increases higher-order aberrations, wavefront-optimized, wavefront-guided, and topography-guided ablations tend to induce fewer higher-order aberrations and may, in principle, be able to reduce preexisting higher-order optical aberrations.

Holland, S, Lin DTC, Tan JC. Topography-guided laser refractive surgery. Curr Opin Ophthalmol. 2013;24(4): 302–309.

Klyce SD, Karon MD, Smolek MK. Advantages and disadvantages of the Zernike expansion for representing wave aberration of the normal and aberrated eye. *J Refract Surg.* 2004; 20(5):S537–S541.

Salmon TO, van de Pol C. Normal-eye Zernike coefficients and root-mean-square wavefront errors. *J Cataract Refract Surg.* 2006;32(12):2064–2074.

Corneal Biomechanics

The cornea consists of collagen fibrils arranged in approximately 200 parallel lamellae that extend from limbus to limbus. The fibrils are oriented at angles to the fibrils in adjacent lamellae. This network of collagen is responsible for the mechanical strength of the cornea. The fibrils are more closely packed in the anterior two-thirds of the cornea and in the axial, or prepupillary, cornea than they are in the peripheral cornea (see BCSC Section 8, *External Disease and Cornea*).

Structural differences between the anterior and posterior stroma affect the biomechanical behavior of the cornea. These include differences in glycosaminoglycans as well as more lamellar interweaving in the anterior corneal stroma; thus, the anterior cornea swells far less than the posterior cornea does. Stress within the tissue is partly related to intraocular pressure (IOP) but not in a linear manner under physiologic conditions (normal IOP range).When the cornea is in a dehydrated state, stress is distributed princi-pally to the posterior layers or uniformly over the entire cornea. When the cornea is edem-atous, the anterior lamellae take up most of the strain. Most keratorefractive procedures alter corneal biomechanical properties either directly (eg, RK weakening the cornea to induce refractive change) or indirectly (eg, excimer laser surgery weakening the cornea by means of tissue removal). The lack of uniformity of biomechanical load throughout the cornea explains the variation in corneal biomechanical response to different keratorefrac-tive procedures. For instance, LASIK has a greater overall effect than does photorefractive keratectomy (PRK) on corneal biomechanics, not only because a lamellar flap is created but also because the laser ablation occurs in the deeper, weaker corneal stroma (a more detailed discussion can be found later in this chapter and in Chapter 5).

Corneal Imaging for Keratorefractive Surgery

Corneal shape, curvature, and thickness profiles can be generated from a variety of technologies such as Placido disk–based systems and elevation-based systems (includ-ing scanning-slit systems and Scheimpflug imaging). Each technology conveys different information about corneal curvature, anatomy, and biomechanical function. In addi-tion, computerized topographic and tomographic systems may display other data: pupil size and location, indices estimating regular and irregular astigmatism, estimates of the probability of having keratoconus, simulated keratometry, and corneal asphericity. Other topography systems may integrate wavefront aberrometry data with topographic data. Although this additional information can be useful in preoperative surgical evaluations, no automated screening system can supplant clinical experience in evaluating corneal imaging.

The degree of asphericity of the cornea can be quantified by determining the Q value, with $Q = 0$ for spherical corneas, $Q < 0$ for prolate corneas (relatively flatter periphery), and $Q > 0$ for oblate corneas (relatively steeper periphery). A normal cornea is prolate, with an asphericity Q value of -0.26. Prolate corneas minimize spherical aberrations by virtue of their relatively flat peripheral curve. Conversely, oblate corneal contours, in which the peripheral cornea is steeper than the center, increase the probability of having induced positive spherical aberrations. After conventional refractive surgery for myopia, with the resulting flattening of the corneal center, corneal asphericity increases in the oblate direc-tion, which may cause degradation of the optics of the eye.

Corneal Topography

Corneal topography provides highly detailed information about corneal curvature. To-pography is evaluated using keratoscopic images, which are captured from Placido disk patterns that are reflected from the tear film overlying the corneal surface and then con-verted to computerized color scales (Fig 1-7). Because the image is generated from the anterior surface of the tear film, irregularities in tear composition or volume can have a major impact on the quality and results of a Placido disk–based system. Because of this effect, reviewing the Placido image (image of the mires) prior to interpreting the maps

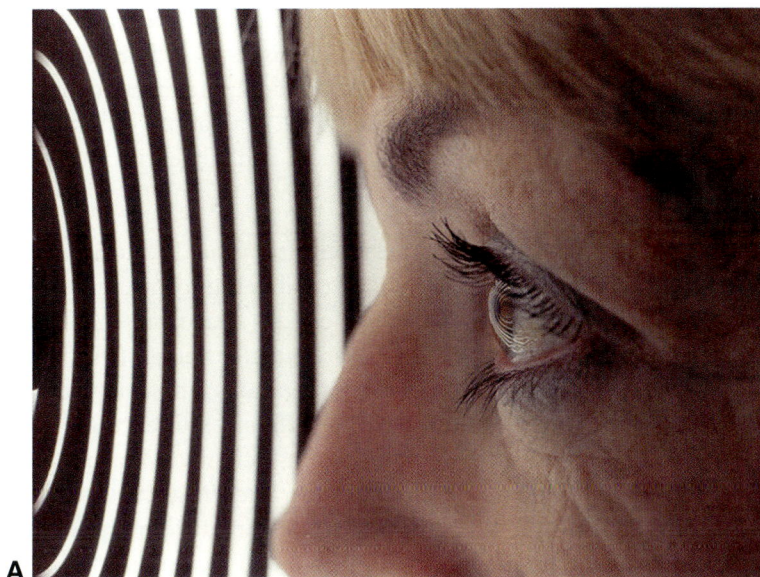

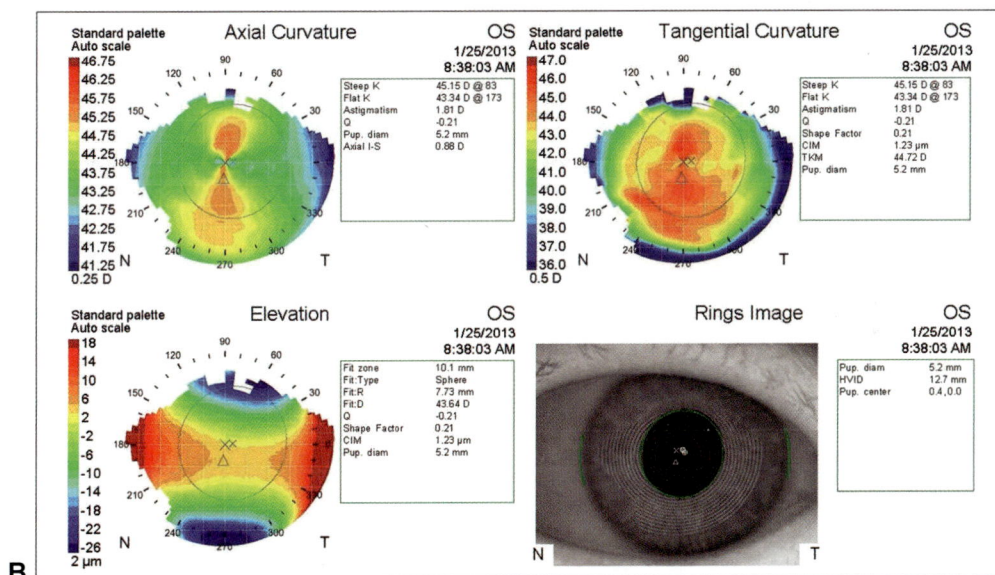

Figure 1-7 Placido imaging of the cornea. **A,** The ring reflections of the Placido imaging device can be seen on this patient's cornea. This image is then captured and analyzed. *(Courtesy of M. Bowes Hamill, MD.)*, **B,** The printout of the captured Placido image is seen in the lower right hand corner of this image with the different calculated color maps displayed in the other corners. *(Courtesy of M. Bowes Hamill, MD.)*

and subsequent numerical data is extremely important. In addition, Placido disk–based systems are referenced from the line that the instrument makes to the corneal surface (termed the *vertex normal*). This line may not necessarily be the patient's line of sight or the visual axis, which may lead to confusion in interpreting topographic maps. For a more extensive discussion of other uses of computerized corneal topography, refer to BCSC Section 3, *Clinical Optics,* and Section 8, *External Disease and Cornea.* Generally, data from the reflection of the mires generated by the topographic instruments are presented not only numerically but—more important for clinical evaluation—also as an image, with corneal curvature typically represented utilizing axial and tangential methods.

Axial power and curvature

Axial power representation derives from the supposition that the cornea is a sphere and that the angle of incidence of the instrument is normal to the cornea. Axial power is based on the concept of "axial distance" (Fig 1-8). As can be seen from the illustration, axial power underestimates steeper curvatures and overestimates flatter curvatures. This representation also is extremely dependent on the reference axis employed—optical or visual. Maps generated from the same cornea but using different reference axes look very different from one another. Axial power representations actually average the corneal powers and thereby provide a "smoother" representation of corneal curvature than does the tangential, or "instantaneous," method. Recall that the curvature and power of the central 1–2 mm of the cornea are generally not well imaged by Placido disk techniques but can be closely approximated by the axial power and curvature indices (formerly called *sagittal curvature*); however, the central measurements are extrapolated and thus are potentially inaccurate. These indices also fail to describe the true shape and power of the peripheral cornea. Topographic maps displaying axial power and curvature provide an intuitive sense of the physiologic flattening of the cornea but do not represent the true refractive power or the true curvature of peripheral regions of the cornea (Fig 1-9).

Instantaneous power and curvature

A second method of describing the corneal curvature on Placido disk–based topography is the *instantaneous radius of curvature* (also called *meridional* or *tangential power*). The

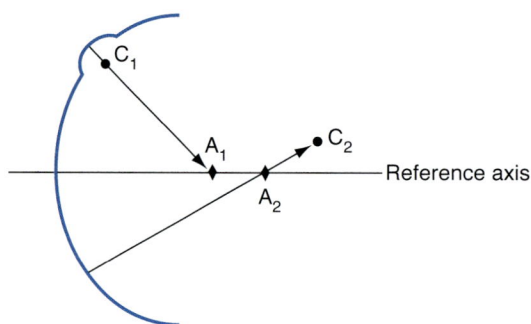

Figure 1-8 Schematic representation of the difference between axial distance (axial curvature) and radius of curvature for 2 points on a curved surface. Points C_1 and C_2 represent the centers of curvature of their respective surface points. Points A_1 and A_2 represent the endpoints of the axial distances for the given axis. As can be seen, local, steeper areas of curvature are underestimated, whereas flatter areas are overestimated. *(Adapted from Roberts C. Corneal topography: a review of terms and concepts. J Cataract Refract Surg. 1996;22(5):624–629, Fig 3.)*

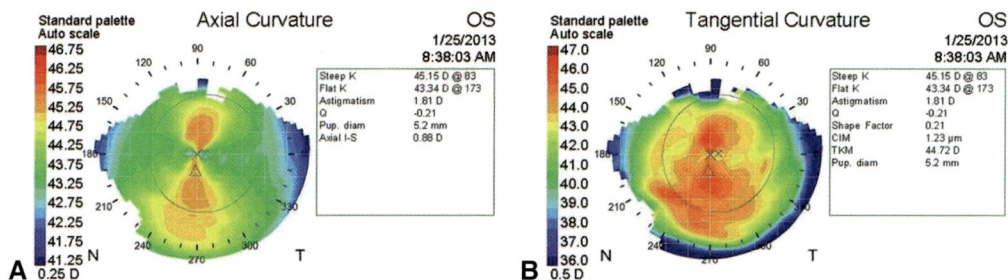

Figure 1-9 Examples of curvature maps. **A,** Axial (sagittal); **B,** instantaneous (tangential). *(Courtesy of J. Bradley Randleman, MD.)*

instantaneous radius of curvature is determined by taking a perpendicular path through the point in question from a plane that intersects the point and the visual axis, while allowing the radius to be the length necessary to correspond to a sphere with the same curvature at that point. The curvature, which is expressed in diopters, is estimated by the difference between the corneal index of refraction and 1.000, divided by this tangentially determined radius. A tangential map typically shows better sensitivity to peripheral changes with less "smoothing" of the curvature than an axial map shows (Fig 1-9). In these maps, diopters are relative units of curvature and are not the equivalent of diopters of corneal power. The potential benefit of this method's increased sensitivity is balanced by its tendency to document excessive detail ("noise"), which may not be clinically relevant.

For routine refractive screening, most surgeons have the topographic output in the axial (sagittal) curvature mode rather than the instantaneous (tangential) mode.

Corneal topography and astigmatism

A normal topographic image of a cornea without astigmatism demonstrates a relatively uniform color pattern centrally with a natural flattening in the periphery (Fig 1-10). *Regular astigmatism* is uniform steepening along a single corneal meridian that can be fully corrected with a cylindrical lens. Topographic imaging of regular astigmatism demonstrates a symmetric "bow-tie" pattern along a single meridian with a straight axis on both sides of center (see Fig 1-10B). The bow-tie pattern on topographic maps is an artifact of Placido-based imaging; that is, because the Placido image cannot detect curvature at the central measurement point, the corneal meridional steepening seems to disappear centrally and become enhanced as the imaging moves farther from center.

Irregular astigmatism is nonuniform corneal steepening from a variety of causes that cannot be corrected by cylindrical lenses. Irregular astigmatism decreases best-corrected visual acuity (BCVA; also called *corrected distance visual acuity, CDVA*) and may reduce contrast sensitivity and increase visual aberrations, depending on the magnitude of irregularity. Rigid gas-permeable and hard contact lenses can correct visual acuity reductions resulting from corneal irregular astigmatism by bridging the irregular corneal surface and the contact lens with the tear film. For more information on irregular astigmatism, see BCSC Section 3, *Clinical Optics.*

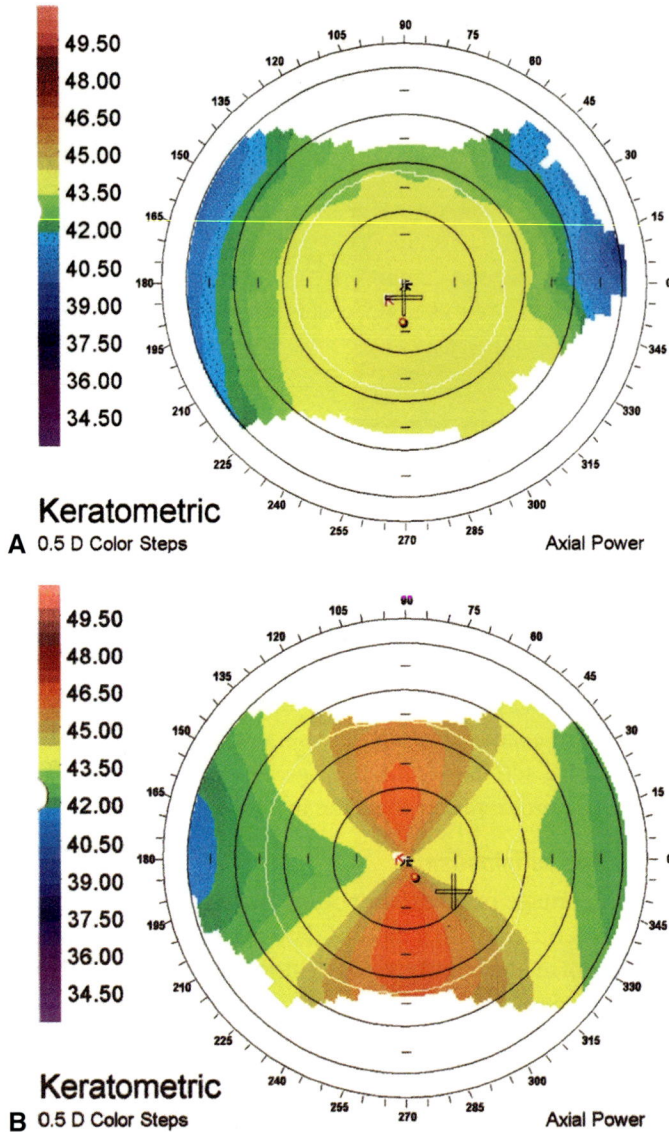

Figure 1-10 Normal corneal topographic patterns. **A,** Round; **B,** symmetric bow tie. *(Courtesy of J. Bradley Randleman, MD.)*

Corneal topography is very helpful in evaluating eyes with irregular astigmatism. Topographic changes include nonorthogonal steep and flat meridians (ie, not 90° apart), Figure 1-11. Asymmetry between the superior and inferior or nasal and temporal halves of the cornea may also be revealed by corneal topography, although these patterns are not necessarily indicative of corneal pathology. In contrast, wavefront analysis can demonstrate higher-order aberrations (such as coma, trefoil, quadrafoil, or secondary astigmatism). The ability to differentiate regular from irregular astigmatism has clinical significance in keratorefractive surgery. Traditional excimer laser ablation can treat

ANSI Z80.23
Std. palette/scale

Axial Curvature

OD

3/18/2013
12:44:08 PM

Steep K	45.98 D @ 156
Flat K	44.40 D @ 66
Astigmatism	1.58 D
Q	-0.42
Shape Factor	0.42
Pup. diam	5.8 mm
0 mm ring	45.92 D
1 mm ring	45.77 D
2 mm ring	45.69 D
3 mm ring	45.51 D
4 mm ring	45.19 D

49.5
49.0
48.5
48.0
47.5
47.0
46.5
46.0
45.5
45.0
44.5
44.0
43.5
43.0
42.5
42.0
41.5
41.0
40.5
40.0
39.5
39.0
38.5
0.5 D

T   N

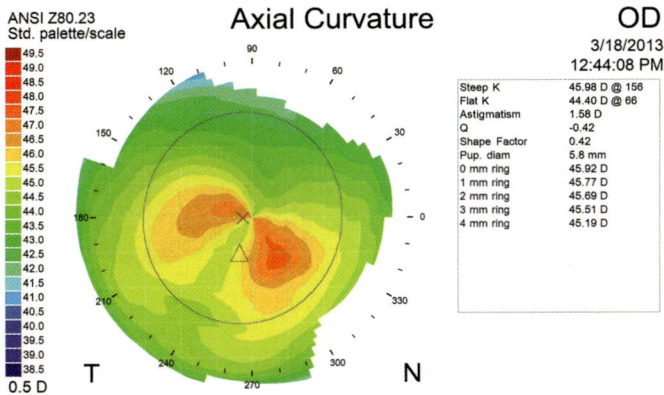

Figure 1-11 A curvature map showing nonorthogonal axes, which may indicate pathology that would contraindicate refractive surgery. *(Courtesy of Gregg J. Berdy, MD.)*

spherocylindrical errors but does not effectively treat irregular astigmatism. Topography-guided ablation may be useful in treating irregular astigmatism not caused by early corneal ectatic disorders.

Limitations of corneal topography

In addition to the limitations of the specific algorithms and the variations in terminology among manufacturers, the accuracy of corneal topography may be affected by other potential problems:

- tear-film effects
- misalignment (misaligned corneal topography may give a false impression of corneal apex decentration suggestive of keratoconus)
- instability (test-to-test variation)
- insensitivity to focus errors
- limited area of coverage (central and limbal)
- decreased accuracy of corneal power simulation measurements (SIM K) after refractive surgical procedures
- decreased accuracy of posterior surface elevation values in the presence of corneal opacities or, often, after refractive surgery (with scanning-slit technology)

Roberts C. Corneal topography: a review of terms and concepts. *J Cataract Refract Surg.* 1996;22(5):624–629.

Corneal Tomography

Whereas surface corneal curvature (power) is best expressed by Placido imaging, overall corneal shape, including spatial thickness profiles, is best expressed by computed tomography. Various imaging systems are available that take multiple slit images and reconstruct them into a corneal-shape profile, including anterior and posterior corneal elevation data (Fig 1-12). These include scanning-slit technology, Scheimpflug-based imaging systems, and anterior segment optical coherence tomography (OCT). To represent

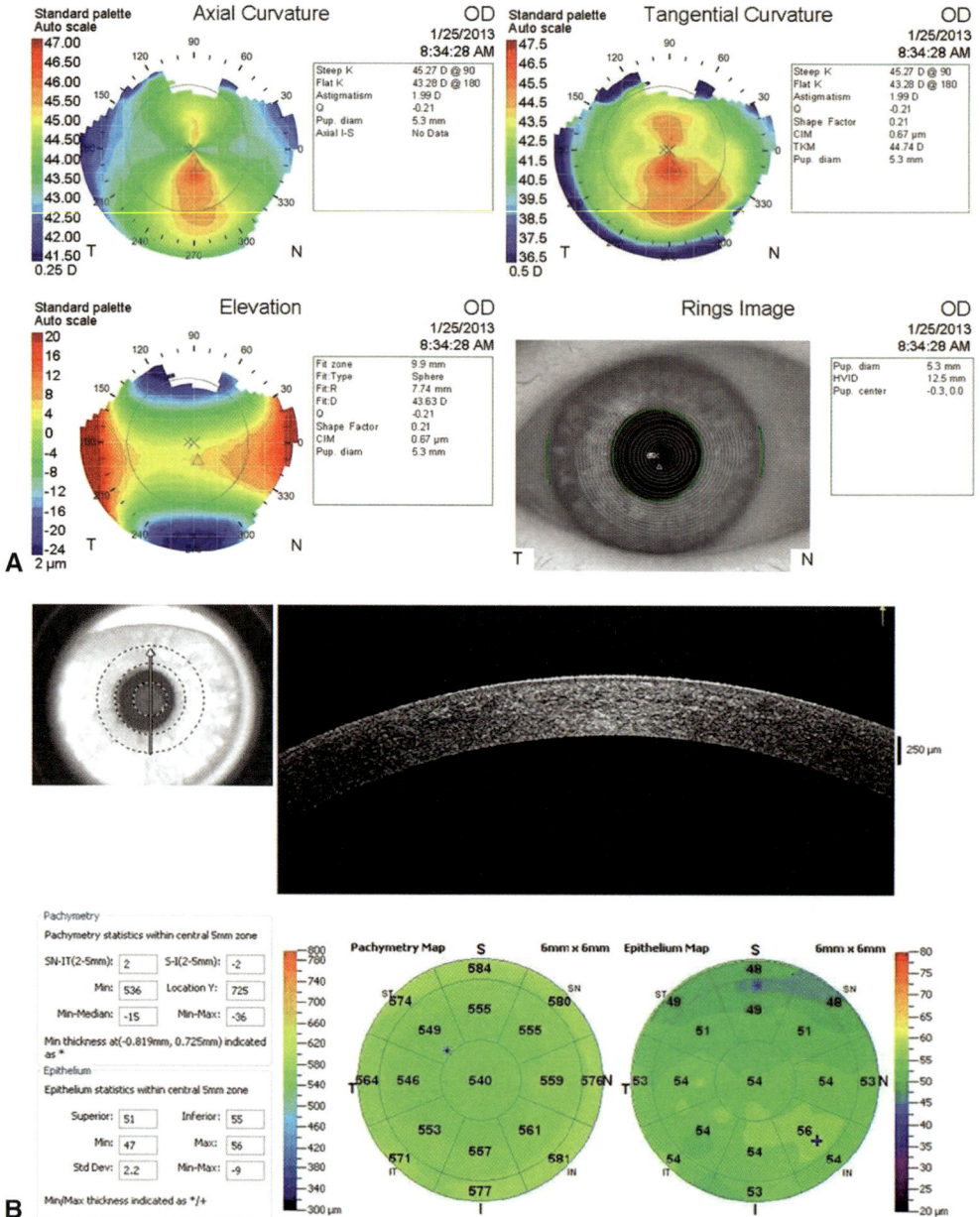

Figure 1-12 Different options for corneal imaging. All images are of the same patient taken at the same visit. **A,** Placido disk–based corneal curvature map showing axial and tangential curvature maps as well as the elevation map and the Placido rings image. Recall that this mapping technology analyzes *only* the surface characteristics of the cornea. **B,** Optical coherence tomography (OCT) image of the same cornea shown in **A.** Note that the corneal thickness profile (of the stroma as well as the epithelium) is well demonstrated, but the overall surface curvature is not. Had this patient previously undergone either LASIK or Descemet membrane–stripping keratoplasty (DSEK), which he has not, the demarcation line would have been well imaged with this technology.

(Continued)

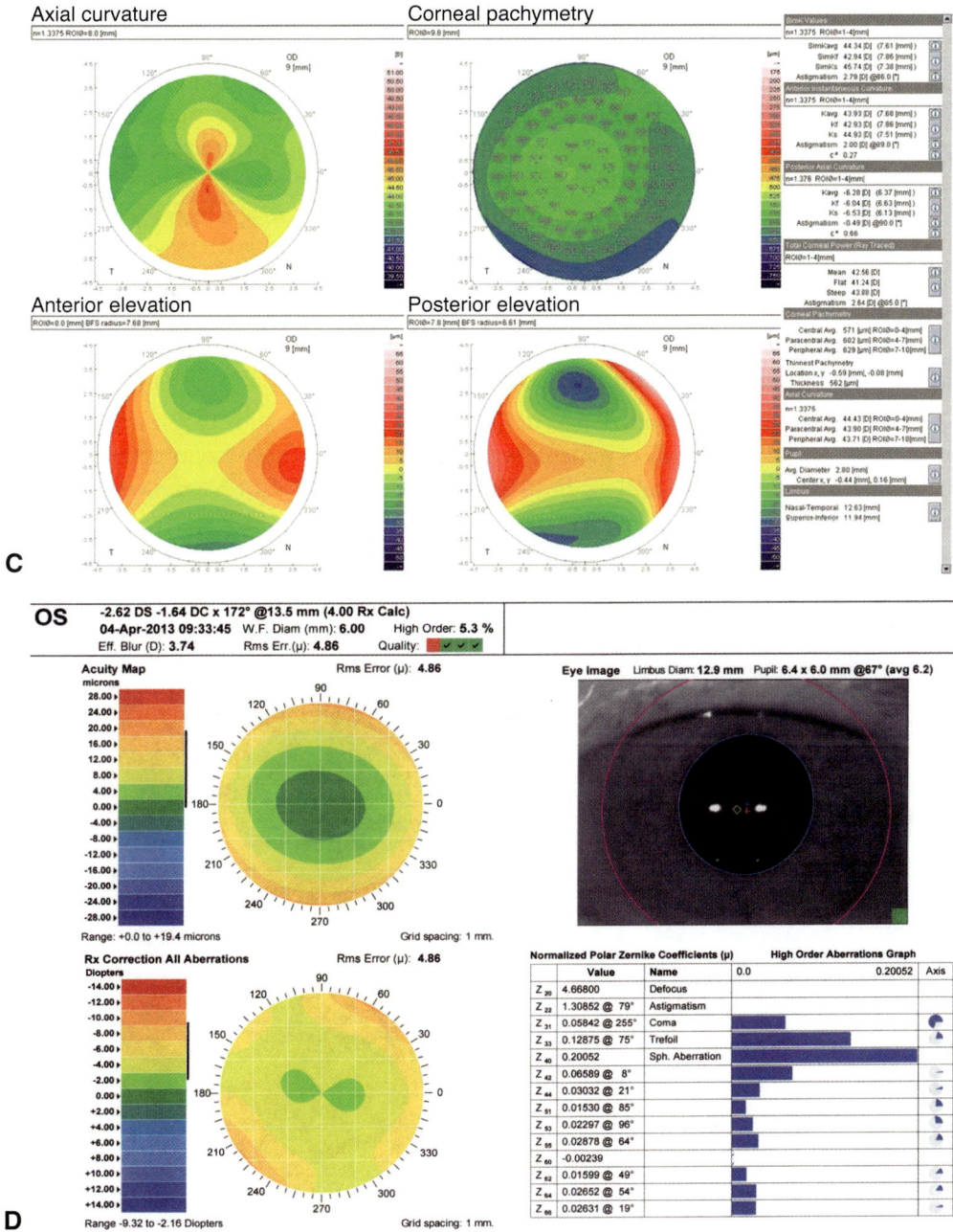

Figure 1-12 *(continued)* **C,** Corneal tomography image using dual Scheimpflug/Placido–based technology of the same patient and eye shown in **A** and **B.** The surface curvature, pachymetry, and anterior and posterior elevation mappings are demonstrated. Numerical values are shown along the right side. **D,** Wavescan image from a device like that illustrated in Fig 1-1A, taken of the fellow eye to that represented in **A, B,** and **C.** Note that this map does not show any corneal surface contours or features but rather provides information about the optics of the entire ocular system. As such, it can provide information on the refractive error and aberrations of the entire eye. *(Courtesy of M. Bowes Hamill, MD.)*

shape directly, color maps may be used to display a *z-height* from an arbitrary plane such as the iris plane; however, in order to be clinically useful, corneal surface maps are plotted to show differences from best-fit spheres or other objects that closely mimic the normal corneal shape (Fig 1-13). In general, each device calculates the best-fit sphere for each map individually. For this reason, comparing elevation maps is not exact because they frequently have different referenced best-fit sphere characteristics.

Elevation-based tomography is especially helpful in refractive surgery for depicting the anterior and posterior surface shapes of the cornea and lens. With such information, alterations to the shape of the ocular structures can be determined with greater accuracy, especially postoperative changes.

Indications for Corneal Imaging in Refractive Surgery

Corneal topography is an essential part of the preoperative evaluation of refractive surgery candidates. About two-thirds of patients with normal corneas have a symmetric astigmatism pattern that is round, oval, or bow-tie shaped (see Fig 1-10). Asymmetric patterns include asymmetric bow-tie patterns, inferior steepening, superior steepening, skewed radial axes, or other nonspecific irregularities.

Corneal topography detects irregular astigmatism, which may result from abnormal tear film, contact lens warpage, keratoconus and other corneal ectatic disorders, corneal surgery, trauma, scarring, and postinflammatory or degenerative conditions. Repeat topographic examinations may be helpful when the underlying etiology is in question, especially in cases of suspicious steepening patterns in patients who wear contact lenses or who have an abnormal tear film. Contact lens wearers often benefit from extended periods without contact lens wear prior to preoperative planning for refractive surgery;

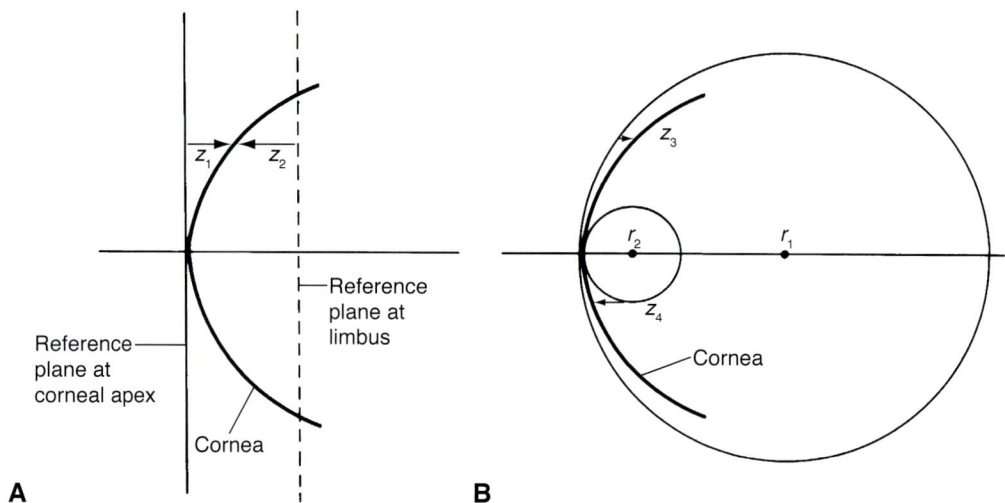

Figure 1-13 Height maps (typically in μm). **A,** Height relative to plane surface; z_1 is below the surface parallel to the corneal apex, and z_2 is above the surface parallel to the corneal limbus. **B,** Height relative to reference sphere; z_3 is below a flat sphere of radius r_1, and z_4 is above a steep sphere of radius r_2. *(Illustration by Christine Gralapp.)*

this period allows the corneal map and refraction to stabilize. Patients with keratoconus or other ectatic disorders are not routinely considered for ablative keratorefractive surgery because the abnormal cornea may exhibit an unpredictable response and/or progressive ectasia. Forme fruste, or subclinical, keratoconus typically is considered a contraindication to ablative refractive surgery. Studies are under way to determine the suitability of some keratorefractive procedures in combination with corneal crosslinking as alternative therapeutic modalities for these patients (see also Chapter 7).

Corneal topography and tomography can also be used to demonstrate the effects of keratorefractive procedures. Preoperative and postoperative maps may be compared to determine the refractive effect achieved (*difference map;* Fig 1-14). Corneal mapping can also help explain unexpected results, including undercorrection and overcorrection, induced astigmatism, and induced aberrations from small optical zones, decentered ablations, or central islands (Fig 1-15).

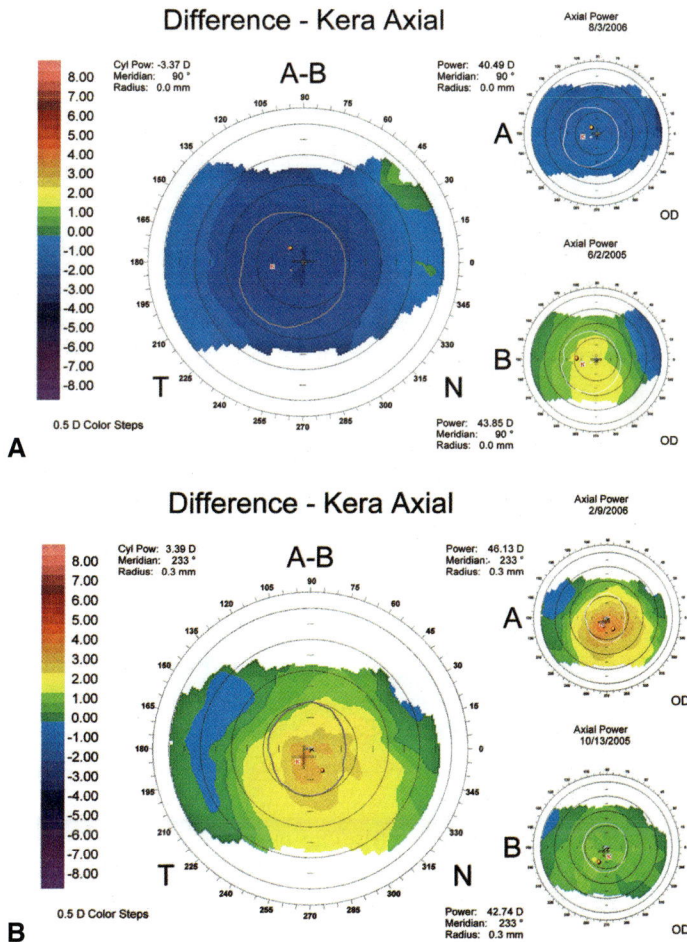

Figure 1-14 Difference maps demonstrating corneal power change before and after myopic **(A)** and hyperopic **(B)** LASIK. *(Courtesy of J. Bradley Randleman, MD.)*

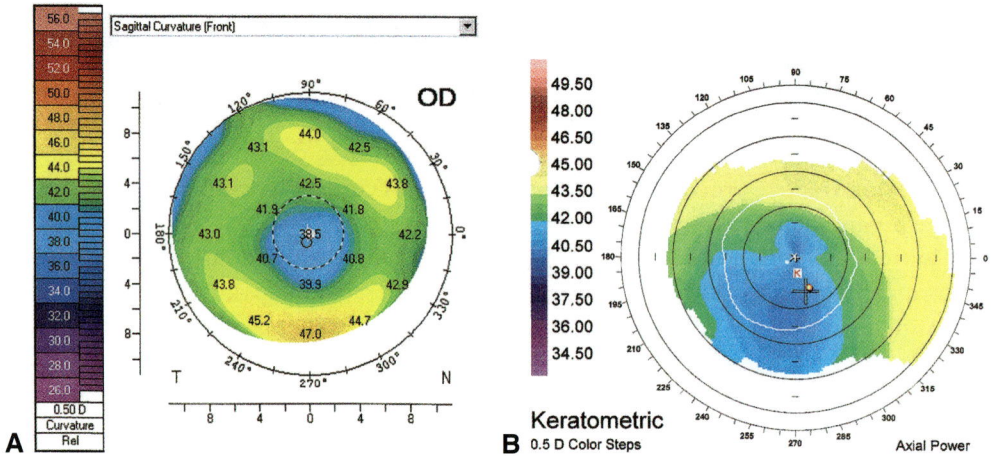

Figure 1-15 Topographic maps showing small optical zone after excimer laser ablation **(A)** and decentered ablation **(B)**. *(Courtesy of J. Bradley Randleman, MD.)*

De Paiva CS, Harris LD, Pflugfelder SC. Keratoconus-like topographic changes in keratoconjunctivitis sicca. *Cornea.* 2003;22(1):22–24.

Rabinowitz YS, Yang H, Brickman Y, et al. Videokeratography database of normal human corneas. *Br J Ophthalmol.* 1996;80(7):610–616.

The Role of Corneal Topography in Refractive Surgery

Corneal topography is one of the key evaluative technologies in refractive surgery, crucial not only in preoperative screening but also in postoperative evaluation of patients with unexpected results. Topographic analysis should be undertaken in all patients being considered for refractive surgery in order to identify patients who should not undergo the procedure. Although refractive surgery has numerous contraindications (see Chapter 2), some of the most important to recognize are the corneal ectatic disorders: keratoconus and pellucid marginal degeneration (see BCSC Section 8, *External Disease and Cornea,* for further discussion).

Keratoconus (KC) and pellucid marginal degeneration (PMD) are generally progressive conditions in which thinning occurs in the central, paracentral, or peripheral cornea, resulting in asymmetric corneal steepening and reduced spectacle-corrected visual acuity. These 2 conditions may be separate entities or different clinical expressions of the same ectatic process; in either case, they are currently contraindications for excimer laser surgery. The topographic pattern in keratoconic eyes usually demonstrates substantial inferonasal or inferotemporal steepening, although severe central and even superior steepening patterns may occur (Fig 1-16). The classic topographic pattern in PMD is inferior steepening, which is most dramatic between the 4 and 8 o'clock positions, with superior flattening. This inferior steepening often extends centrally, coming together in what has been described as a "crab-claw" shape (see Chapter 10, Fig 10-2). There may be substantial overlap in the topographic patterns of KC and PMD.

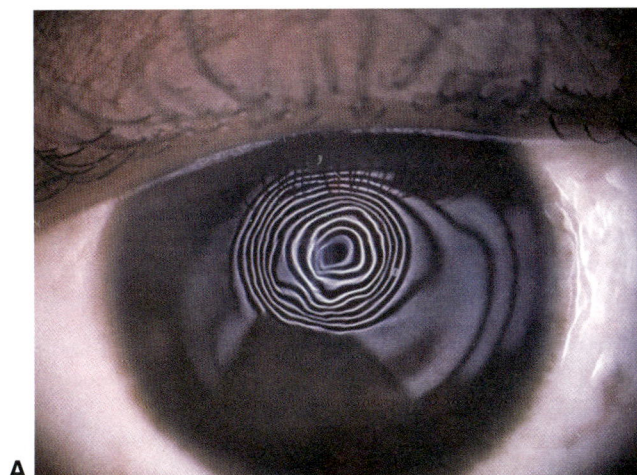

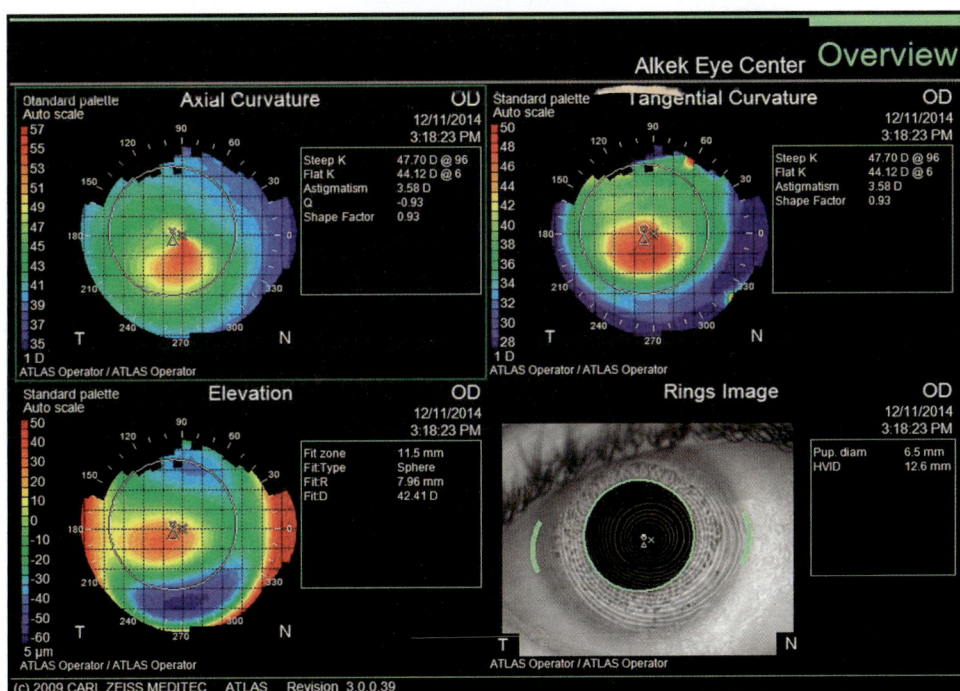

Figure 1-16 Corneal topography in keratoconus. Placido imaging showing distorted corneal mires **(A)** and axial and elevation topography in keratoconus **(B)**. *(Courtesy of M. Bowes Hamill, MD.)*

The patient who poses the greatest difficulty in preoperative evaluation for refractive surgery is the one in whom KC ultimately develops but who shows no obvious clinical signs at the time of examination. Corneal topography may reveal subtle abnormalities that should alert the surgeon to this problem. Although newer screening indices take into account various topographic and corneal biomechanical factors that may indicate a higher likelihood of subclinical KC, none of these indices is definitive. In addition to topographic metrics, substantial displacement of the thinnest area of the cornea from the center as revealed by corneal tomography is also suggestive of KC. Normal corneas are substantially thicker peripherally than centrally (by approximately 50–60 µm), and corneas that are not thicker peripherally suggest an ectatic disorder. Newer technologies such as high-resolution anterior segment OCT, ultra-high-frequency ultrasound, and hysteresis analysis may be helpful as screening tests for keratoconus by aiding in evaluating the relative position of the posterior and anterior apex, epithelial thickness, and corneal biomechanical properties; however, these technologies have yet to be validated.

Ambrósio R Jr, Alonso RS, Luz A, Coca Velarde LG. Corneal-thickness spatial profile and corneal-volume distribution: tomographic indices to detect keratoconus. *J Cataract Refract Surg.* 2006;32(11):1851–1859.

Lee BW, Jurkunas UV, Harissi-Dagher M, Poothullil AM, Tobaigy FM, Azar DT. Ectatic disorders associated with a claw-shaped pattern on corneal topography. *Am J Ophthalmol.* 2007;144(1):154–156.

Rabinowitz YS. Videokeratographic indices to aid in screening for keratoconus. *J Refract Surg.* 1995;11(5):371–379.

Rabinowitz YS, McDonnell PJ. Computer-assisted corneal topography in keratoconus. *Refract Corneal Surg.* 1989;5(6):400–408.

Corneal Effects of Keratorefractive Surgery

All keratorefractive procedures induce refractive changes by altering corneal curvature; however, the method by which the alteration is accomplished varies by procedure and by the refractive error being treated. Treatment of myopia requires a *flattening,* or decrease, in central corneal curvature, whereas treatment of hyperopia requires a *steepening,* or increase, in central corneal curvature. Corneal refractive procedures can be performed using a variety of techniques, including incisional, tissue addition or subtraction, alloplastic material addition, collagen shrinkage, and laser ablation (see the section Laser Biophysics for discussion of laser ablation).

Overall patient satisfaction after refractive surgery depends largely on the successful correction of refractive error and creation of a corneal shape that maximizes visual quality. The natural shape of the cornea is *prolate,* or steeper centrally than peripherally. In contrast, an *oblate* cornea is steeper peripherally than centrally. The natural prolate corneal shape results in an aspheric optical system, which reduces spherical aberration and therefore minimizes fluctuations in refractive error as the pupil changes size. Oblate corneas, such as those resulting from myopic treatments, increase spherical aberration. Common concerns in patients with substantial spherical aberration include glare, halos, and decreased night vision.

Incisional Techniques

Incisions perpendicular to the corneal surface alter its shape, depending on the direction, depth, location, length, and number of incisions (see Chapter 4). All incisions cause a

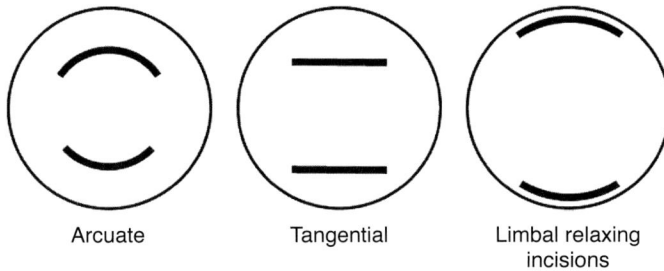

Arcuate   Tangential   Limbal relaxing
incisions

Figure 1-17 Schematic diagrams of incisions used in astigmatic keratotomy. Flattening is induced in the axis of the incisions (at 90° in this case), and steepening is induced 90° away from the incisions (at 180° in this case). *(Illustrations by Cyndie C. H. Wooley.)*

local flattening of the cornea. Radial incisions lead to flattening in both the meridian of the incision and the one 90° away. Tangential (arcuate or linear) incisions lead to flattening in the meridian of the incision and steepening in the meridian 90° away that may be equal to or less than the magnitude of the decrease in the primary meridian (Fig 1-17); this phenomenon is known as *coupling* (see Chapter 3, Fig 3-3).

Reducing the optical zone of the radial incisions increases their effect; similarly, by placing tangential incisions closer to the visual axis, the greater is the effect. In addition, increasing in the length of tangential incision, up to 3 clock-hours, increases the effect.

For optimum effect, an incision should be 85%–90% deep to retain an intact posterior lamella and maximum anterior bowing of the other lamellae. Nomograms for number of incisions and optical zone size can be calculated using finite element analysis, but surgical nomograms are typically generated empirically (eg, see Chapter 3, Table 3-1). The important variables for radial and astigmatic surgery include patient age and the number, depth, and length of incisions. The same incision has greater effect in older patients than it does in younger patients. IOP and preoperative corneal curvature are not significant predictors of effect.

Rowsey JJ. Ten caveats in refractive surgery. *Ophthalmology.* 1983;90(2):148–155.

Tissue Addition or Subtraction Techniques

With the exception of laser ablation techniques (discussed in the section Laser Biophysics), lamellar procedures that alter corneal shape through tissue addition or subtraction are primarily of historical interest only. *Keratomileusis* for myopia was originated by Barraquer as "carving" of the anterior surface of the cornea. It is defined as a method to modify the spherical or meridional surface of a healthy cornea by tissue subtraction. *Epikeratoplasty* (sometimes called *epikeratophakia*) adds a precision lathed lenticule of donor tissue to the corneal surface to induce hyperopic or myopic changes. *Keratophakia* requires the addition of a tissue lenticule or synthetic inlay intrastromally (see Chapter 4). There is, however, recurring interest in femtosecond laser techniques to excise intrastromal lenticules to alter corneal curvature without the need for excimer laser ablation. These procedures are termed *refractive lenticule extraction (ReLEx), femtosecond lenticule extraction*

(FLEx), and *small-incision lenticule extraction (SMILE).* For more detailed discussion of these procedures, see Chapter 12.

Alloplastic Material Addition Techniques

The shape of the cornea can be altered by adding alloplastic material such as hydrogel on the surface or into the corneal stroma to modify the anterior shape or refractive index of the cornea. For example, the 2 arc segments of an intrastromal corneal ring can be placed in 2 pockets of the stroma to directly reshape the surface contour according to the profile and location of the individual rings (Fig 1-18). In addition to altering the shape or curvature of the cornea, new inlay materials and designs have been developed that alter the optical function of the cornea—specifically the KAMRA corneal inlay (AcuFocus Inc, Irvine, CA), for presbyopia, approved in 2015, and the Raindrop (ReVision Optics, Inc, Lake Forest, CA), approved in 2016. For further discussion, see Chapter 4.

Collagen Shrinkage Techniques

Alteration in corneal biomechanics can also be achieved by collagen shrinkage. Heating collagen to a critical temperature of 58°–76°C causes it to shrink, inducing changes in the corneal curvature. *Thermokeratoplasty* and *conductive keratoplasty (CK)* are avoided in the central cornea because of scarring but can be used in the midperiphery to cause local collagen contraction with concurrent central corneal steepening (Fig 1-19; see also Chapter 7).

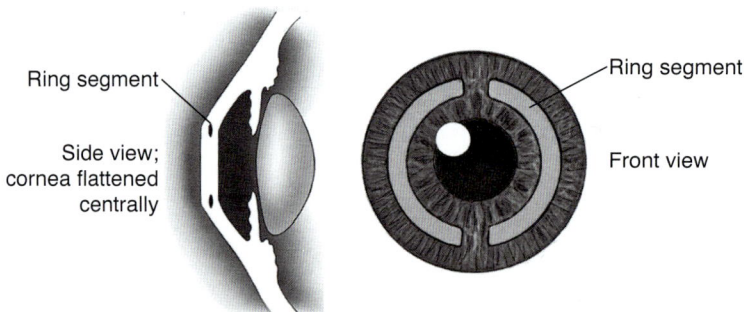

Figure 1-18 Schematic illustrations showing placement of intrastromal corneal ring segments. *(Illustrations by Jeanne Koelling.)*

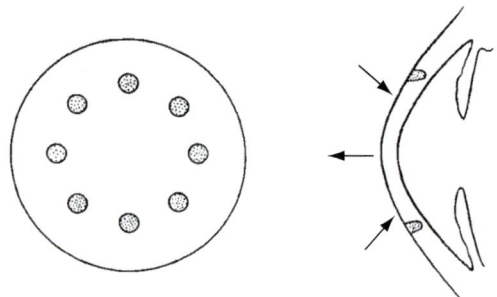

Figure 1-19 Schematic diagrams of thermo-keratoplasty and conductive keratoplasty. Heat shrinks the peripheral cornea, causing central steepening *(arrows).*

Laser Biophysics

Laser–Tissue Interactions

Three different types of laser–tissue interactions are used in keratorefractive surgery: photoablative, photodisruptive, and photothermal. *Photoablation,* the most important laser–tissue interaction in refractive surgery, breaks chemical bonds using excimer (from "*exci*ted di*mer*") lasers or other lasers of the appropriate wavelength. Laser energy of 4 eV per photon or greater is sufficient to break carbon–nitrogen or carbon–carbon tissue bonds. Argon-fluoride (ArF) lasers are excimer lasers that use electrical energy to stimulate argon to form dimers with fluorine gas. They generate a wavelength of 193 nm with 6.4 eV per photon. The 193-nm light is in the ultraviolet C (high ultraviolet) range, approaching the wavelength of x-rays. In addition to having high energy per photon, light at this end of the electromagnetic spectrum has very low tissue penetrance and thus is suitable for operating on the surface of tissue. This laser energy is capable of great precision, with little thermal spread in tissue; moreover, its lack of penetrance or lethality to cells makes the 193-nm laser nonmutagenic, enhancing its safety. (DNA mutagenicity occurs in the range of 250 nm.) Solid-state lasers have been designed to generate wavelengths of light near 193 nm without the need to use toxic gas, but the technical difficulties in manufacturing these lasers have limited their clinical use.

The femtosecond laser is approved by the US Food and Drug Administration (FDA) for creating flaps for LASIK and for the SMILE procedure. It may also be used to create channels for intrastromal ring segments and for lamellar keratoplasty and PKP. It uses a 1053-nm infrared beam that causes *photodisruption,* a process by which tissue is transformed into plasma, and the subsequent high pressure and temperature generated lead to rapid tissue expansion and formation of microscopic cavities within the corneal stroma. Contiguous photodisruption allows creation of the corneal flap, lenticule of tissue, channel, or keratoplasty incision.

Photothermal effects are achieved by focusing a Ho:YAG laser with a wavelength of 2.13 μm into the anterior stroma. The beam's energy is absorbed by water in the cornea, and the resulting heat causes local collagen shrinkage and subsequent surface flattening. This technique is FDA approved for low hyperopia but not commonly used.

Fundamentals of Excimer Laser Photoablation

All photoablative procedures result in the removal of corneal tissue. The amount of tissue removed centrally for myopic treatments using a broad beam laser is estimated by the *Munnerlyn formula:*

$$\text{Ablation Depth (μm)} \approx \frac{\text{Degree of Myopia (D)} \times \text{(Optical Zone Diameter)}^2 \text{ (mm)}}{3}$$

Clinical experience has confirmed that the effective change is independent of the initial curvature of the cornea. The Munnerlyn formula highlights some of the problems and limitations of laser vision correction. The amount of ablation increases by the square of the optical zone, but the complications of glare, halos, and regression increase when the optical zone decreases. To reduce these adverse effects, the optical zone should be 6 mm or larger.

With surface ablation, the laser treatment is applied to the Bowman layer and the anterior stroma, LASIK, on the other hand, combines an initial lamellar incision with ablation of the cornea, typically in the stromal bed (see Chapter 5 for further details of surgical technique). Theoretical limits for residual posterior cornea apply the same as they do for PRK. Flaps range in thickness from ultrathin (80–100 μm) to standard (120–180 μm). The thickness and diameter of the LASIK flap depend on instrumentation, corneal diameter, corneal curvature, and corneal thickness.

Treatments for myopia flatten the cornea by removing central corneal tissue, whereas those for hyperopia steepen the cornea by removing a doughnut-shaped portion of midperipheral tissue. Some lasers use a multizone treatment algorithm to conserve tissue by employing several concentric optical zones to achieve the total correction required. This method can provide the full correction centrally, while the tapering peripheral zones reduce symptoms and allow higher degrees of myopia to be treated. For an extreme example, 12.00 D of myopia can be treated as follows: 6.00 D are corrected with a 4.5-mm optical zone, 3.00 D with a 5.5-mm optical zone, and 3.00 D with a 6.5-mm optical zone (Fig 1-20). Thus, the total 12.00 D correction is achieved in the center using a shallower ablation depth than would be necessary for a single pass (103 μm instead of 169 μm). For hyperopia, surface ablation and LASIK use a similar formula to determine the maximum ablation depth, but the ablation zone is much larger than the optical zone. The zone of maximal ablation coincides with the outer edge of the optical zone. A transition zone of ablated cornea is necessary to blend the edge of the optical zone with the peripheral cornea.

Care must be taken to ensure that enough stromal tissue remains after creation of the LASIK flap and ablation to maintain adequate corneal structure. The historical standard has been to leave a minimum of 250 μm of tissue in the stromal bed, although the exact amount of remaining tissue required to ensure biomechanical stability is not known and likely varies among individuals. See Chapters 2 and 5 for further discussion of these issues.

Types of Photoablative Lasers

Photoablative lasers can be subdivided into broad-beam lasers, scanning-slit lasers, and flying spot lasers. *Broad-beam lasers* have larger-diameter beams and slower repetition rates and rely on optics or mirrors to create a smooth and homogeneous multimode laser beam of up to approximately 7 mm in diameter. These lasers have very high energy per pulse and require a small number of pulses to ablate the cornea. *Scanning-slit lasers* generate a narrow-slit laser beam that is scanned over the surface of the tissue to alter the photoablation profile,

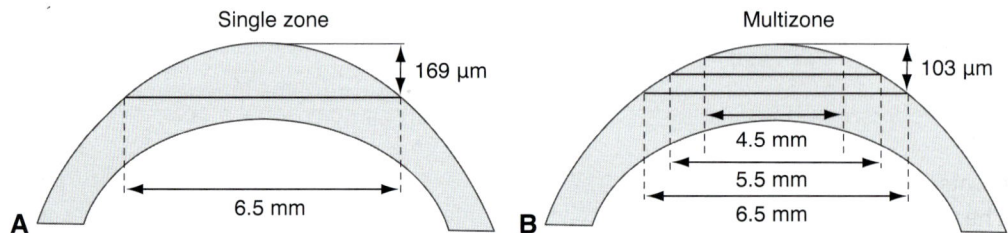

Figure 1-20 Diagrammatic comparison of single and multizone keratectomies. **A,** Depth of ablation required to correct 12.00 D of myopia in a single pass. **B,** Depiction of how the use of multiple zones reduces the ablation depth required. *(Illustrations by Cyndie C. H. Wooley.)*

thus improving the smoothness of the ablated cornea and allowing for larger-diameter abla-tion zones. *Flying spot lasers* use smaller-diameter beams (approximately 0.5–2.0 mm) that are scanned at a higher repetition rate; they require use of a tracking mechanism for precise placement of the desired pattern of ablation. Broad-beam lasers and some scanning-slit lasers require a mechanical iris diaphragm or ablatable mask to create the desired shape in the cornea, whereas the rest of the scanning-slit lasers and the flying spot lasers use a pattern projected onto the surface to guide the ablation profile without masking. The majority of excimer lasers in current clinical use some form of variable or flying spot ablation profile.

Wavefront-optimized and wavefront-guided laser ablations

Because conventional laser treatment profiles have small blend zones and create a more oblate corneal shape postoperatively following myopic corrections, they are likely to in-duce some degree of higher-order aberration, especially spherical aberration and coma. These aberrations occur because the corneal curvature is relatively more angled peripher-ally in relation to laser pulses emanating from the central location; thus, the pulses hitting the peripheral cornea are relatively less effective than are the central pulses.

Wavefront-optimized laser ablation improves the postoperative corneal shape by tak-ing the curvature of the cornea into account and increasing the number of peripheral pulses; this approach minimizes the induction of higher-order aberrations and often re-sults in better-quality vision and fewer night-vision concerns due to maintenance of a more prolate corneal shape. As in conventional procedures, the patient's refraction alone is used to program the wavefront-optimized laser ablation. This technology does not di-rectly address preexisting higher-order aberrations; however, recent studies have found that the vast majority of patients do not have substantial preoperative higher-order aber-rations. It also has the advantage of being quicker than wavefront-guided technology and avoids the additional expense of the aberrometer.

In *wavefront-guided laser ablation,* information obtained from a wavefront-sensing aberrometer (which quantifies the aberrations) is transferred electronically to the treat-ment laser to program the ablation. This process is distinct from those in conventional excimer laser and wavefront-optimized laser treatments, in which the subjective refrac-tion alone is used to program the laser ablation. The wavefront-guided laser attempts to treat both lower-order (ie, myopia or hyperopia and/or astigmatism) and higher-order aberrations by applying complex ablation patterns to the cornea to correct the wavefront deviations. The correction of higher-order aberrations requires non–radially symmetric patterns of ablation (which are often much smaller in magnitude than ablations needed to correct defocus and astigmatism). The difference between the desired and the actual wavefront is used to generate a 3-dimensional map of the planned ablation. Accurate reg-istration is required to ensure that the ablation treatment actually delivered to the cornea matches the intended pattern. Such registration is achieved by using marks at the limbus before obtaining the wavefront patterns or by iris registration, which matches reference points in the natural iris pattern to compensate for cyclotorsion and pupil centroid shift. The wavefront-guided laser then uses a pupil-tracking system, which helps maintain cen-tration during treatment and allows accurate delivery of the customized ablation profile.

The results for both wavefront-optimized and wavefront-guided ablations for myo-pia, hyperopia, and astigmatism are excellent, with well over 90% of eyes achieving 20/40 or better uncorrected distance visual acuity (UCVA; also called *uncorrected distance visual acuity, UDVA*). Although most visual acuity parameters are similar between conventional and customized treatments (including both wavefront-optimized and wavefront-guided treatments), the majority of recent reports demonstrate improved vision quality when customized treatment profiles are used. Outcomes with wavefront-optimized treatments are similar to those of wavefront-guided treatments for most patients, with the exception of patients with substantial preoperative higher-order aberrations.

Topography-guided laser ablations

Topography-guided lasers are similar in concept to wavefront-guided lasers, but they link the treatment to the corneal topography rather than to the total wavefront data. Although experience is still early, these instruments may offer significant benefit in the treatment of highly aberrated eyes, such as eyes with previous RK or PKP.

Myrowitz EH, Chuck RS. A comparison of wavefront-optimized and wavefront-guided ablations. *Curr Opin Ophthalmol.* 2009;20(4):247–250.

Netto MV, Dupps W Jr, Wilson SE. Wavefront-guided ablation: evidence for efficacy compared to traditional ablation. *Am J Ophthalmol.* 2006;141(2):360–368.

Padmanabhan P, Mrochen M, Basuthkar S, Viswanathan D, Joseph R. Wavefront-guided versus wavefront-optimized laser in situ keratomileusis: contralateral comparative study. *J Cataract Refract Surg.* 2008;34(3):389–397.

Pasquali T, Krueger R. Topography-guided laser refractive surgery. *Curr Opin Ophthalmol.* 2012;23(4):264–268.

Perez-Straziota CE, Randleman JB, Stulting RD. Visual acuity and higher-order aberrations with wavefront-guided and wavefront-optimized laser in situ keratomileusis. *J Cataract Refract Surg.* 2010;36(3):437–441.

Schallhorn SC, Farjo AA, Huang D, et al; American Academy of Ophthalmology. Wavefront-guided LASIK for the correction of primary myopia and astigmatism: a report by the American Academy of Ophthalmology. *Ophthalmology.* 2008;115(7):1249–1261.

Schallhorn SC, Tanzer DJ, Kaupp SE, Brown M, Malady SE. Comparison of night driving performance after wavefront-guided and conventional LASIK for moderate myopia. *Ophthalmology.* 2009;116(4):702–709.

Stonecipher KG, Kezirian GM. Wavefront-optimized versus wavefront-guided LASIK for myopic astigmatism with the ALLEGRETTO WAVE: three-month results of a prospective FDA trial. *J Refract Surg.* 2008;24(4):S424–S430.

Corneal Wound Healing

All forms of keratorefractive surgery are exquisitely dependent on corneal wound healing to achieve the desired results. Satisfactory results require either modifying or reducing wound healing or exploiting normal wound healing for the benefit of the patient. For example, astigmatic keratotomy requires initial weakening of the cornea followed by permanent corneal healing, with replacement of the epithelial plugs with collagen and remodeling of the collagen to ensure stability and avoid long-term hyperopic drift. PRK requires the epithelium to heal quickly, and with minimal stimulation of the underlying keratocytes, to avoid corneal scarring and haze. Lamellar keratoplasty requires intact epithelium and healthy endothelium early in the postoperative period to seal the flap. Later, the cornea must heal in the periphery to secure the flap in place and avoid late-term displacement while minimizing irregular astigmatism; also, the cornea must remain devoid of significant healing centrally to maintain a clear visual axis. In addition to stromal healing, regeneration of the corneal nerves is crucial to a normal ocular surface and good visual function. Delay or difficulty in re-innervation can lead to problems with corneal sensation and tear-film stability and to dry eye symptoms.

The understanding of corneal wound healing has advanced tremendously with recognition of the multiple factors involved in the cascade of events initiated by corneal wounding. The cascade is somewhat dependent on the nature of the injury. Injury to the epithelium can lead to loss of underlying keratocytes from apoptosis. The remaining keratocytes respond by generating new glycosaminoglycans and collagen, to a degree dependent on the duration of the epithelial defect and the depth of the stromal injury. Corneal haze is localized in the subepithelial anterior stroma and may persist for several years after surface ablation. Clinically significant haze, however, is present in only a small percentage of eyes. The tendency toward haze formation is greater with deeper ablations, increased surface irregularity, and prolonged absence of the epithelium. Despite loss of the Bowman layer, normal or even enhanced numbers of hemidesmosomes and anchoring fibrils form to secure the epithelium to the stroma.

Controversy persists over the value of different drugs for modulating wound healing in surface ablation. Typically, clinicians in the United States use corticosteroids in a tapering manner following surgery to reduce inflammation. Mitomycin C has been applied to the stromal bed after excimer surface ablation to attempt to decrease haze formation (see Chapters 5 and 6). Vitamin C has been postulated to play a role in protecting the cornea from ultraviolet light damage by the excimer laser, but no randomized, prospective clinical trial has yet been performed. Various growth factors that have been found to promote wound healing after PRK, including transforming growth factor β, may be useful in the future.

Haze formation does not seem to occur in the central flap interface after LASIK, which may be related either to lack of significant epithelial injury and consequent subcellular signaling or to maintenance of some intact surface neurons. LASIK shows very little long-term evidence of healing between the disrupted lamellae and only typical stromal healing at the peripheral wound. The lamellae are initially held in position by negative stromal pressure generated by the endothelial cells aided by an intact epithelial surface. Even years after treatment, the lamellar interface can be broken and the flap lifted, indicating that only a minimal amount of healing occurs. LASIK flaps can also be dislodged secondary to trauma many years postoperatively.

Dupps WJ Jr, Wilson SE. Biomechanics and wound healing in the cornea. *Exp Eye Res.* 2006; 83(4):709–720.

Majmudar PA, Schallhorn SC, Cason JB, et al. Mitomycin-C in corneal surface excimer laser ablation techniques: a report by the American Academy of Ophthalmology. *Ophthalmology.* 2015;122(6):1085–1095.

Netto MV, Mohan RR, Sinha S, Sharma A, Dupps W, Wilson SE. Stromal haze, myofibroblasts, and surface irregularity after PRK. *Exp Eye Res.* 2006;82(5):788–797. Epub 2005 Nov 21.

Schmack I, Dawson DG, McCarey BE, Waring GO III, Grossniklaus HE, Edelhauser HF. Cohesive tensile strength of human LASIK wounds with histologic, ultrastructural, and clinical correlations. *J Refract Surg.* 2005;21(5):433–445.

CHAPTER 2

Patient Evaluation

The preoperative patient evaluation is perhaps the most critical component in achieving successful outcomes after refractive surgery. It is during this encounter that the surgeon develops an impression as to whether the patient is a good candidate for refractive surgery. Perhaps the most important goal of this evaluation, however, is to identify who should *not* have refractive surgery.

Patient History

The evaluation actually begins before the physician sees the patient. Technicians or refractive surgical coordinators who interact with a patient may get a sense of the patient's goals and expectations for refractive surgery. If the patient is particularly quarrelsome about the time or date of the appointment or argues about cost, the surgeon should be informed. Such a patient may not be a good candidate for surgery.

Important parts of the preoperative refractive surgery evaluation include an assessment of the patient's expectations; the social, medical, and ocular history; manifest and cycloplegic refractions; a complete ophthalmic evaluation, including slit-lamp and fundus examinations; and ancillary testing (Table 2-1). If the patient is a good candidate for surgery, the surgeon should discuss the benefits, risks, and alternatives with the patient as part of the informed consent process. (See "Discussion of Findings and Informed Consent" later in this chapter.)

Because accurate test results are crucial to the success of refractive surgery, the refractive surgeon must closely supervise office staff members who are performing the various tests (eg, corneal topography or pachymetry) during the preoperative evaluation. Likewise, the surgeon should make sure the instruments used in the evaluation are properly calibrated, as miscalibrated instruments can result in faulty data and poor surgical results.

Patient Expectations

One of the most important aspects of the entire evaluation is assessing the patient's expectations. Inappropriate patient expectations are probably the leading cause of patient dissatisfaction after refractive surgery. The results may be exactly what the surgeon expected, but if those expectations were not conveyed adequately to the patient before surgery, the patient may be disappointed.

The surgeon should explore expectations relating to both the refractive result (eg, uncorrected visual acuity [UCVA; also called *uncorrected distance visual acuity, UDVA*])

Table 2-1 Important Parts of the Preoperative Refractive Surgery Evaluation

Patient expectations and motivations
Assessment of specific patient expectations
Discussion of uncorrected distance versus reading vision

History
Social history, including vision requirements of profession and hobbies, tobacco and alcohol use
Medical history, including systemic medications and diseases such as diabetes mellitus and
    rheumatologic diseases
Ocular history, including history of contact lens wear

Ophthalmic examination
Uncorrected near and distance vision, ocular dominance
Manifest refraction (pushing plus)
Monovision demonstration, if indicated
External evaluation
Pupillary evaluation
Motility
Slit-lamp examination, including intraocular pressure measurement
Corneal topography
Wavefront analysis, if indicated
Pachymetry
Cycloplegic refraction (refining sphere, not cylinder)
Dilated fundus examination

Informed consent
Discussion of findings
Discussion of medical and surgical alternatives and risks
Answering of patient questions
Having patient read informed consent document when undilated and unsedated, ideally before
    the day of procedure, and sign prior to surgery

---

and the emotional result (eg, improved self-esteem). Patients need to understand that they should not expect refractive surgery to improve their best-corrected visual acuity (BCVA; also called *corrected distance visual acuity, CDVA*). In addition, they need to realize that refractive surgery will not alter the course of eventual presbyopia, nor will it prevent potential future ocular problems such as cataract, glaucoma, or retinal detachment. If the patient has clearly unrealistic goals, such as a guarantee of 20/20 uncorrected visual acuity or perfect uncorrected reading *and* distance vision, even though he or she has presbyopia, the patient may need to be told that refractive surgery cannot currently fulfill his or her needs. The refractive surgeon should exclude such patients.

Social History

An accurate social and occupational history can uncover specific vision requirements of the patient's profession. Certain occupations require that best vision be at a specific distance. For example, to avoid wearing glasses at the pulpit, a minister may desire that best uncorrected vision be at arm's length. Military personnel, firefighters, or police officers may have restrictions on minimum UCVA and BCVA and on the type of refractive surgery allowed. Knowledge of a patient's recreational activities may help guide the surgeon to the most appropriate refractive procedure or determine whether that patient is even a good candidate for refractive surgery. For example, a surface laser procedure may be preferable to a lamellar procedure for a patient who is active and at high risk of ocular trauma. Someone with highly myopic and presbyopic vision who is used to examining objects a few inches from the eyes without the use of glasses (eg, jeweler or stamp collector) may be dissatisfied with postoperative emmetropia. Tobacco and alcohol use should be documented.

Medical History

The medical history should include systemic conditions, prior surgical procedures, and current and prior medications. Certain systemic conditions, such as connective tissue disorders and diabetes mellitus, can lead to poor healing after refractive surgery. An immunocompromised state—for example, from cancer or human immunodeficiency virus infection and acquired immunodeficiency syndrome—may increase the risk of infection after refractive surgery (see Chapter 10). Medications that affect healing or the ability to fight infection, such as systemic corticosteroids or chemotherapeutic drugs, should be specifically noted. The use of corticosteroids increases the risk of cataract development, which could compromise the long-term postoperative visual outcome. Use of certain medications—for example, isotretinoin and amiodarone—traditionally has been thought to increase the risk of poor results with photorefractive keratectomy (PRK) and laser in situ keratomileusis (LASIK) due to a potentially increased risk of poor corneal healing; however, there is no evidence for this association in the peer-reviewed literature. Previous use of isotretinoin can damage the meibomian glands and predispose a patient to dry-eye symptoms postoperatively. Because of a possible increased risk of delayed epithelial healing, caution needs to be taken with patients using sumatriptan who are undergoing PRK or LASIK and with patients using hormone replacement therapy or antihistamines who are undergoing PRK.

Although laser manufacturers do not recommend excimer laser surgery for patients with cardiac pacemakers and implanted defibrillators, many such patients have undergone the surgery without problems. It may be best to check with the pacemaker and defibrillator manufacturer before laser surgery. Refractive surgery is also generally contraindicated in pregnant and breastfeeding women because of possible changes in refraction and corneal hydration status. Many surgeons recommend waiting at least 3 months after delivery and cessation of breastfeeding before performing the refractive surgery evaluation and procedure.

O'Doherty MA, O'Doherty JV, O'Keefe M. Outcome of LASIK for myopia in women on hormone replacement therapy. *J Refract Surg*. 2006;22(4):350–353.

Pertinent Ocular History

The ocular history should focus on previous and current eye problems, such as dry-eye symptoms, blepharitis, recurrent erosions, glaucoma, and retinal tears or detachments. In addition, potentially recurrent conditions, such as ocular herpes simplex virus infection, should be recognized so that preventive measures can be instituted. Ocular medications should be noted. Prior ocular surgical procedures, such as radial keratotomy or penetrating keratoplasty, may affect clinical decision making in refractive surgery. A personal or family history of keratoconus may eliminate a patient from refractive surgery consideration. A history of previous methods of optical correction, such as glasses and contact lenses, should be taken. The stability of the current refraction is a very important consideration. A significant change in prescription for glasses or contact lenses is generally thought to be greater than 0.50 D in either sphere or cylinder within the past year. A contact lens history should be taken. Information gathered should include the type of lenses used (eg, soft, rigid gas-permeable [RGP], polymethyl methacrylate [PMMA]); the wearing schedule (eg, daily-wear disposable, daily-wear frequent replacement, overnight wear indicating number of nights worn in a row); the type of cleaning and disinfecting agents used; and the age of the lenses.

Because contact lens wear can change the shape of the cornea (corneal warpage), it is recommended that patients discontinue contact lens wear before the refractive surgery evaluation as well as before the surgery. The exact length of time the patient should be without contact lens wear has not been established. Current clinical practice typically involves discontinuation of soft contact lenses for at least 3 days to 2 weeks (toric lenses may require longer) and of rigid contact lenses for at least 2–3 weeks, but it may take months for the corneal curvature to return to normal in some long-term rigid contact lens wearers. For this reason, some surgeons keep patients out of rigid contact lenses for 1 month for every decade of contact lens wear. Before being considered for refractive surgery, patients with irregular or unstable corneas should discontinue wearing their contact lenses for a longer period and then be reevaluated every few weeks until the refraction and corneal topography stabilize. For patients who wear RGP contact lenses and find glasses a hardship, some surgeons suggest changing to soft contact lenses for a period to aid stabilization and regularization of the corneal curvature.

Bower KS, Woreta F. Update on contraindications for laser-assisted in situ keratomileusis and photorefractive keratectomy. *Curr Opin Ophthalmol.* 2014;25(4):251–257.

de Rojas Silva V, Rodríguez-Conde R, Cobo-Soriano R, Beltrán J, Llovet F, Baviera J. Laser in situ keratomileusis in patients with a history of ocular herpes. *J Cataract Refract Surg.* 2007;33(11):1855–1859.

Patient Age, Presbyopia, and Monovision

The age of a patient is a consideration in predicting postoperative patient satisfaction. The loss of near vision with aging should be discussed with all patients. Before 40 years of age, individuals with emmetropia generally do not require reading adds to see a near target. After this age, patients need to understand that if their eyes are made emmetropic through refractive surgery, they will require reading glasses for near vision. They must also understand that "near vision" tasks include all tasks performed up close, such as applying makeup, shaving, or seeing the computer or cell phone screen—not just "reading." These points cannot be overemphasized for patients with myopia who are approaching 40 years of age. Before refractive surgery, these patients can read well with and without their glasses. Some may even read well with their contact lenses. If their eyes are made emmetropic after surgery, many will not read well without reading glasses. The patient needs to understand this phenomenon and must be willing to accept this result before undergoing any refractive surgery that aims for emmetropia. In patients who wear glasses, a trial with contact lenses will simulate vision following refractive surgery, and approximate the patient's reading ability after surgery.

A discussion of monovision (ie, 1 eye corrected for distance and the other eye for near/intermediate vision) often fits well into the evaluation at this point. The alternative of monovision correction should be discussed with all patients in the age groups approaching or affected by presbyopia. Many patients have successfully used monovision in contact lenses and want it after refractive surgery. Others have never tried it but would like to, and still others have no interest. If a patient has not used monovision before but is interested, the attempted surgical result should first be demonstrated with glasses or temporary contact lenses at near and distance. Generally, the dominant eye is corrected for distance, and the nondominant eye is corrected to approximately –1.50 to –1.75 D. For most patients, such refraction allows good uncorrected distance and near vision without intolerable anisometropia. Some surgeons prefer a "mini-monovision" procedure, whereby the near-vision eye is corrected to approximately –0.75 D, which allows some near vision with better distance vision and less anisometropia. The exact amount of monovision depends on the desires of the patient. Higher amounts of monovision (up to –2.50 D) can be used successfully in selected patients who want excellent postoperative near vision. However, in some patients with a higher degree of postoperative myopia, improving near vision may lead to unwanted adverse effects of loss of depth perception and anisometropia. It is advisable to have a patient simulate monovision with contact lenses before surgery (generally about 5 days to 1 week, but practices are variable) to ensure that distance and near vision, as well as stereovision, are acceptable and that no muscle imbalance is present, especially with higher degrees of monovision.

Although typically the nondominant eye is corrected for near, some patients prefer that the dominant eye be corrected for near. Of several methods for testing ocular dominance, one of the simplest is to have the patient point to a distant object, such as a small letter on an eye chart. Alternatively, the patient can make an "okay sign" with 1 hand and look at the examiner through the opening, and then close each eye to determine which eye he or she was using when pointing; this is the dominant eye.

Examination

Uncorrected Visual Acuity and Manifest and Cycloplegic Refraction

The refractive elements of the preoperative examination are extremely critical because they directly determine the amount of surgery to be performed. Visual acuity at distance and near should be measured. The current glasses prescription and visual acuity with those glasses should also be determined, and a manifest refraction should be performed. The sharpest visual acuity with the least amount of minus ("pushing plus") should be the final endpoint (see BCSC Section 3, *Clinical Optics*). The duochrome test should not be used as the final endpoint because it tends to overminus patients. Document the best visual acuity obtainable, even if it is better than 20/20. An automated refraction with an autorefractor or wavefront aberrometer may be helpful in providing a starting point for the manifest refraction.

A cycloplegic refraction is also necessary. Sufficient waiting time must be allowed between the time the patient's eyes are dilated with cycloplegic eye drops and measurement of the refraction. Tropicamide, 1%, or cyclopentolate, 1%, are the most commonly used cycloplegic drops. For full cycloplegia, waiting at least 30 minutes (with tropicamide, 1%) or 60 minutes (with cyclopentolate, 1%) is recommended. The cycloplegic refraction should refine the sphere and not the cylinder from the manifest refraction, as it is done to neutralize accommodation. For eyes with greater than 5.00 D of refractive error, a vertex distance measurement should be performed to obtain the most accurate refraction.

When the difference between the manifest and cycloplegic refractions is large (eg, >0.50 D), a postcycloplegic manifest refraction may be helpful to recheck the original. In patients with myopia, such a large difference is often caused by an overminused manifest refraction. In patients with hyperopia, substantial latent hyperopia may be present, in which case the surgeon and patient need to decide exactly how much hyperopia to treat. If there is significant latent hyperopia, a pushed-plus spectacle or contact lens correction can be worn for several weeks or months preoperatively to reduce the postoperative adjustment that may result from treating the true refraction.

Refractive surgeons have their own preferences for whether to program the laser using the manifest or cycloplegic refraction, based on their individual nomogram and technique and on the patient's age. Many surgeons plan their laser input according to the manifest refraction, especially for younger patients, if that refraction has been performed with a careful pushed-plus technique.

Pupillary Examination

After the manifest refraction (but before dilating eye drops are administered), the external and anterior segment examinations are performed. Specific attention should be given to the pupillary examination. The pupil size should be evaluated in bright room light and under dim illumination, and the surgeon should look for an afferent pupillary defect. Various techniques are available for measuring pupil size in dim illumination, including use of a near card with pupil sizes on the edge (with the patient fixating at distance), or a pupillometer. The dim-light measurement should be taken using an amount of light entering the eye that closely approximates the amount entering during normal nighttime activities, such as night driving; it should not necessarily be done under completely dark conditions.

Pupil measurements should be standardized as much as possible. Measuring the low-light pupil diameter preoperatively and using that measurement to direct surgery remains a controversial approach. Conventional wisdom suggests that the optical zone should be larger than the pupil diameter to minimize vision disturbances such as glare and halos. Recent evidence, however, does not support an association between preoperative pupil size and an increased incidence of either glare or halo concerns 1 year postoperatively. It is not clear, therefore, that pupil size can be used to predict which patients are more likely to have such symptoms. However, a thorough and documented discussion with the patient is required. The size of the effective optical zone—which is related to the ablation profile and the level of refractive error—may be more important in minimizing visual adverse effects than is the low-light pupil diameter.

When asked, patients often note that they had glare under dim-light conditions even before undergoing refractive surgery. Thus, it is helpful for patients to become aware of their glare and halo symptoms preoperatively, as this knowledge may minimize postoperative concerns or misunderstanding.

Chan A, Manche EE. Effect of preoperative pupil size on quality of vision after wavefront-guided LASIK. *Ophthalmology.* 2011;118(4):736–741.

Edwards JD, Burka JM, Bower KS, Stutzman RD, Sediq DA, Rabin JC. Effect of brimonidine tartrate 0.15% on night-vision difficulty and contrast testing after refractive surgery. *J Cataract Refract Surg.* 2008;34(9):1538–1541.

Pop M, Payette Y. Risk factors for night vision complaints after LASIK for myopia. *Ophthalmology.* 2004;111(1):3–10.

Schallhorn SC, Kaupp SE, Tanzer DJ, Tidwell J, Laurent J, Bourque LB. Pupil size and quality of vision after LASIK. *Ophthalmology.* 2003;110(8):1606–1614.

Schmidt GW, Yoon M, McGwin G, Lee PP, McLeod SD. Evaluation of the relationship between ablation diameter, pupil size, and visual function with vision-specific quality-of-life measures after laser in situ keratomileusis. *Arch Ophthalmol.* 2007;125(8):1037–1042.

Ocular Motility, Confrontation Fields, and Ocular Anatomy

Ocular motility should be carefully evaluated prior to surgery. In patients with asymptomatic tropia or phoria, symptoms may develop after refractive surgery if the change in refraction causes the motility status to break down. If there is a history of strabismus (see Chapter 10) or a concern about ocular alignment postoperatively, a trial with contact lenses before surgery should be considered. A sensory motor evaluation can be obtained preoperatively if strabismus is an issue. Confrontation field tests should be performed as part of the basic ophthalmic examination.

The general anatomy of the orbits should also be assessed. Patients with small palpebral fissures and/or large brows may not be ideal candidates for LASIK because there may be inadequate exposure and difficulty in achieving suction with the microkeratome or femtosecond laser suction ring.

Intraocular Pressure

The intraocular pressure (IOP) should be checked after the manifest refraction is completed and corneal topography measurements are taken. Patients with glaucoma (see Chapter 10) should be advised that during certain refractive surgery procedures, the IOP is dramatically elevated, potentially aggravating optic nerve damage. Also, topical corticosteroids are used after most refractive surgery procedures and, after a surface ablation procedure, may be used for months. Long-term use of topical corticosteroids may cause marked elevation of IOP in corticosteroid responders.

Samuelson TW. Refractive surgery in glaucoma. *Curr Opin Ophthalmol.* 2004;15(2):112–118.

Slit-Lamp Examination

A complete slit-lamp examination of the eyelids and anterior segment should be performed. The conjunctiva should be examined specifically for scarring, conjunctivochalasis, or chemosis, which may cause problems with microkeratome suction. The cornea should be evaluated for surface abnormalities such as decreased tear breakup time (Fig 2-1) and punctate epithelial erosions (Fig 2-2). Significant blepharitis (Fig 2-3), meibomitis, and dry-eye syndrome should be addressed before refractive surgery, as they are associated with increased postoperative discomfort and decreased vision, and dry-eye symptoms frequently increase postoperatively. A careful examination for epithelial basement membrane dystrophy (Fig 2-4) is required, because its presence increases the risk of flap complications during LASIK. Patients with epithelial basement membrane dystrophy are not ideal candidates for LASIK and may be better candidates for surface ablation, because removal of the abnormal epithelium may be palliative. Signs of keratoconus, such as corneal

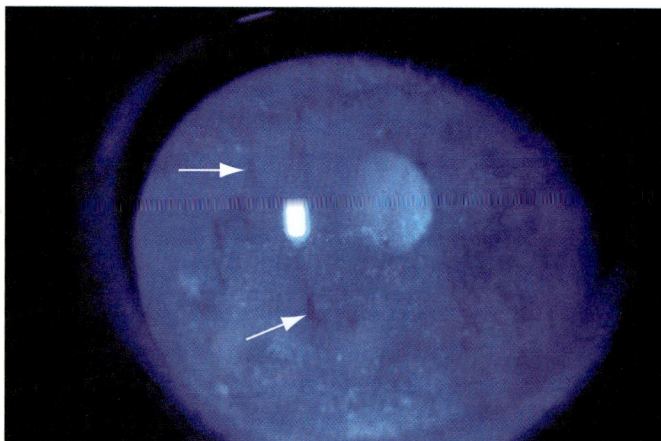

Figure 2-1 Slit-lamp photograph showing decreased tear breakup time. After instillation of fluorescein dye, the patient keeps the eye open for 10 seconds, and the tear film is examined with cobalt blue light. Breaks, or dry spots, in the tear film *(arrows)* are visible in this image. Punctate epithelial erosions are also present. *(Courtesy of Christopher J. Rapuano, MD.)*

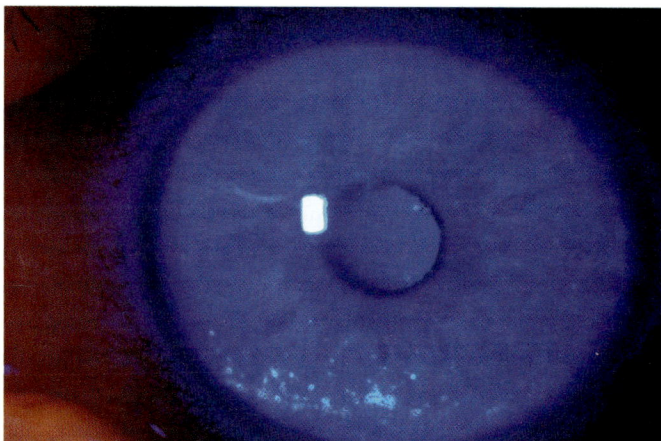

Figure 2-2 Slit-lamp photograph, showing punctate epithelial erosions. Inferior punctate fluorescein staining is noted in this image from a patient with moderately dry eyes. *(Courtesy of Christopher J. Rapuano, MD.)*

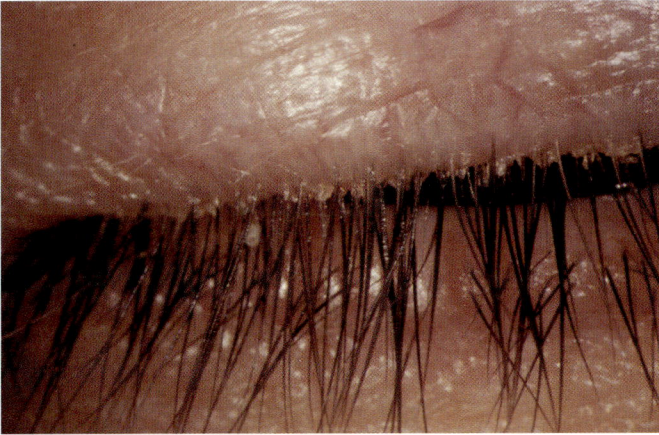

Figure 2-3 Example of blepharitis. Moderate crusting at the base of the lashes is shown in this image of a patient with seborrheic blepharitis. *(Courtesy of Christopher J. Rapuano, MD.)*

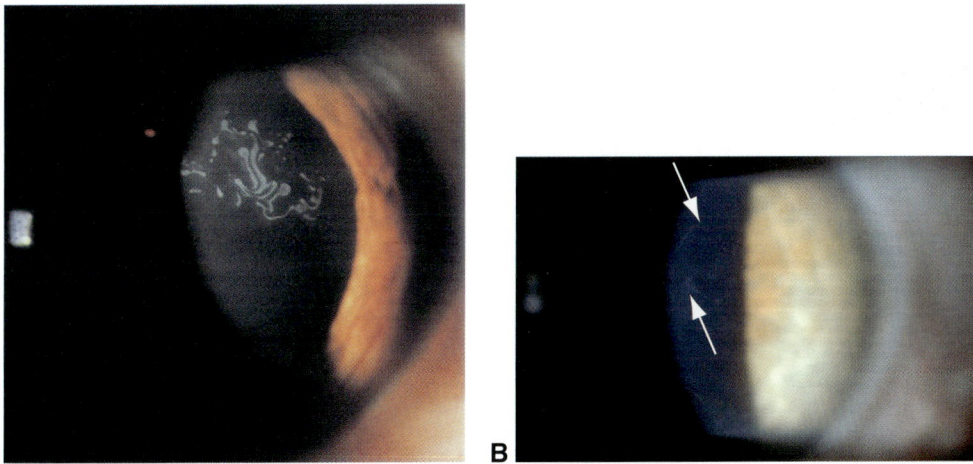

Figure 2-4 Images of epithelial basement membrane dystrophy. Epithelial map changes can be obvious **(A)** or more subtle **(B)**. *Arrows* show geographic map lines. *(Part A courtesy of Vincent P. deLuise, MD; part B courtesy of Christopher J. Rapuano, MD.)*

thinning and steepening, may also be found. Keratoconus is typically a contraindication to incisional or ablative refractive surgery (see Chapter 10). The endothelium should be examined carefully for signs of cornea guttata and other dystrophies. Poor visual results have been reported in patients with cornea guttata and a family history of Fuchs dystrophy. Corneal edema is generally considered a contraindication to refractive surgery. The deposits of granular and Avellino corneal dystrophies may increase substantially in size and number in the flap interface after LASIK, resulting in poor vision.

The anterior chamber, iris, and crystalline lens should also be examined. A shallow anterior chamber depth may be a contraindication for insertion of certain phakic intraocular lenses (PIOLs) (see Chapter 8). Careful evaluation of the crystalline lens for clarity is essential in both the undilated and dilated state, especially in patients more than 50 years of age. Surgeons should be wary of progressive myopia due to nuclear sclerosis. Patients with mild lens changes that are visually insignificant should be informed of these findings and advised that the changes may become more significant in the future, independent of refractive surgery. They should also be told that IOL power calculations may be less accurate when performed after keratorefractive surgery. In patients with moderate lens opacities, cataract extraction may be the best form of refractive surgery.

Kim TI, Kim T, Kim SW, Kim EK. Comparison of corneal deposits after LASIK and PRK in eyes with granular corneal dystrophy type II. *J Refract Surg.* 2008;24(4):392–395.

Moshirfar M, Feiz V, Feilmeier MR, Kang PC. Laser in situ keratomileusis in patients with corneal guttata and family history of Fuchs' endothelial dystrophy. *J Cataract Refract Surg.* 2005; 31(12):2281–2286.

Dilated Fundus Examination

A dilated fundus examination before refractive surgery is made to ensure that the posterior segment is normal. Special attention should be given to the macula, optic nerve (glaucoma, optic nerve drusen), and peripheral retina (retinal breaks, detachment). Patients and surgeons should realize that highly myopic eyes are naturally at increased risk of retinal detachment (see Chapter 10), unrelated to refractive surgery. The patient should be evaluated by a retinal specialist if any concerning retinal pathology is discovered.

Alió JL, Grzybowski A, El Aswad A, Romaniuk D. Refractive lens exchange. *Surv Ophthalmol.* 2014;59(6):579–598.

Packard R. Refractive lens exchange for myopia: a new perspective? *Curr Opin Ophthalmol.* 2005;16(1):53–56.

Ancillary Tests

Corneal Topography

The corneal curvature must be evaluated. Although manual keratometry readings can be quite informative, they have largely been replaced by computerized corneal topographic analyses. Several different methods are available to analyze the corneal curvature, including Placido disk-based topography, scanning slit-beam imaging, rotating Scheimpflug photography, high-frequency ultrasound, and optical coherence tomography (OCT) techniques. (See also the discussion of corneal topography in Chapter 1.) These techniques image the cornea and provide color maps showing corneal power and/or elevation. Patients with visually significant irregular astigmatism are generally not good candidates for corneal refractive surgery. Early keratoconus, pellucid marginal degeneration (Fig 2-5), and contact lens warpage are potential causes of visually significant irregular astigmatism. Irregular astigmatism secondary to contact lens warpage usually reverses over time, although the reversal may take months. Serial corneal topographic studies should be performed to document the resolution of visually significant irregular astigmatism before any refractive surgery is undertaken.

Unusually steep or unusually flat corneas can increase the risk of poor flap creation with the microkeratome. Femtosecond laser flap creation theoretically may avoid these

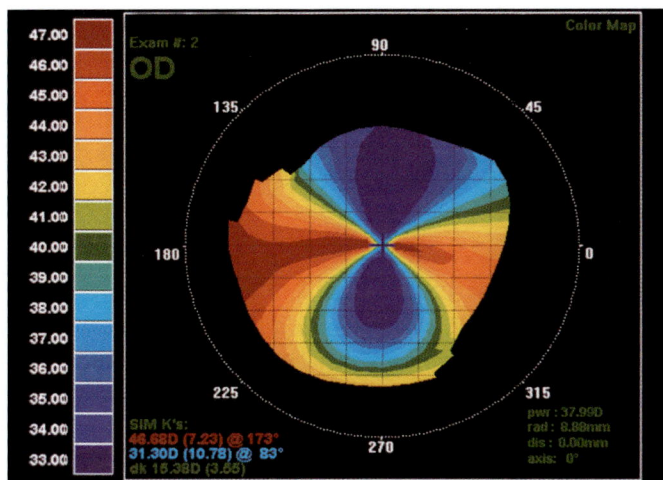

Figure 2-5 A corneal topographic map of the typical irregular against-the-rule astigmatism found in eyes with pellucid marginal degeneration. Note that the steepening nasally and temporally connects inferiorly. *(Courtesy of Christopher J. Rapuano, MD.)*

risks. When keratometric or corneal topographic measurements reveal an amount or an axis of astigmatism that differs significantly from that determined through refraction, the refraction should be rechecked for accuracy. Lenticular astigmatism or posterior corneal curvature may account for the difference between refractive and keratometric or topographic astigmatism. Most surgeons will treat the amount and axis of the refractive astigmatism, as long as the patient understands that after any future cataract surgery, some astigmatism may reappear (after the astigmatism contributed by the natural lens has been eliminated).

Pachymetry

Corneal thickness is an important criterion for determining adequacy for keratorefractive surgery. Corneal pachymetry is usually measured with ultrasound; however, certain non–Placido disk corneal topography and OCT systems can also be used if properly calibrated. Some systems provide a map showing the relative thickness of the cornea at various locations. The accuracy of the pachymetry measurements of scanning-slit systems decreases markedly for eyes that have undergone keratorefractive surgery. Because the thinnest part of the cornea is typically located centrally, a central measurement should always be taken. The thickness of the cornea is an important factor in determining whether the patient is a candidate for refractive surgery and identifying the optimal refractive procedure. In a study of 896 eyes undergoing LASIK, the mean central corneal thickness was 550 μm ± 33 μm (range, 472–651 μm). It has been suggested that an unusually thin cornea (beyond 2 standard deviations) indicates that the patient may not be ideal for any refractive surgery. Many surgeons would not consider LASIK refractive surgery if the central corneal thickness is less than 480 μm, even if the calculated residual stromal bed (RSB) is thicker than 250 μm. If LASIK is performed and results in a relatively thin RSB—for example, around 250 μm—future enhancement surgery that further thins the stromal bed may not be possible. If there is suspicion that endothelial integrity is causing an abnormally thick cornea, specular microscopy may be helpful in assessing the health of the endothelium.

Price FW Jr, Koller DL, Price MO. Central corneal pachymetry in patients undergoing laser in situ keratomileusis. *Ophthalmology.* 1999;106(11):2216–2220.

Wavefront Analysis

Wavefront analysis is a technique that can provide an objective refraction measurement (see also discussion of this topic in Chapters 1 and 5). Certain excimer lasers can use this wavefront analysis information directly to guide the ablation, a procedure called *wavefront-guided,* or *custom, ablation.* Some surgeons use wavefront analysis to document levels of preoperative higher-order aberrations. Refraction data from the wavefront analysis unit can also be used to refine the manifest refraction. If the manifest refraction and the wavefront analysis refraction are very dissimilar, the patient may not be a good candidate for wavefront treatment. Note that a custom wavefront ablation generally removes more tissue than does a standard ablation in the same eye.

Calculation of Residual Stromal Bed Thickness After LASIK

A lamellar laser refractive procedure such as LASIK involves creation of a corneal flap, ablation of the stromal bed, and replacement of the flap. The strength and integrity of the cornea postoperatively depend greatly on the thickness of the RSB. Thickness of the RSB is calculated by subtracting the sum of the flap thickness and the calculated laser ablation depth from the preoperative corneal thickness. For example, if the central corneal thickness is 550 μm, the flap thickness is estimated to be 140 μm, and the ablation depth for the patient's refraction is 50 μm, the RSB would be 550 μm – (140 μm + 50 μm) = 360 μm. When the surgeon determines the RSB, the amount of tissue removed should be based on the actual intended refractive correction, not on the nomogram-adjusted number entered into the laser computer. For example, if a patient with –10.00 D myopia that is being fully corrected, the amount of tissue removed is 128 μm for a 6.5-mm ablation zone for a broad-beam laser. Even if the surgeon usually takes off 15% of the refraction for a conventional ablation and enters that number into the laser computer, approximately 128 μm of tissue will be removed, not 85% of 128 μm.

Most surgeons believe the RSB should be at least 250 μm. Others want the RSB to be greater than 50% of the original corneal thickness. If the calculation reveals a thinner RSB than desired, LASIK may not be the best surgical option. In these cases, a surface ablation procedure may be a better option, as this will result in a thicker RSB postoperatively.

Discussion of Findings and Informed Consent

After completing the evaluation, the surgeon must analyze the information and discuss the findings with the patient. If the patient is a candidate for refractive surgery, the discussion must include the risks and benefits of the medical and surgical alternatives. (Table 2-2 provides an overview of the most common refractive surgery procedures, their

Table 2-2 Limitations of the Most Common Refractive Surgery Procedures

Procedure	Typical Spherical Range	Typical Cylinder Range	Limitations
LASIK	−10.00 to +4.00 D	Up to 4.00 D	Thin corneas (thin residual stromal bed); epithelial basement membrane dystrophy; small palpebral fissures; preoperative severe dry eye; certain medications. Flat and steep corneas may predispose to flap complications. Wavefront-guided ablations may have more restricted FDA-approved treatment parameters.
Surface ablation	−10.00 to +4.00 D	Up to 4.00 D	Preoperative severe dry eye syndrome; certain medications. Postoperative haze may occur at high end of treatment range but range may be extended with the use of mitomycin C. There is prolonged vision-recovery time and more postoperative discomfort compared with LASIK.
Intrastromal corneal ring segments	−1.00 to −4.00 D	None	Not FDA approved to correct cylinder; glare symptoms; white opacities at edge of ring segments; not after radial keratotomy
Intrastromal corneal ring segments	FDA approved to treat myopia in keratoconus	NA	Approved for patients 21 years or older; contact lens intolerance; corneal thickness ≥450 µm at incision site; no corneal scarring
Phakic intraocular lenses	−3.00 to −20.00 D	None	FDA approved for myopia; intraocular surgery; long-term complications such as glaucoma, iritis, cataract, pupil distortion, corneal edema
Refractive lens exchange	All ranges	Up to 3.00 D	Not FDA approved; same complications as with cataract extraction with a lens implant

FDA = US Food and Drug Administration; LASIK = laser in situ keratomileusis; NA = not applicable.

typical refractive ranges, and their key limitations.) Significant aspects of this discussion are the expected visual acuity results for the amount of refractive error (including the need for distance and/or reading glasses, the chance of needing an enhancement, and whether maximal surgery is being performed during the initial procedure), the risk of decreased BCVA or severe vision loss, the adverse effects of glare and halos or dry eyes, the change in vision quality, and the rare need to revise a corneal flap (eg, for flap displacement, significant striae, or epithelial ingrowth). The patient should understand that the laser ablation may be aborted if there is an incomplete, decentered, or buttonholed flap. The pros and cons of surgery on 1 eye versus both eyes on the same day should also be discussed, and patients should be allowed to decide which is best for them. Although the consequences of bilateral infection are higher with bilateral surgery, serial unilateral surgery may result in temporary anisometropia and is more inconvenient. Nonsurgical alternatives, such as glasses and contact lenses, should also be discussed.

If a patient is considering refractive surgery, he or she should be given the informed consent document to take home and review. The patient should be given an opportunity to discuss any questions related to the surgery or the informed consent form with the surgeon preoperatively. The consent form should be signed before surgery and never when the patient is dilated and/or sedated. For sample informed consent forms, see the website of the Ophthalmic Mutual Insurance Company (OMIC; www.omic.com /risk-management/consent-forms/).

CHAPTER 3

Incisional Corneal Surgery

▶ *This chapter includes a related video, which can be accessed by scanning the QR code provided in the text or going to www.aao.org/bcscvideo_section13.*

Incisional refractive surgery for treatment of myopia has largely been replaced by other modalities, but is still used for treatment of primary astigmatism during cataract surgery and residual astigmatism after both cataract and keratorefractive surgery (limbal relaxing incisions) and following penetrating keratoplasty (arcuate keratotomy). In fact, the use of incisional surgery, both traditional and intrastromal, has increased significantly with the advent of refractive cataract surgery utilizing femtosecond laser platforms and multifocal lens implants.

The history of incisional keratotomy dates back to the 1890s. Lans examined astigmatic changes induced in rabbits after partial-thickness corneal incisions and thermal cautery. Sato made significant contributions to incisional refractive surgery in the 1930s and 1940s. He observed central corneal flattening and improvement in vision after the healing of spontaneous ruptures of the Descemet membrane (corneal hydrops) in patients with advanced keratoconus, which led him to develop a technique to induce artificial ruptures of the Descemet membrane. His long-term results in humans were poor, because incisions were made posteriorly through the Descemet layer, leading to endothelial cell failure and corneal edema in 75% of patients. In the 1960s and 1970s, Fyodorov, using radial incisions on the anterior cornea, established that the diameter of the central optical clear zone was inversely related to the amount of refractive correction: smaller central clear zones yield greater myopic corrections.

Incisional Correction of Myopia

Radial Keratotomy in the United States

Radial keratotomy (RK) is now largely considered an obsolete procedure, but it did play an important role in the history of refractive surgery. RK differs from surface ablation/photorefractive keratectomy (PRK) and laser in situ keratomileusis (LASIK) in that it does not involve removal of tissue from the central cornea; rather, there is a redistribution of power from the center to the periphery.

To evaluate the safety and efficacy of RK, the Prospective Evaluation of Radial Kera-totomy (PERK) study was undertaken in 1982 for patients with myopia from −2.00 D to −8.75 D (mean, −3.875 D). The sole surgical variable was the diameter of the central optical clear zone (3.00, 3.50, or 4.00 mm), based on the level of preoperative myopia. Ten years after the procedure, 53% of the 435 study patients had 20/20 or better uncorrected visual acuity (UCVA; also called *uncorrected distance visual acuity, UDVA*) and 85% had 20/40 or better. In addition, the older the patient, the greater the effect achieved with the same surgical technique. The most important finding in the 10-year PERK study was the continuing long-term instability of the procedure. A hyperopic shift of 1.00 D or greater was found in 43% of eyes between 6 months and 10 years postoperatively.

> Waring GO III, Lynn MJ, McDonnell PJ; PERK Study Group. Results of the Prospective Evaluation of Radial Keratotomy (PERK) study 10 years after surgery. *Arch Ophthalmol.* 1994;112(10):1298–1308.

Surgical technique

Radial corneal incisions sever collagen fibrils in the corneal stroma. This produces a wound gape with midperipheral bulging of the cornea, compensatory central corneal flat-tening, and decreased refractive power, thereby decreasing myopia (Fig 3-1).

The design of the diamond-blade knife (angle and sharpness of cutting edge, width of blade, and design of footplate) influenced both the depth and the contour of incisions. The ideal depth of RK incisions is 85%–90% of the corneal thickness.

Postoperative refraction, visual acuity, and corneal topography

Radial keratotomy changes not only the curvature of the central cornea but also its overall topography, creating an oblate cornea—flatter in the center and steeper in the periphery. The procedure reduces myopia but increases spherical aberration. The result is less cor-relation among refraction, central keratometry, and UCVA, presumably because the new corneal curvature creates a more complex, multifocal optical system. The effect is that keratometric readings, which sample a limited number of points approximately 3.0 mm

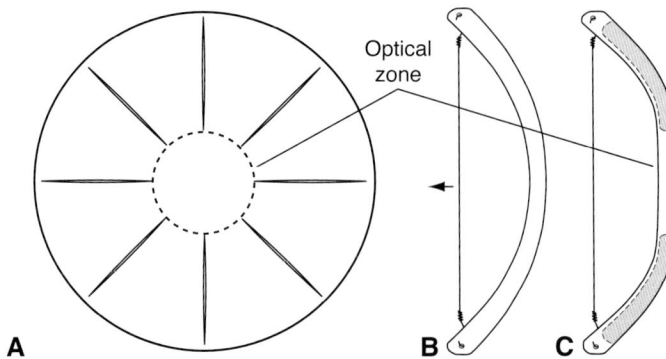

Figure 3-1 Schematic diagrams of the effect of radial incisions. **A,** 8-incision radial keratotomy (RK) with circular central optical zone *(dashed circle),* which shows the limit of the inner inci-sion length. **B,** Cross-sectional view of the cornea, pre-RK. **C,** After RK the corneal periphery is steepened and the center flattens. Flattening is induced in the central cornea. *(Modified from Trout-man RC, Buzard KA. Corneal Astigmatism: Etiology, Prevention, and Management. St Louis: Mosby-Year Book; 1992.)*

apart, might show degrees of astigmatism that differ from those detected by refraction. Also, central corneal flattening affects intraocular lens (IOL) power calculations for cataract surgery (discussed later in this chapter and in Chapter 11).

Stability of refraction

Most eyes were generally stable by 3 months after RK surgery. However, diurnal fluctuation of vision and a progressive flattening effect after surgery have been known to persist, resulting in refractive instability.

Diurnal fluctuation of vision occurs due to hypoxic edema of the incisions with the eyelids closed during sleep. This edema causes flattening of the cornea (and hyperopic shift) upon awakening, followed by steepening later in the day. In a subset of the PERK study at 10 years, the mean change in the spherical equivalent of refraction between the morning (waking) and evening examinations was an increase of 0.31 ± 0.58 D in minus power.

The *progressive flattening effect of surgery* was one of the major untoward results described in the PERK study. Greater hyperopic shift was noted with smaller optical zones. The potential stabilizing effect of corneal crosslinking (CCL) is currently being studied.

Elbaz U, Yeung SN, Ziai S, Lichtinger AD, et al. Collagen crosslinking after radial keratotomy. *Cornea.* 2014;33(2):131–136.

Mazzotta C, Baiocchi S, Denaro R, Tosi GM, Caporossi T. Corneal collagen cross-linking to stop corneal ectasia exacerbated by radial keratotomy. *Cornea.* 2011;30(2):225–228.

Complications

After RK surgery, 1%–3% of eyes experienced loss of 2 or more lines of Snellen visual acuity. This effect was due to induction of irregular astigmatism from hypertrophic scarring, intersecting radial and transverse incisions (Fig 3-2), and central clear zones smaller than 3.0 mm.

Many patients reported the appearance of starburst, glare, or halo effects around lights at night after RK. Treatment with drugs that promote pupillary constriction, such as pilocarpine, or decrease pupillary dilation, such as brimonidine may be able to reduce symptoms by keeping the pupillary diameter within the central optical clear zone. Other complications included fluctuation in vision and loss of best-corrected visual acuity (BCVA; also called *corrected distance visual acuity, CDVA*), induced astigmatism due to

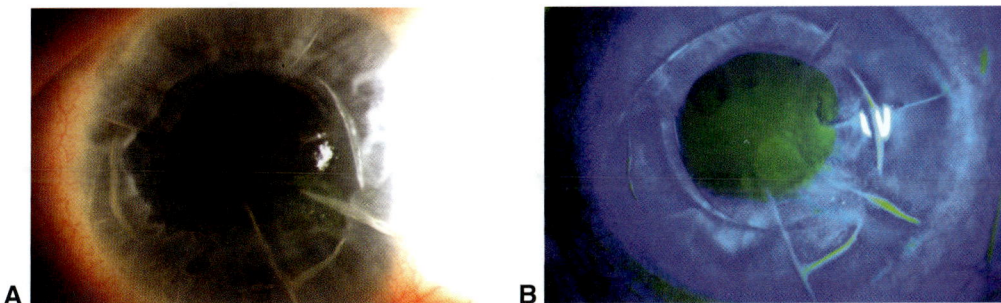

Figure 3-2 **A,** Crossed RK and arcuate keratotomy incisions with epithelial plugs in a patient who had intraoperative corneal perforation. **B,** Fluorescein study demonstrates gaping of the incisions, causing persistent ocular irritation. *(Courtesy of Jayne S. Weiss, MD.)*

epithelial plugs and wound gape (see Fig 3-2), vascularization of stromal scars, and non-progressive endothelial disruption beneath the incisions.

Potentially blinding complications occurred only rarely after RK. These included perforation of the cornea, which can lead to endophthalmitis, epithelial downgrowth, and traumatic cataract. The postoperative use of contact lenses often resulted in vascularization of the incisions, with subsequent scarring and irregular astigmatism. Radial keratotomy incisions remain a point of weakness, and rupture of RK wounds secondary to blunt trauma has been reported up to 13 years after the procedure.

Ocular surgery after radial keratotomy

It is not uncommon for RK patients to present years later with hyperopia. LASIK and PRK have been shown to be effective in correcting hyperopia and myopia after RK. However, surface ablation may be preferred, as creation of a LASIK flap may result in irregular astigmatism, splaying of the incisions, epithelial ingrowth, as well as loss of sections of the flap, which can be challenging to treat. Surface ablation avoids the LASIK-related risks after RK but increases the risk of postoperative corneal haze. The off-label use (in the United States) of mitomycin C, 0.02% (0.2 mg/mL) applied to the stroma after laser ablation for 12–30 seconds, has dramatically reduced corneal haze after RK and other prior corneal surgical procedures (eg, corneal transplant and LASIK). The drug should be copiously irrigated from the eye so that toxic effects are reduced.

Patients undergoing laser vision correction for refractive errors after RK need to understand that laser correction will not remove scars caused by RK incisions, so glare or fluctuation symptoms may remain after the laser surgery. In addition, some patients may still experience continued hyperopic progression.

In patients with endothelial dystrophy, corneal infection, irregular astigmatism, severe visual fluctuations, or starburst effects, keratoplasty may be needed to restore visual functioning. It should be avoided if the patient's visual problems can be corrected with glasses or contact lenses (see the section Corneal Transplantation After Refractive Surgery in Chapter 11). If keratoplasty is deemed necessary, before trephination the RK incisions may need to be stabilized with sutures outside the trephine cut. This minimizes the chance of their opening and allows adequate suturing of the donor corneal graft to the recipient bed.

Cataract extraction with IOL implantation may lead to variable results after RK. In the early postoperative period, corneal edema may result in temporary hyperopia. In addition, IOL power calculation may be problematic and may result in ametropia. Calculation of implant power for cataract surgery after RK should be done by first using a third-generation formula (eg, Haigis, Hoffer Q, Holladay 2, or SRK/T) rather than a regression formula (eg, SRK I or SRK II) and then choosing the highest resulting IOL power. Keratometric power is determined in 1 of 3 ways: direct measurement using corneal topography; application of pre-RK keratometry value minus the refractive change; or adjustment of the base curve of a plano contact lens by the overrefraction (see the section Eyes With No Preoperative Information in Chapter 11).

A useful online resource for calculating IOL power in a post-RK patient is the post–refractive surgery IOL power calculator available on the website of the American Society of Cataract and Refractive Surgery (ASCRS), www.ascrs.org, and directly at http://iolcalc .ascrs.org (see Chapter 11). In addition, modalities such as intraoperative wavefront aberrometry can be used to obtain real-time IOL calculations that may help improve refractive outcomes.

Incision placement and construction is vital when performing cataract surgery in the post-RK patient. Scleral tunnel incisions are often preferred, because clear corneal incisions increase the risk of the blade transecting the RK incision, which can induce irregular astigmatism. To help reduce preoperative corneal astigmatism, the surgeon may consider placing the incision in the steep astigmatic meridian of the cornea; in addition, toric IOLs can be used in patients with regular astigmatism but multifocal IOLs should be avoided. At the conclusion of surgery, care should be taken to prevent overhydrating the cataract incisions to avoid rupture of the RK incisions.

Anbar R, Malta JB, Barbosa JB, Leoratti MC, Beer S, Campos M. Photorefractive keratectomy with mitomycin-C for consecutive hyperopia after radial keratotomy. *Cornea*. 2009;28(4): 371–374.

Chen M. An evaluation of the accuracy of the ORange (Gen II) by comparing it to the IOLMaster in the prediction of postoperative refraction. *Clin Ophthalmol*. 2012;6:397–401.

Hemmati HD, Gologorsky D, Pineda R. Intraoperative wavefront aberrometry in cataract surgery. *Semin Ophthalmol*. 2012;27(5–6):100–106.

Hill WE, Byrne SF. Complex axial length measurements and unusual IOL power calculations. *Focal Points: Clinical Modules for Ophthalmologists*. San Francisco: American Academy of Ophthalmology; 2004, module 9.

Joyal H, Grégoire J, Faucher A. Photorefractive keratectomy to correct hyperopic shift after radial keratotomy. *J Cataract Refract Surg*. 2003;29(8):1502–1506.

Linebarger EJ, Hardten DR, Lindstrom RL. Laser-assisted in situ keratomileusis for correction of secondary hyperopia after radial keratotomy. *Int Ophthalmol Clin*. 2000;40(3):125–132.

Majmudar PA, Schallhorn SC, Cason JB, et al. Mitomycin-C in corneal surface excimer laser ablation techniques: a report by the American Academy of Ophthalmology. *Ophthalmology*. 2015;122(6):1085–1095.

Nassaralla BA, McLeod SD, Nassaralla JJ Jr. Prophylactic mitomycin C to inhibit corneal haze after photorefractive keratectomy for residual myopia following radial keratotomy. *J Refract Surg*. 2007;23(3):226–232.

Salamon SA, Hjortdal JO, Ehlers N. Refractive results of radial keratotomy: a ten-year retrospective study. *Acta Ophthalmol Scand*. 2000;78(5):566–568.

Seitz B, Langenbucher A. Intraocular lens calculations status after corneal refractive surgery. *Curr Opin Ophthalmol*. 2000;11(1):35–46.

Shammas. HJ. Intraocular lens power calculation in patients with prior refractive surgery. *Focal Points: Clinical Modules for Ophthalmologists*. San Francisco: American Academy of Ophthalmology; 2013, module 6.

Wang Ll, Hill WE, Koch DD. Evaluation of intraocular lens power prediction methods using the American Society of Cataract and Refractive Surgeons Post-Keratorefractive Intraocular Lens Power Calculator. *J Cataract Refract Surg*. 2010;36(9):1466–1473.

Incisional Correction of Astigmatism

Several techniques of incisional surgery have been used to correct astigmatism, including tangential (transverse/straight) keratotomy and arcuate (curved) keratotomy (AK), in which incisions are typically placed in the cornea at the 7-mm optical zone; and limbal relaxing incisions (LRIs), which are placed at the limbus. Tangential keratotomy was used in the past in combination with RK to correct myopic astigmatism, but now is seldom used. AK is used to correct post-keratoplasty astigmatism. Along with LRIs, AK is used to correct astigmatism during or after cataract surgery and IOL implantation, as well as after refractive surgery procedures such as LASIK and PRK (Video 3-1). Several femtosecond laser platforms have been approved for incisional keratotomies when used for capsulotomy and phacofragmentation of the crystalline lens.

VIDEO 3-1 Femtosecond laser-assisted astigmatic keratotomy.
Courtesy of George O. Waring IV, MD.
Access all Section 13 videos at www.aao.org/bcscvideo_section13.

Coupling

When a single meridian is flattened as a result of an astigmatic incision, a compensatory steepening occurs in the meridian 90° away. This phenomenon is known as *coupling* (Fig 3-3). When the coupling ratio (the amount of flattening in the meridian of the incision divided by the induced steepening in the opposite meridian) is 1.0, the spherical equivalent remains unchanged. When there is a coupling ratio greater than 1.0, a hyperopic shift occurs. The type of incision (arcuate versus tangential) and the length and number of parallel incisions can influence the coupling ratio. Long, straight, and tangential incisions tend to induce a coupling ratio greater than 1.0, unlike short, arcuate incisions. When a correction is less than 2.00 D of astigmatism, the coupling ratio is typically 1.0; however, when a correction is greater than 2.00 D of astigmatism, the ratio tends to be greater than 1.0. In general, LRIs do not change the spherical equivalent.

Rowsey JJ, Fouraker BD. Corneal coupling principles. *Int Ophthalmol Clin.* 1996;36(4):29–38.

Arcuate Keratotomy and Limbal Relaxing Incisions

AK is an incisional surgical procedure in which arcuate incisions of approximately 95% depth are made in the steep meridians of the midperipheral cornea at the 7–9-mm

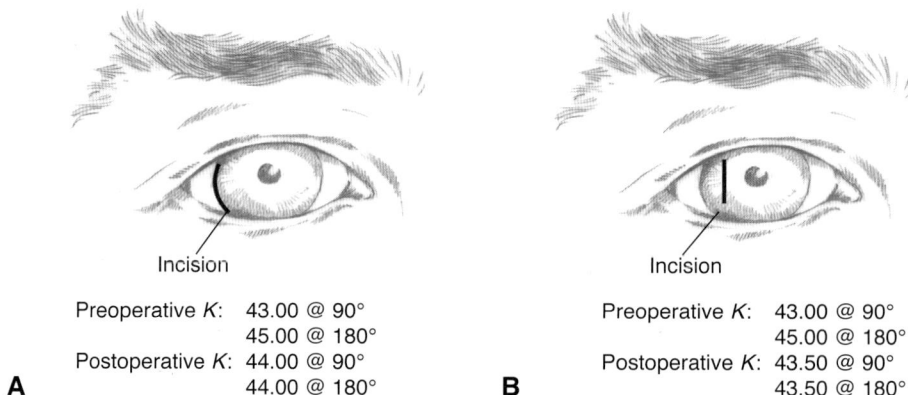

A

Incision

Preoperative *K*: 43.00 @ 90°
              45.00 @ 180°
Postoperative *K*: 44.00 @ 90°
              44.00 @ 180°

B

Incision

Preoperative *K*: 43.00 @ 90°
              45.00 @ 180°
Postoperative *K*: 43.50 @ 90°
              43.50 @ 180°

Figure 3-3 Coupling effect of astigmatic incisions. **A,** A limbal relaxing incision has a coupling ratio of 1.0, and the spherical equivalent and average corneal power are not changed. **B,** A transverse incision has a coupling ratio greater than 1.0, which causes a hyperopic change in refraction by making the average corneal power flatter. *(Illustration by Cyndie C. H. Wooley.)*

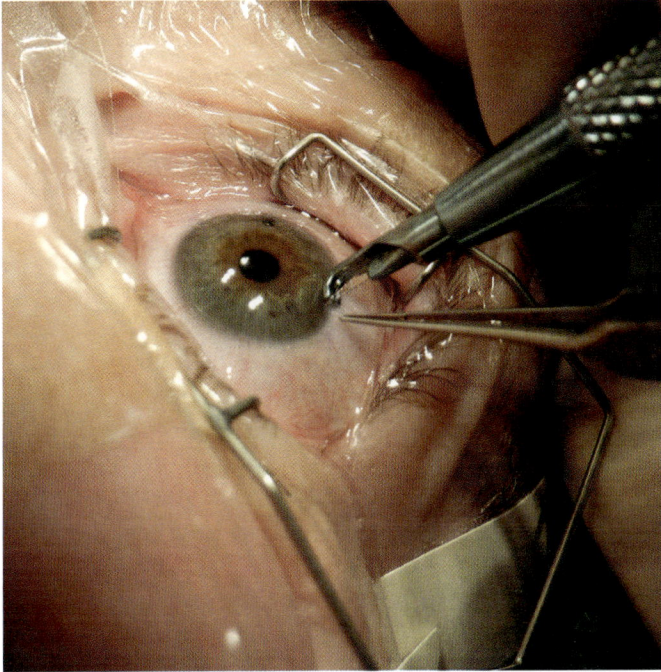

Figure 3-4 Limbal relaxing incision. A relaxing incision is made at the limbus with the use of a diamond knife. The coupling ratio is typically 1.0 and does not change the spherical equivalent. *(Courtesy of Brian S. Boxer Wachler, MD.)*

optical zone. LRIs are incisions set at approximately 600 µm depth, or 50 µm less than the thinnest pachymetry measurement at the limbus. They are placed just anterior to the limbus (Fig 3-4). AKs differ from LRIs by their midperipheral location and greater relative corneal depth. However, AKs and LRIs are similar in that both have coupling ratios of 1.0 and therefore correct astigmatism without inducing a substantial hyperopic shift. Increasing the length of an LRI increases the magnitude of the astigmatic correction. For AK, the amount of cylindrical correction is increased by increasing the length or depth of the incision, using multiple incisions, or reducing the optical zone (Table 3-1). Older patient age is associated with increased effect of astigmatic incisions.

Instrumentation

The instruments used in AKs and LRIs are similar. Adjustable diamond blades are more often used in AKs. Preset diamond blades are more often used in LRI surgical procedures (Fig 3-5), although adjustable blades may be used. The femtosecond laser has been adapted to create peripheral arcuate incisions. These incisions may be titratable, as only part of the incision may be opened initially, followed by a larger area later if there is a need for greater astigmatic correction.

Surgical Techniques

With any astigmatism correction system, accurate determination of the steep meridian is essential. The plus cylinder axis of the manifest refraction is used, as this accounts for

Table 3-1 Sample Nomogram for Limbal Relaxing Incisions to Correct Keratometric Astigmatism During Cataract Surgery

Preoperative Astigmatism (D)	Age (Years)	Number	Length (Degrees)
With-the-rule			
0.75–1.00	<65	2	45
	≥65	1	45
1.01–1.50	<65	2	60
	≥65	2	45 (or 1 × 60)
>1.50	<65	2	80
	≥65	2	60
Against-the-rule/oblique[a]			
1.00–1.25[b]	–	1	35
1.26–2.00	–	1	45
>2.00	–	2	45

[a] Combined with temporal corneal incision.

[b] Especially if cataract incision is not directly centered on the steep meridian.

From Wang L, Misra M, Koch DD. Peripheral corneal relaxing incisions combined with cataract surgery. *J Cataract Refract Surg.* 2003;29(4):712–722.

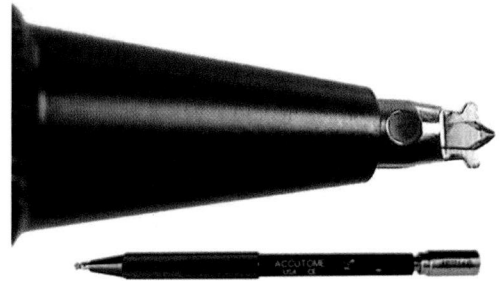

Figure 3-5 600-μm preset diamond knife for creating limbal relaxing incision.

corneal and lenticular astigmatism, which are "manifest" in the refraction. If the crystalline lens is to be removed at the time of the astigmatic incisional surgery (ie, LRI), the correction should be based on the steep meridian and magnitude as measured with corneal topography or keratometry. Intraoperative keratoscopy/aberrometry can be helpful in determining incision location and effect. The amount of treatment for a given degree of astigmatism employing LRIs can be determined from one of several nomograms, such as the one shown in Table 3-1.

It is prudent to make reference marks, using a surgical marking pen, with the patient sitting up, preferably at the slit lamp (Fig 3-6). Marking with the patient in this position avoids reference-mark error due to cyclotorsion of the eyes. Studies have demonstrated that up to 15° of cyclotorsion can occur when patients move from an upright to a supine position. Concomitantly, during cataract surgery, AK incisions may be placed in pairs along the steep meridian, usually between the 7-mm and 9-mm optical zone and, because of induced glare and aberrations, no closer than 3.5 mm from the center of the pupil. LRIs are placed in the peripheral cornea, near the limbus. AK incisions used to correct post–penetrating keratoplasty astigmatism are often made in the graft or in the graft–host

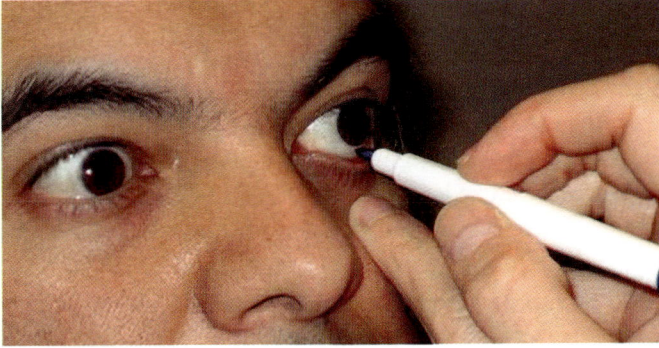

Figure 3-6 Marking the 6 o'clock axis of the limbus while the patient is sitting upright and looking straight ahead.

junction, but care must be taken to avoid perforation. When AK incisions are made in the host, the effect is significantly reduced. AK incisions in a corneal graft may require compression sutures at the meridian 90° away, and an initial overcorrection is desired in order to compensate for wound healing.

> Nichamin LD. Nomogram for limbal relaxing incisions. *J Cataract Refract Surg.* 2006;32(9): 1048.

Outcomes

The outcome of AK and LRI surgery depends on several variables, including patient age; the distance separating the incision pairs (optical zone); and the length, depth, and number of incisions. Few large prospective trials have been performed. The Astigmatism Reduction Clinical Trial (ARC-T) of AK, which used a 7-mm optical zone and varying arc lengths, showed a reduction in astigmatism of 1.6 ± 1.1 D in patients with preoperative, naturally occurring astigmatism of 2.8 ± 1.2 D. Other studies of AKs have shown a final UCVA of 20/40 in 65%–80% of eyes. Overcorrections have been reported in 4%–20% of patients.

Studies of LRIs are limited, but these incisions are frequently used with seemingly good results in astigmatic patients undergoing cataract surgery. One study showed an absolute change in refractive astigmatism of 1.72 ± 0.81 D after LRIs in patients with mixed astigmatism. Astigmatism was decreased by 0.91 D, or 44%, in another series of LRIs in 22 eyes of 13 patients. Incisions in the horizontal meridian have been reported to cause approximately twice as much astigmatic correction as those in the vertical meridian (see Table 3-1).

> Faktorovich EG, Maloney RK, Price FW Jr. Effect of astigmatic keratotomy on spherical equivalent: results of the Astigmatism Reduction Clinical Trial. *Am J Ophthalmol.* 1999; 127(3):260–269.
> Price FW, Grene RB, Marks RG, Gonzales JS; ARC-T Study Group. Astigmatism Reduction Clinical Trial: a multicenter prospective evaluation of the predictability of arcuate keratotomy. Evaluation of surgical nomogram predictability. *Arch Ophthalmol.* 1995;113(3): 277–282.

Complications

Irregular astigmatism may occur after either AKs or LRIs; however, it is more common with AKs than with LRIs, presumably because LRIs are farther from the corneal center, thus mitigating any effects of irregular incisions. Off-axis AKs can lead to undercorrection or even worsening of preexisting astigmatism. To avoid creating an edge of cornea that swells and cannot be epithelialized, arcuate incisions and LRIs should not intersect other incisions (see Fig 3-2). Corneal infection and perforation have been reported.

Ocular Surgery After Arcuate Keratotomy and Limbal Relaxing Incisions

AK and LRIs can be combined with or performed after cataract surgery, PRK, and LASIK surgery. Better predictability can be obtained if astigmatic correction is performed after refractive stability is achieved. Penetrating keratoplasty can be done after extensive AK, but the wounds may have to be sutured before trephination, as discussed earlier for RK. A prerequisite for combining LRIs with cataract surgery is the use of astigmatically predictable phacoemulsification.

Bains KC, Hamill MB. Refractive enhancement of pseudophakic patients. *Focal Points: Clinical Modules for Ophthalmologists.* San Francisco: American Academy of Ophthalmology; 2014, module 11.

Bayramlar HH, Dağlioğlu MC, Borazan M. Limbal relaxing incisions for primary mixed astigmatism and mixed astigmatism after cataract surgery. *J Cataract Refract Surg.* 2003; 29(4):723–728.

Budak K, Yilmaz G, Aslan BS, Duman S. Limbal relaxing incisions in congenital astigmatism: 6 month follow-up. *J Cataract Refract Surg.* 2001;27(5):715–719.

Dick HB, Gerste RD, Schultz T. Femtosecond laser-assisted cataract surgery. *Focal Points: Clinical Modules for Ophthalmologists.* San Francisco: American Academy of Ophthalmology; 2015, module 4.

Gills JP. Treating astigmatism at the time of cataract surgery. *Curr Opin Ophthalmol.* 2002; 13(1):2–6.

Nichamin LD. Astigmatism control. *Ophthalmol Clin North Am.* 2006;19(4):485–493.

Rao SN, Konowal A, Murchison AE, Epstein RJ. Enlargement of the temporal clear corneal cataract incision to treat preexisting astigmatism. *J Refract Surg.* 2002;18(4):463–467.

Rubenstein JB, Raciti M. Management of astigmatism: LRIs. *Int Ophthalmol Clin.* 2012;52(2): 31–40.

Tejedor J, Murube J. Choosing the location of corneal incision based on preexisting astigmatism in phacoemulsification. *Am J Ophthalmol.* 2005;139(5):767–776.

Yeu E, Rubenstein JB. Management of stigmatism in Lens-Based Surgery. *Focal Points: Clinical Modules for Ophthalmologists.* San Francisco: American Academy of Ophthalmology; 2008, module 2.

CHAPTER 4

Onlays and Inlays

▶ *This chapter includes a related video, which can be accessed by scanning the QR code provided in the text or going to www.aao.org/bcscvideo_section13.*

Refractive errors, including presbyopia, may be treated by placing preformed tissue or synthetic material onto or into the cornea. This approach alters the optical power of the cornea by changing the shape of the anterior corneal surface or by creating a lens with a higher index of refraction than the corneal stroma that is then implanted within the cornea. Intracorneal inlays with small apertures that use the pinhole effect to increase depth of focus have been developed. Tissue addition procedures, such as epikeratoplasty, have fallen out of favor because of the poor predictability of the refractive and visual results, loss of best-corrected visual acuity (BCVA; also called *corrected distance visual acuity, CDVA*), and difficulty of obtaining donor tissue. Compared with donor tissue, synthetic material can be shaped more precisely, and it can be mass-produced. Because of problems with reepithelialization when synthetic material is placed on top of the cornea, synthetic material generally has to be placed within the corneal stroma. This placement requires a partial or complete lamellar dissection using specialized instruments. Early work using lenticules made of glass and plastic resulted in necrosis of the overlying stroma because glass and plastic are impermeable to water, oxygen, and nutrients. Current techniques use lenticule inlays made of more permeable substances such as hydrogel, with or without microperforations in the lenticule, to increase the transmission of nutrients. Another category of corneal inlays are corneal ring segments made of polymethyl methacrylate (PMMA). Because the ring segments are narrow, the overlying stroma can receive nutrients from surrounding tissue.

Keratophakia

In keratophakia, a plus-powered lens is placed intrastromally to increase the curvature of the anterior cornea to correct hyperopia and presbyopia. After a central lamellar keratectomy is performed with a microkeratome or femtosecond laser, the flap is lifted, the lenticule is placed onto the host bed, and the flap is replaced and adheres without sutures. Lenticules can be prepared from either donor cornea or synthetic material; these types are referred to as homoplastic and alloplastic lenticules, respectively.

Homoplastic Corneal Inlays

A homoplastic inlay is created from a donor cornea by a lamellar keratectomy after removal of the epithelium and Bowman layer. The lenticule (fresh or frozen) is then shaped into a lens using an automated lathe. The lens can be preserved fresh in refrigerated tissue-culture medium, frozen at subzero temperatures, or freeze-dried.

Keratophakia has been used to correct aphakia and hyperopia of up to 20.00 D, but few studies on this procedure have been published. Troutman and colleagues reported on 32 eyes treated with homoplastic keratophakia, 29 of which also underwent cataract extraction. Even for procedures done by experienced surgeons, refractive predictability was still low: the eyes of 25% of patients were more than 3.00 D from the intended correction. Complications included irregular lamellar resection, wound dehiscence, and postoperative corneal edema. Although the procedure was originally intended to be used in conjunction with cataract extraction for the correction of aphakia, the complexity of the procedure and the unpredictable refractive results could not compete—in the early 1980s—with aphakic contact lenses or the improved technology of intraocular lens (IOL) implantation. Homoplastic keratophakia using tissue from stromal lenticule extraction has been suggested, however, for treating hyperopia, presbyopia, and ectatic corneal diseases.

Ganesh S, Brar S, Rao PA. Cryopreservation of extracted corneal lenticules after small incision lenticule extraction for potential use in human subjects. *Cornea.* 2014;33(12): 1355–1362.

Lim CH, Riau AK, Lwin NC, Chaurasia SS, Tan DT, Mehta JS. LASIK following small incision lenticule extraction (SMILE) lenticule re-implantation: a feasibility study of a novel method for treatment of presbyopia. *PLoS One.* 2013;8(12):e83046. www.ncbi.nlm.nih.gov /pmc/articles/PMC3859649/. Accessed November 6, 2016.

Sun L, Yao P, Li M, Shen Y, Zhao J, Zhou X. The safety and predictability of implanting autologous lenticule obtained by SMILE for hyperopia. *J Refract Surg.* 2015;31(6):374–379.

Alloplastic Corneal Inlays

Alloplastic inlays offer several potential advantages over homoplastic inlays, such as the ability to be accurately mass-produced in a wide range of sizes and powers. Synthetic material may have optical properties that are superior to those of tissue lenses.

For insertion of the inlay, a laser in situ keratomileusis (LASIK)–type flap or a stromal pocket dissection can be performed; such procedures are technically easier than a complete lamellar keratectomy. Experiments performed in the early 1980s resulted in corneal opacities, nonhealing epithelial erosions, and diurnal fluctuation in vision because fluid and nutrients were blocked from reaching the anterior cornea. Thus, to allow for the transfer of fluid and nutrients to the anterior cornea, either permeable materials were used or microperforations were incorporated into the inlays. Because of work performed by Knowles and others, most subsequent studies used water-permeable hydrogel implants. Hydrogel lenses have an index of refraction similar to that of the corneal stroma, so these lenses have little intrinsic optical power when implanted. To be effective, hydrogel inlays must change the curvature of the anterior cornea. Other mechanisms of action include inlays with refractive power and small aperture inlays. Four different presbyopic inlays have been developed and are currently in investigational studies.

In 2015, the US Food and Drug Administration (FDA) approved the KAMRA corneal inlay (AcuFocus Inc, Irvine, CA). This small-aperture inlay is indicated for the improvement of near vision in presbyopic patients who require near correction. This device is an ultrathin (5-μm), biocompatible polymer that is microperforated to allow improved nutrient flow. The 3.8-mm-diameter inlay has a central aperture of 1.6 mm and is generally implanted in the nondominant eye (Fig 4-1). The surgeon places the inlay into an intrastromal pocket created by femtosecond laser, using a spot and line separation of 6 × 6 μm or less. The inlay should be placed at a depth equal to or greater than 200 μm, centered on the patient-fixated, coaxially sighted corneal light reflex. Although the inlay has no refractive power, the central aperture functions as a pinhole to increase depth of focus and improve near vision without changing distance vision. (See Corneal Inlays in Chapter 9.)

In the FDA study, an average gain of 3 lines of uncorrected near vision in the implanted eye was observed at 12 months. With a 6 × 6 spot and line separation in the FDA study, 95% of eyes achieved the primary efficacy endpoint of 20/40 or better uncorrected near acuity, and a primary safety endpoint of 0.0% eyes having greater than or equal to 2 lines of persistent loss of BCVA. Rare but reported complications include refractive instability, decentration, and haze. In the FDA study with a 6 × 6 spot and line separation, 2.9% of inlays were removed, and all eyes with removals returned to their preoperative BCVA.

Ismail MM. Correction of hyperopia with intracorneal implants. *J Cataract Refract Surg.* 2002; 28(3):527–530.

Knowles WF. Effect of intralamellar plastic membranes on corneal physiology. *Am J Ophthalmol.* 1961;51:1146–1156.

Waring GO IV. Correction of presbyopia with a small aperture corneal inlay. *J Refract Surg.* 2011;27(11):842–845.

Whitman J, Dougherty PJ, Parkhurst GD, et al. Treatment of presbyopia in emmetropes using a shape-changing corneal inlay: 1-year clinical outcomes. *Ophthalmology.* 2016;123(3): 466–475.

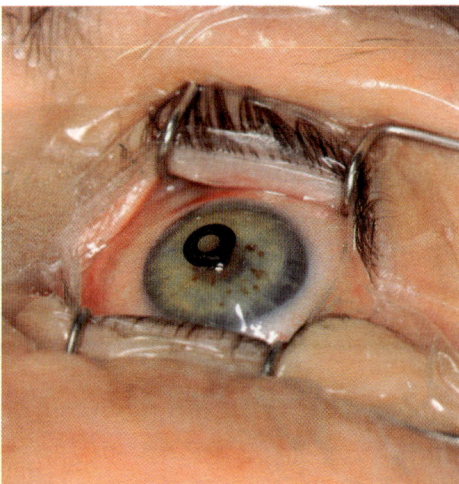
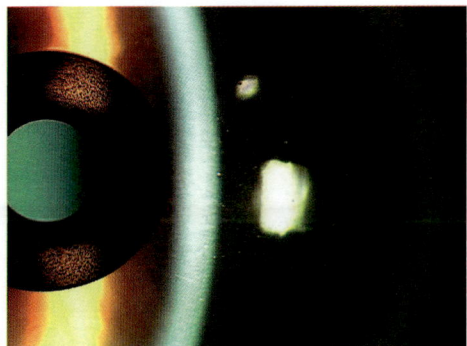

A **B**

Figure 4-1 Small-aperture corneal inlay for the surgical treatment of presbyopia. **A,** The inlay is surgically implanted into a stromal pocket in the nondominant eye. **B,** Slit-lamp photograph of a small-aperture inlay. *(Courtesy of George O. Waring IV, MD.)*

Epikeratoplasty

Epikeratoplasty involved suturing a preformed homoplastic lenticule directly onto the Bowman layer of the host cornea (see Fig 4-1). Because no viable cells existed in the donor tissue, classic graft rejection did not occur. Epikeratoplasty was originally intended to create a "living contact lens" for patients with aphakia who were unable to wear contact lenses. Indications for this procedure were later expanded to include hyperopia, myopia, and keratoconus, but problems such as adherence of the grafted tissue, infection, epithelial ingrowth into the bed, poor predictability of results, and corneal edema have relegated epikeratoplasty to a historical footnote. In treating patients with these conditions, surgeons need to approach corneal refractive surgery with caution.

> Werblin TP, Kaufman HE, Friedlander MH, Sehon KL, McDonald MB, Granet NS. A prospective study of the use of hyperopic epikeratophakia grafts for the correction of aphakia in adults. *Ophthalmology.* 1981;88(11):1137–1140.

Intrastromal Corneal Ring Segments

Background

Intrastromal corneal ring segments (ICRS) can treat low degrees of myopia by displacing the lamellar bundles and shortening the corneal arc length. However, the main indication for ICRS placement is keratoconus and other forms of ectatic corneal diseases. These circular arcs, made of PMMA, are placed in the posterior midperipheral corneal stroma in a lamellar channel (Figs 4-2, 4-3). The thicker the segment is, the greater will be the flattening of the central cornea and the reduction in myopia. Ferrara rings (Ferrara Ophthalmics, Belo Horizonte, Brazil) or Kerarings (Mediphacos, Belo Horizonte,

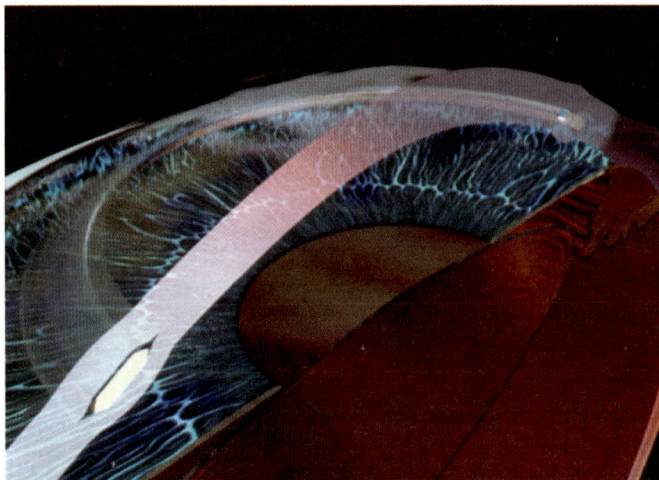

Figure 4-2 Rendering of a cross section of the cornea with an intrastromal corneal ring segment. The ring segment displaces the lamellar bundles, thereby shortening the corneal arc length and reducing the myopia. *(Courtesy of Addition Technology.)*

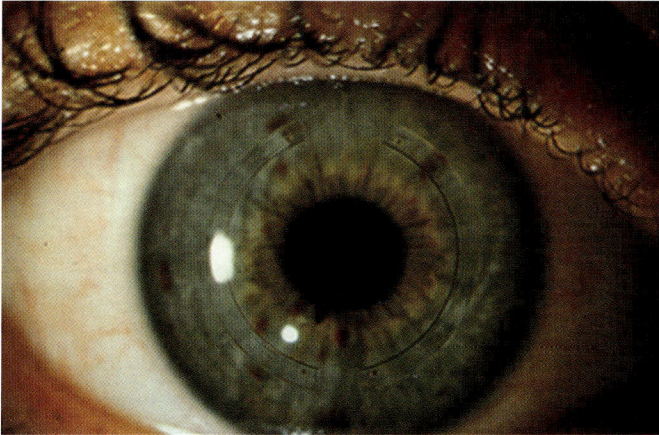

Figure 4-3 Clinical photograph showing ring segments implanted in an eye to treat low myopia. Note the vertical placement of the ring segments with a clear central zone. *(Courtesy of Steven C. Schallhorn, MD.)*

Brazil) have a smaller optical zone and a greater flattening effect than do Intacs (Oasis Medical, San Dimas, CA). This section focuses on Intacs because Ferrara-type rings, although commonly used internationally, are not FDA approved for use in the United States.

Treatment using ring segments has several potential advantages over other forms of refractive surgery. The ring segments can be explanted, making the refractive result of the procedure potentially reversible, and they can be replaced with ring segments of a different thickness to titrate the refractive result. Intacs are FDA approved to treat myopia at levels ranging from –1.00 to –3.00 D spherical equivalent; they are not approved for patients with astigmatism. However, Intacs surgery is no longer commonly performed for myopia because the results are not as predictable as are those with ablative corneal surgery.

Intacs are typically contraindicated in

- patients with collagen vascular, autoimmune, or immunodeficiency diseases
- pregnant or breastfeeding women
- patients who may be predisposed to future complications because of the presence of ocular conditions (such as herpetic keratitis, recurrent corneal erosion syndrome, and corneal dystrophy)

Instrumentation

Initially, a 1-piece 360° Intacs ring was used in the procedure, but it proved difficult to insert. The design was later changed to 2 segments of 150° arc each. The segments have a fixed inner diameter of 6.80 mm and an outer diameter of 8.10 mm, and they are available in various thicknesses: 0.210, 0.250, 0.275, 0.300, 0.325, 0.350, 0.400, and 0.450 mm. The degree of correction achieved is related to the thickness of the ring segments; thicker ring segments are used for greater correction. Manually operated surgical equipment or a femtosecond laser can be used to create the channels.

Technique

The procedure involves creating a lamellar channel at approximately 68%–70% stromal depth, followed by insertion of the ring segments. The geometric center of the cornea is marked with a blunt hook. An ultrasound pachymeter is used to measure the thickness of the cornea over the entry mark. A diamond knife is set to 68%–70% of the stromal depth and then used to create a 1.0-mm radial incision. Specially designed mechanical instruments are then used to create the channels for the segments by blunt separation of the collagen lamellae (Fig 4-4). Similar entry incisions and channels may be created using a femtosecond laser (Video 4-1). The channels are created in an arc pattern at the desired inner and outer diameters. Once the channels are created, specialized forceps are used to insert the first ring segment and rotate it into position, followed by similar insertion and rotation of the second segment. Tissue glue or 1 or 2 10-0 nylon sutures may be used to close the radial incision at the corneal surface.

VIDEO 4-1 Implantation of asymmetric corneal ring segments for the surgical management of keratoconus.
Courtesy of George O. Waring IV, MD.
Access all Section 13 videos at www.aao.org/bcscvideo_section13.

Outcomes

Food and Drug Administration clinical trials provided the most complete outcome analysis of Intacs for myopia. A total of 452 patients enrolled in these trials. Patients received 0.25-, 0.30-, or 0.35-mm ring segments to correct an average preoperative mean spherical equivalent of –2.240 D (range, –0.750 to –4.125 D). At 12 months postoperatively, 97% of treated eyes had 20/40 or better uncorrected vision and 74% had achieved 20/20 or better. In addition, 69% and 92% of eyes were within ±0.50 and 1.00 D of emmetropia, respectively. These clinical outcomes were similar to early results with photorefractive keratectomy (PRK) and LASIK, although excimer laser studies generally treated a broader range of preoperative myopia.

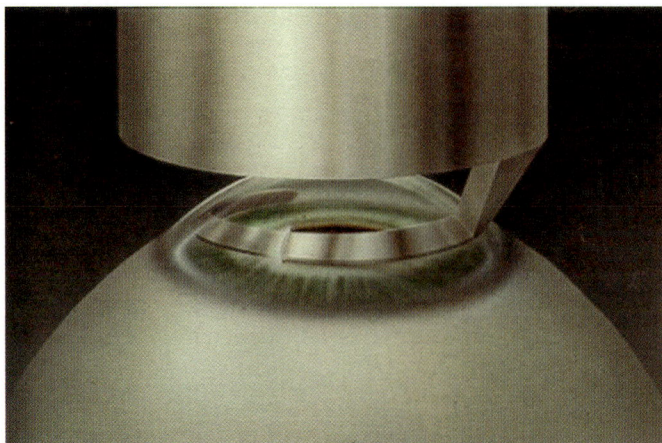

Figure 4-4 Rendering of the Intacs dissector tool as it is being rotated to create the intrastromal channel. *(Courtesy of Addition Technology.)*

Additional FDA approval was later granted to include intermediate segment sizes of 0.275 and 0.325 mm. Internationally, CE (Conformité Européene) marking status (similar in concept to US FDA approval) was extended to thicker segment sizes. In 2000, Colin found that Intacs implantation compared favorably with PRK for treating low myopia, although it induced greater astigmatism.

The removal or exchange rate varies between 3% and 15%. A common reason for a ring segment exchange is residual myopia. Ring segment removal is most often performed because of disabling vision symptoms such as glare, double vision, and photophobia. Few complications are associated with ring segment removal. In a series of 684 eyes that received Intacs, 46 (6.7%) underwent their removal. Most patients returned to their original preoperative myopia by 3 months postremoval (73% returned to within 0.50 D of preoperative mean spherical equivalent). No patient had a loss of BCVA of more than 2 lines. However, up to 15% of patients reported new or worsening symptoms after removal.

Intracorneal Ring Segments and Keratoconus

In the past, very few surgical options other than penetrating and lamellar keratoplasty were available for the treatment of keratoconus. Excimer laser procedures, which correct ametropia by removing tissue, are generally not recommended for treating keratoconus because of the risk of exacerbating corneal structural weakening and ectasia.

In 2004, Intacs received a *Humanitarian Device Exemption* from the FDA for use in reducing or eliminating myopia and astigmatism in certain patients with keratoconus, specifically those who can no longer achieve adequate vision with their contact lenses or glasses (Fig 4-5). The intent was to restore functional vision and defer the need for a corneal transplant. Labeled selection criteria for patients include

- progressive deterioration in vision such that the patient can no longer achieve adequate functional vision on a daily basis with contact lenses or glasses
- age 21 years or older

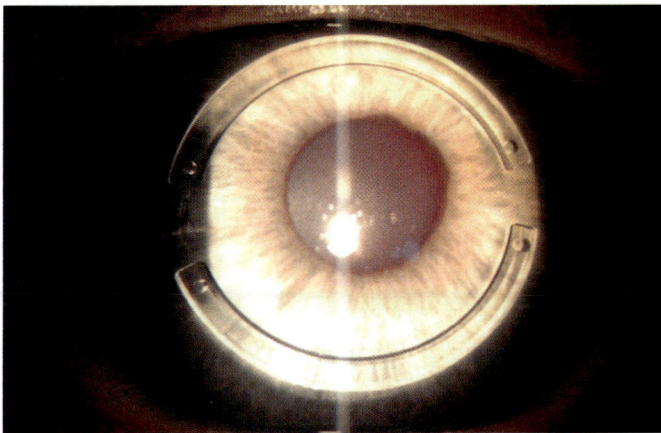

Figure 4-5 Slit-lamp biomicroscopy of the cornea immediately after symmetric intracorneal ring segment implantation for the surgical management of keratoconus. *(Courtesy of George O. Waring IV, MD.)*

- clear central corneas
- a corneal thickness of 450 μm or greater at the proposed incision site
- a lack of options other than corneal transplantation for improving functional vision

Although these are FDA labeling parameters, many surgeons perform Intacs insertion outside these criteria. In one study of 26 keratoconus patients, the ring segments were oriented horizontally, with a thick ring (0.450 mm) placed in the inferior cornea and a thinner one (0.250 mm) in the superior cornea. In another study of 50 patients (74 eyes), the orientation of the ring segments was adjusted according to the refractive cylinder. On the basis of the level of myopia, either the 0.300-mm ring or the 0.350-mm ring (the largest available in the United States at that time) was placed inferiorly, and the 0.250-mm ring was placed superiorly. Patients had mild to severe keratoconus with or without scarring. A superficial channel with perforation of the Bowman layer in 1 eye was the only operative complication. A total of 6 rings were explanted for segment migration and externalization (1 ring) and foreign-body sensation (5 rings).

The improvement in vision was significant. With an average follow-up period of 9 months, the mean uncorrected visual acuity (UCVA); also called *uncorrected distance visual acuity, UDVA*) improved from approximately 20/200 (1.05 logMAR [base 10 logarithm of the minimum angle of resolution]) to 20/80 (0.61 logMAR) (P <.01). The mean BCVA also improved, from approximately 20/50 (0.41 logMAR) to 20/32 (0.24 logMAR) (P <.01). Most patients still required optical correction to achieve their best-corrected vision. Eyes with corneal scarring had a similar improvement in UCVA and BCVA. Inferior steepening was reduced on topography as was coma. The dioptric power of the inferior cornea relative to the superior (I–S value) was reduced from a preoperative mean of 25.62 to 6.60 postoperatively.

A study evaluating the long-term stability of Intacs in keratoconus found that in nearly 93% of patients with documented progression of keratoconus pre-Intacs, there was no further progression of keratoconus between 1 and 5 years after Intacs implantation. In addition, no statistically significant differences were noted in mean steep, flat, and average keratometry readings; manifest refraction spherical equivalent; and UCVA and BCVA (P >.05) between 1 and 5 years postimplantation.

Number of Segments

Although most surgeons implant 2 Intacs segments, the use of only 1 segment may be indicated. If the steep area is peripheral (similar to pellucid marginal degeneration), it may be preferable to place 1 segment instead of 2 segments because the keratoconic cornea has 2 optical areas of distortion within the pupil: a steep lower area and a flat upper area. For peripheral keratoconus, it is better to flatten the steep area and steepen the flat area than to flatten the entire cornea. Single-segment placement can achieve that result (Fig 4-6). When a single segment is placed, it flattens the adjacent cornea but causes steepening of the cornea 180° away—the "beanbag effect" (ie, when one sits on a beanbag, it flattens in one area and pops up in another area). This effect may yield a more physiologic improvement than would the global flattening effect from the use of double segments. Intacs treatment can also be combined with corneal crosslinking for improved corneal strength and phakic IOL implantation to improve refractive error (see Chapter 7).

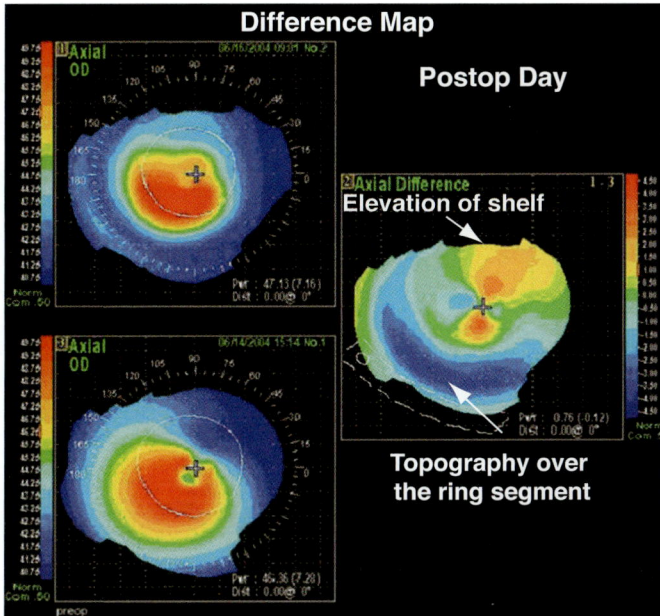

Figure 4-6 Corneal topography analysis before and after single-segment Intacs placement. The preoperative topography (lower left) shows oblique steepening, and the postoperative topography (upper left) shows contraction of a steep cone after a single-segment Intacs was placed outside the cone. The difference map (subtraction of preoperative and postoperative topography) (right) shows topography over the ring segment (blue) and steepening in the overly flat area (red). The apex of the cornea has moved more centrally. *(Courtesy of Brian S. Boxer Wachler, MD.)*

Bedi R, Touboul D, Pinsard L, Colin J. Refractive and topographic stability of Intacs in eyes with progressive keratoconus: five-year follow-up. *J Refract Surg.* 2012;28(6):392–396.

Ertan A, Karacal H, Kamburoğlu G. Refractive and topographic results of transepithelial cross-linking treatment in eyes with Intacs. *Cornea.* 2009;28(7):719–723.

Sharma M, Boxer Wachler BS. Comparison of single-segment and double-segment Intacs for keratoconus and post-LASIK ectasia. *Am J Ophthalmol.* 2006;141(5):891–895.

Wollensak G, Spörl E, Seiler T. Riboflavin/ultraviolet-A-induced collagen crosslinking for the treatment of keratoconus. *Am J Ophthalmol.* 2003;135(5):620–627.

Complications

The loss of BCVA (≥2 lines of vision) after intracorneal ring segment insertion has been found to be approximately 1% at 1 year postoperatively. Adverse events (defined as events that, if left untreated, could be serious or result in permanent sequelae) have been reported to occur in approximately 1% of patients. Reported adverse events include

- anterior chamber perforation
- microbial keratitis
- implant extrusion (Fig 4-7)
- shallow ring segment placement
- corneal thinning over Intacs (Fig 4-8)

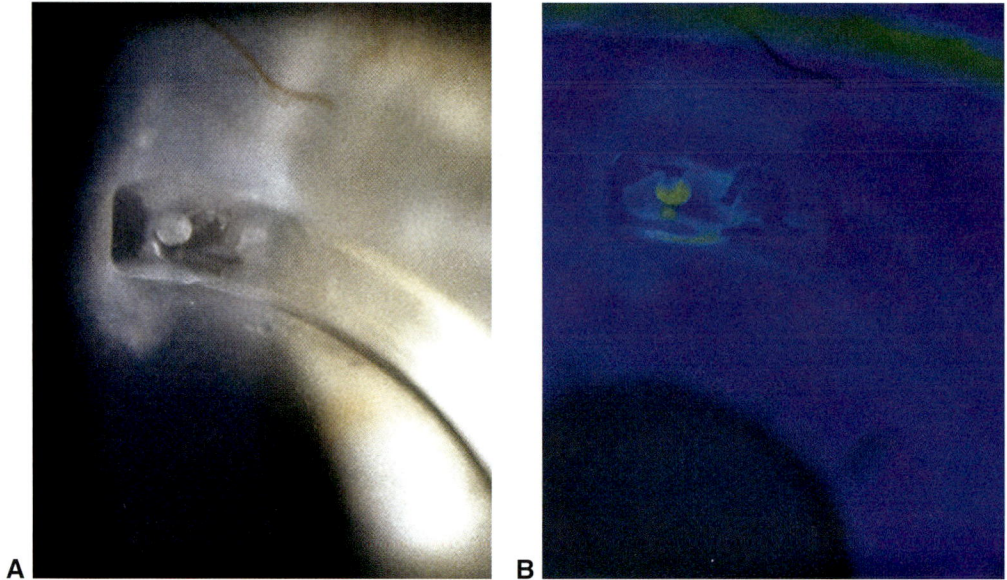

Figure 4-7 Slit-lamp images of an adverse event of Intacs placement: extrusion of the ring segment. **A,** Tip extrusion. **B,** Tip extrusion easily seen with fluorescein dye. *(Courtesy of Brian S. Boxer Wachler, MD.)*

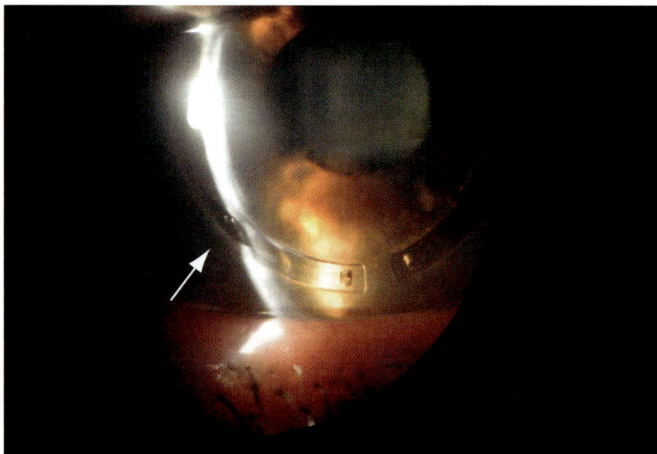

Figure 4-8 Image of an adverse event of Intacs: corneal thinning over the ring segment *(arrow)* after excessive use of a nonsteroidal anti-inflammatory drug. *(Courtesy of Brian S. Boxer Wachler, MD.)*

Ocular complications (defined as clinically significant events that do not result in permanent sequelae) have been reported in 11% of patients at 12 months postoperatively. These complications include

- reduced corneal sensitivity (5.5%)
- induced astigmatism between 1.00 and 2.00 D (3.7%)
- deep neovascularization at the incision site (1.2%)

- persistent epithelial defect (0.2%)
- iritis/uveitis (0.2%)

Visual symptoms rated as severe and always present have been reported in approximately 14% of patients and may be related to large pupil diameter. These complications include

- difficulty with night vision (4.8%)
- blurred vision (2.9%)
- diplopia (1.6%)
- glare (1.3%)
- halos (1.3%)
- fluctuating distance vision (1.0%)
- fluctuating near vision (0.3%)
- photophobia (0.3%)

Fine white deposits occur frequently within the lamellar ring channels after Intacs placement (Fig 4-9). The incidence and density of the deposits increase with the thickness of the ring segment and the duration of implantation. Deposits do not seem to alter the optical performance of the ring segments or to cause corneal thinning or necrosis, although some patients are bothered by their appearance.

Intacs achieve the best results in eyes with mild to moderate keratoconus. The goals are generally to improve vision and reduce distortions and are determined on the basis of the degree of keratoconus. For example, a patient with mild keratoconus and a BCVA of 20/30 may have the goal of improved quality of vision in glasses or soft contact lenses. However, a contact lens–intolerant patient with more advanced keratoconus and a BCVA of 20/60 may have the goal of improved ability to wear a rigid gas-permeable (RGP) contact lens. For some advanced cases of keratoconus, such as eyes with keratometry values

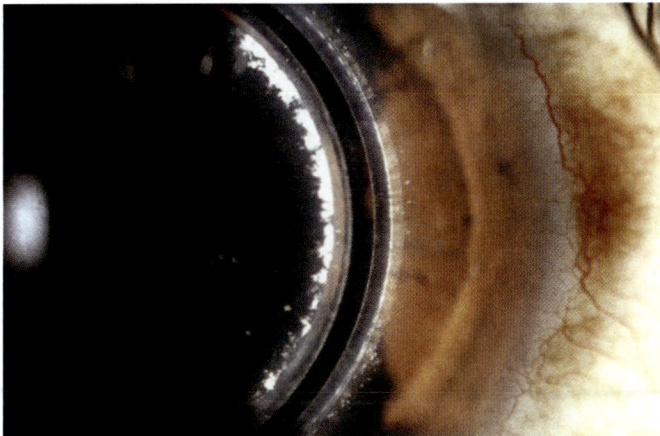

Figure 4-9 Clinical photograph showing grade 4 deposits around ring segments. The deposits can be graded on a scale from 0 (no deposits) to 4 (confluent deposits). These channel deposits are typically not apparent until weeks or months after surgery. Although the corneal opacities may cause cosmetic concerns, they usually do not cause other ocular problems. *(Courtesy of Addition Technology.)*

greater than 60.00 D, the likelihood of functional improvement of vision is lower than for eyes with flatter keratometry values. In such cases, despite the use of Intacs, a corneal transplant may be unavoidable. If required, penetrating or lamellar keratoplasty may be performed after Intacs placement.

Ectasia After LASIK

Ring segments have also been used for the postoperative management of corneal ectasia after LASIK. As in the treatment of keratoconus, few surgical options are available to treat corneal ectasia. Use of an excimer laser to remove additional tissue is generally considered contraindicated. A lamellar graft or penetrating keratoplasty may result in significant morbidity, such as irregular astigmatism, delayed recovery of vision, and tissue rejection. In limited early trials that used Intacs to treat post-LASIK ectasia, myopia was reduced and UCVA was improved. However, the long-term effect of such an approach for managing post-LASIK ectasia is still being evaluated. Use of Intacs for post-LASIK ectasia is an off-label treatment, and care should be taken with implantation in the presence of a lamellar interface.

Kymionis GD, Tsiklis NS, Pallikaris AI, et al. Long-term follow-up of Intacs for post-LASIK corneal ectasia. *Ophthalmology.* 2006;113(11):1909–1917.

Rabinowitz Y. INTACS for keratoconus and ectasia after LASIK. *Int Ophthalmol Clin.* 2013; 53(1):27–39.

Other Considerations With Intrastromal Corneal Ring Segments and LASIK

Corneal ring segments have been used to correct residual myopia following LASIK with good initial results. In such cases, a nomogram adjustment is necessary to reduce the risk of overcorrection. This procedure may be useful in patients whose stromal bed is not sufficient to support a second excimer laser ablation.

Conversely, after ring segments have been removed from patients whose vision did not improve satisfactorily (eg, due to undercorrection or induced astigmatism), LASIK has been performed with good success. The flap is created in a plane superficial to the previous ring segment channel.

Orthokeratology

Orthokeratology, or corneal refractive therapy, refers to the overnight use of RGP contact lenses to temporarily reduce myopia. The goal of this nonsurgical method of temporary myopia reduction is to achieve functional UCVA during the day. The contact lens is fitted at a base curve that is flatter than the corneal curvature. Temporary corneal flattening results from the flattening of corneal epithelium. Use of the lens is intended for the temporary reduction of naturally occurring myopia between –0.50 and –6.00 D of sphere, with up to 1.75 D of astigmatism.

Orthokeratology is most appropriate for highly motivated patients with low myopia who do not want refractive surgery but who want to avoid use of contact lenses and glasses during the day. These contact lenses do not treat astigmatism or hyperopia. Prospective patients should be informed that in clinical trials, approximately one-third of patients discontinued contact lens use, and most patients (75%) experienced discomfort at some point during contact lens wear. Complications of orthokeratology include induced astigmatism, induced higher-order aberrations, recurrent erosions, and infectious keratitis. Infectious keratitis—the most serious complication—can be bilateral and seems to be more common in children and teenagers. Pathogens implicated include *Pseudomonas, Acanthamoeba, Staphylococcus,* and *Nocardia* species.

The prevalence and incidence of complications associated with orthokeratology, such as bacterial and parasitic keratitis, have not been determined. Sufficiently large, well-designed, controlled studies are needed to provide a more reliable measure of the risks of treatment and to identify risk factors for complications. See BCSC Section 3, *Clinical Optics,* for further discussion of orthokeratology.

Berntsen DA, Barr JT, Mitchell GL. The effect of overnight contact lens corneal reshaping on higher-order aberrations and best-corrected visual acuity. *Optom Vis Sci.* 2005;82(6): 490–497.

Mascai MS. Corneal ulcers in two children wearing Paragon corneal refractive therapy lenses. *Eye Contact Lens.* 2005;31(1):9–11.

Premarket Approval. Paragon CRT. PMA P870024/S043. US Food and Drug Administration website. Updated November 7, 2016. Available at https://goo.gl/7sOAnM. Accessed November 7, 2016.

Saviola JF. The current FDA view on overnight orthokeratology: how we got here and where we are going. *Cornea.* 2005;24(7):770–771.

Schein OD. Microbial keratitis associated with overnight orthokeratology: what we need to know. *Cornea.* 2005;24(7):767–769.

Van Meter WS, Musch DC, Jacobs DS, et al. Safety of overnight orthokeratology for myopia: a report by the American Academy of Ophthalmology. *Ophthalmology.* 2008;115(12): 2301–2313.

Watt K, Swarbrick HA. Microbial keratitis in overnight orthokeratology: review of the first 50 cases. *Eye Contact Lens.* 2005;31(5):201–208.

CHAPTER 5

Photoablation: Techniques and Outcomes

▶ *This chapter includes related videos, which can be accessed by scanning the QR codes provided in the text or going to www.aao.org/bcscvideo_section13.*

The 193-nm argon-fluoride (ArF) excimer laser treats refractive error by ablating the anterior corneal stroma to create a new radius of curvature. Two major refractive surgical techniques use excimer laser ablation. In *surface ablation* techniques, including photorefractive keratectomy (PRK), laser subepithelial keratomileusis (LASEK), and epipolis laser in situ keratomileusis (epi-LASIK), the Bowman layer is exposed either by debriding the epithelium through various methods or by loosening and moving, but attempting to preserve, the epithelium. In LASIK, the excimer laser ablation is performed under a lamellar flap that is created with either a mechanical microkeratome or a femtosecond laser. Excimer laser ablation algorithms can be classified generally as conventional, wavefront-optimized, wavefront-guided, and topography-guided.

Excimer Laser

Background

The excimer laser uses a high-voltage electrical charge to transiently combine atoms of excited argon and fluorine; when the molecule, or dimer, reverts to its separate atoms, a charged photon is emitted. The word *excimer* comes from "*exc*ited d*imer.*" Srinivasan, an IBM engineer, was studying the far-ultraviolet (UV; 193-nm) ArF excimer laser for photoetching of computer chips. He and Trokel, an ophthalmologist, not only showed that the excimer laser could remove corneal tissue precisely with minimal adjacent corneal damage—*photoablation*—but they also recognized its potential use for refractive and therapeutic corneal surgery.

Photoablation, the removal of corneal tissue with minimal adjacent corneal damage, occurs because the cornea has an extremely high absorption coefficient at 193 nm. A single 193-nm photon has sufficient energy to directly break carbon–carbon and carbon–nitrogen bonds that form the peptide backbone of the corneal collagen molecules. Excimer laser radiation ruptures the collagen polymer into small fragments, expelling a discrete volume and depth of corneal tissue from the surface with each pulse of the laser (Fig 5-1) without significantly damaging adjacent tissue.

Surface Ablation

Surface ablation procedures were initially performed as PRK, the sculpting of the de-epithelialized corneal stroma to alter refractive power, and they underwent extensive pre-clinical investigation before being applied to sighted human eyes. Results of early animal studies provided evidence of relatively normal wound healing in laser-ablated corneas.

The popularity of PRK decreased in the late 1990s when LASIK began to be performed because of LASIK's faster recovery of vision and decreased postoperative discomfort. Although more LASIK than surface ablation procedures are still performed, the number of

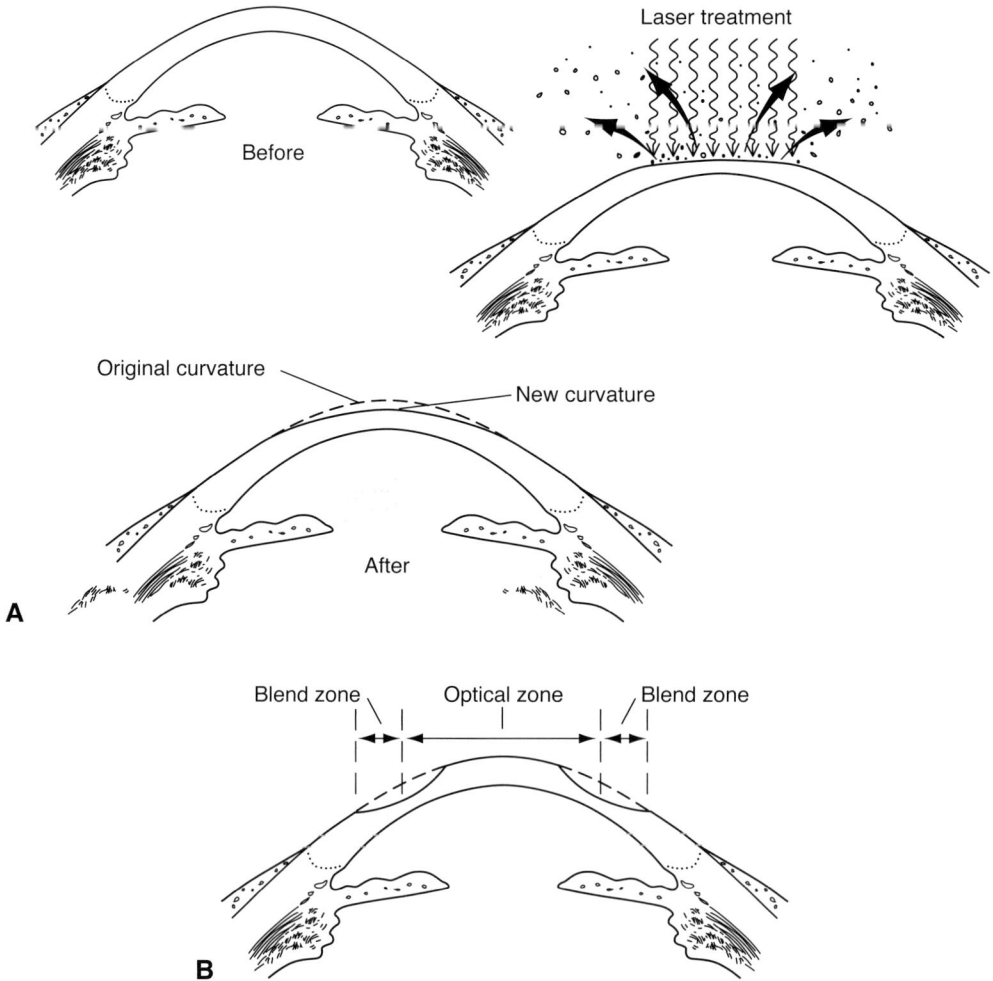

Figure 5-1 Schematic representations of corneal recontouring by the excimer laser for a myopic ablation. **A,** Correction of myopia by flattening the central cornea. **B,** Correction of hyperopia by steepening the central corneal optical zone and blending the periphery.

(Continued)

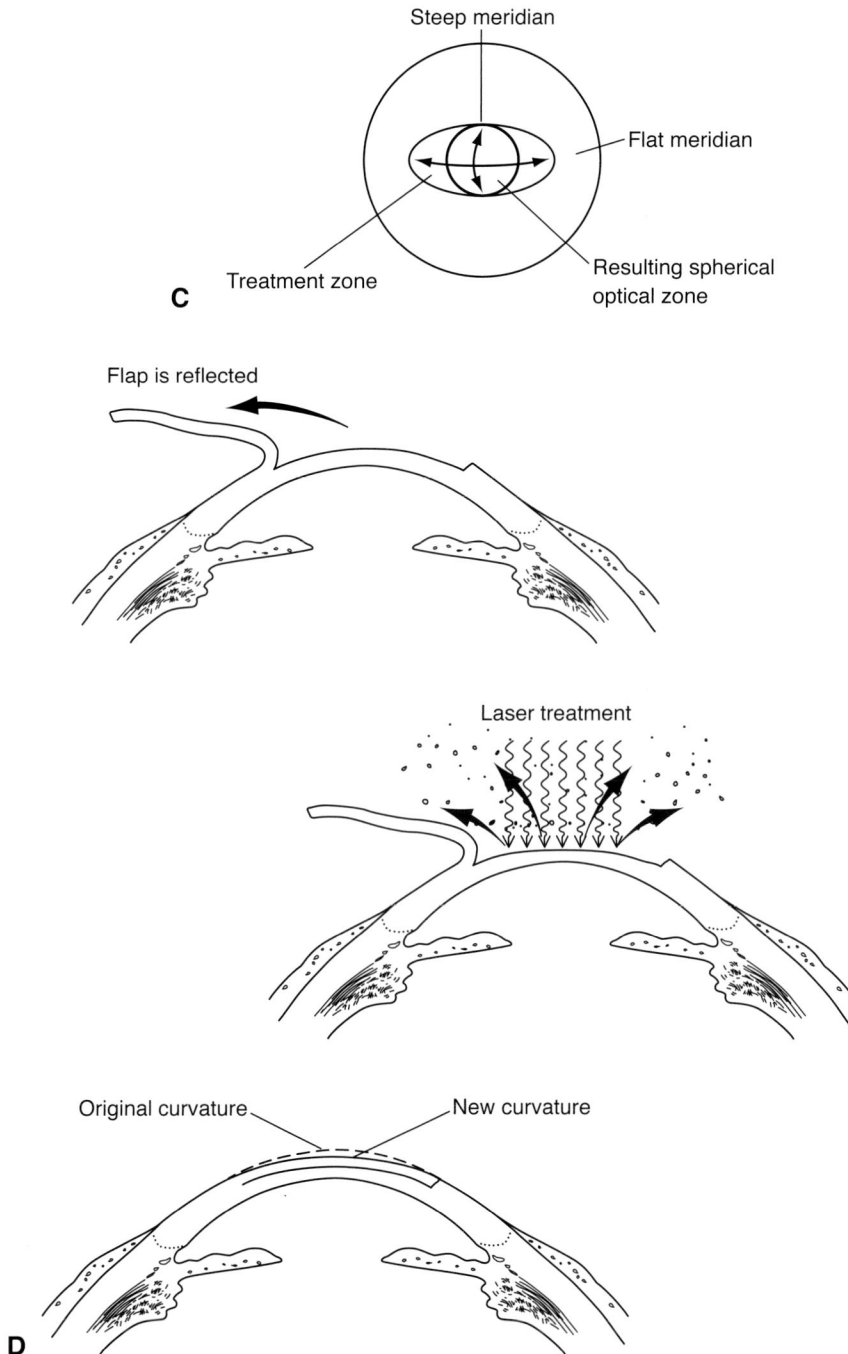

Figure 5-1 *(continued)* **C,** Correction of astigmatism by differential tissue removal 90° apart. Note that in correction of myopic astigmatism, the steeper meridian with more tissue removal corresponds to the smaller dimension of the ellipse. **D,** In LASIK, a flap is reflected back, the excimer laser ablation is performed on the exposed stromal bed, and the flap is then replaced. The altered corneal contour of the bed causes the same alteration in the anterior surface of the flap. *(Illustrations by Jeanne Koelling.)*

surface ablations has increased in recent years. PRK remains an especially attractive alternative for specific indications, including irregular or thin corneas; epithelial basement membrane disease (often called *map-dot-fingerprint dystrophy*); previous corneal surgery, such as penetrating keratoplasty (PKP) and radial keratotomy (RK); and treatment of some LASIK flap complications, such as incomplete or buttonholed flaps. Surface ablation eliminates the potential for stromal flap–related complications and may have a decreased incidence of postoperative dry eye as compared to LASIK. Corneal haze, the major risk of PRK, decreased markedly with the use of adjunctive mitomycin C; subsequently, the use of PRK for higher levels of myopia has increased.

Majmudar PA, Forstot SL, Dennis RF, et al. Topical mitomycin-C for subepithelial fibrosis after refractive corneal surgery. *Ophthalmology.* 2000;107(1):89–94.

Srinivasan R. Ablation of polymers and biological tissue by ultraviolet lasers. *Science.* 1986; 234(4776):559–565.

Trokel SL, Srinivasan R, Braren B. Excimer laser surgery of the cornea. *Am J Ophthalmol.* 1983; 96(6):710–715.

LASIK

The term *keratomileusis* comes from the Greek words for "cornea" *(kerato)* and "to carve" *(mileusis). Laser in situ keratomileusis,* which combines keratomileusis with excimer laser stromal ablation, is currently the most frequently performed keratorefractive procedure because of its safety, efficacy, quick recovery of vision, and minimal patient discomfort. LASIK combines 2 refractive technologies: excimer laser stromal ablation and creation of a stromal flap.

Wavefront-Guided, Wavefront-Optimized, and Topography-Guided Ablations

Conventional excimer laser ablation treats lower-order, or spherocylindrical, aberrations such as myopia, hyperopia, and astigmatism. These lower-order aberrations constitute approximately 90% of all aberrations. Higher-order aberrations make up the remainder; such aberrations cannot be treated with glasses. Some ophthalmologists feel that small amounts of higher-order aberrations, which are commonly found in patients with excellent uncorrected vision, may not adversely affect their vision. Higher-order aberrations are also a by-product of excimer laser ablation. Some higher-order aberrations can cause symptoms—such as loss of contrast sensitivity and nighttime halos and glare—that decrease the quality of vision. The aberrations most commonly associated with these visual concerns are spherical aberration and coma. See Chapter 1 for more detailed discussion of higher-order aberrations.

In an effort to reduce preexisting aberrations and minimize the induction of new aberrations, *wavefront-guided* ablation creates ablation profiles that are customized for individual patients. In addition to addressing higher-order aberrations, wavefront-guided treatments can correct the lower-order aberrations of spherical error and astigmatism.

Wavefront-optimized lasers do not use patient-specific wavefront data. Instead, they adjust the ablation profile of conventional treatments to create a more prolate shape with the additional peripheral ablation in the myopic patient, thereby reducing spherical aberration; however, they have no effect on other higher-order aberrations.

Compared with conventional excimer laser ablation, wavefront-guided ablations and wavefront-optimized ablations appear to offer better contrast sensitivity and induce fewer postoperative higher-order aberrations. Although advances in aberrometry and registration systems have led to improved outcomes, patients who undergo photoablation may still have more higher-order aberrations postoperatively than they did preoperatively. Wavefront-guided ablations in general remove more tissue than conventional ablations.

Wavefront-guided ablation appears to have clear-cut benefit compared with wavefront-optimized ablation only for patients with significant preoperative higher-order aberrations. The procedure is not suitable for all patients and may be inappropriate for use after cataract surgery, particularly with multifocal intraocular lenses. Intraocular lenses, especially multifocal intraocular lenses, interfere with capturing the wavefront scan and could result in the delivery of an inaccurate treatment. In addition, wavefront data may be impossible to obtain in highly irregular corneas or in eyes with small pupils.

Topography-guided ablations have recently been approved by the US Food and Drug Administration (FDA). Topography-guided systems use corneal topography data to create ablation profiles that treat existing corneal shape irregularities and optimize corneal curvature. Topography-guided ablations have gained traction outside the US in the treatment of corneas with irregular surfaces, such as those with small or decentered optical zones from prior excimer ablations, LASIK flap complications, or post-RK corneal irregularities. Data from a recent FDA clinical trial, demonstrated that topography-guided ablations may result in excellent outcomes for even routine laser vision correction cases in previously unoperated eyes.

Nuijts RM, Nabar VA, Hament WJ, Eggink FA. Wavefront-guided versus standard laser in situ keratomileusis to correct low to moderate myopia. *J Cataract Refract Surg.* 2002;28(11): 1907–1913.

Stonecipher KG, Kezirian GM. Wavefront-optimized versus wavefront-guided LASIK for myopic astigmatism with the ALLEGRETTO WAVE: three-month results of a prospective FDA trial. *J Refract Surg.* 2008;24(4):S424–S430.

Stulting RD, Fant BS PharmD; T-CAT Study Group. Results of topography-guided laser in situ keratomileusis custom ablation treatment with a refractive excimer laser. *J Cataract Refract Surg.* 2016;42(1):11–18.

Patient Selection for Photoablation

The preoperative evaluation of patients considering refractive surgery is presented in detail in Chapter 2. Table 5-1 lists relative contraindications to photoablation.

Special Considerations for Surface Ablation

In general, any condition that significantly delays epithelial healing is a relative contraindication to surface ablation. Although keloid scar formation was listed as a contraindication to PRK in FDA trials, 1 study found that African Americans with a history of keloid formation did well after PRK, and keloid formation is no longer considered a contraindication to surface ablation or LASIK. Historically, patients taking isotretinoin or amiodarone

Table 5-1 Relative Contraindications to Excimer Laser Photoablation

Connective tissue disease
  Rheumatoid arthritis
  Sjögren syndrome
  Systemic lupus erythematosus
  Granulomatosis with polyangiitis (Wegener granulomatosis)
Corneal ectatic disorders
Corneal stromal dystrophies
Diabetic retinopathy
Dry eye syndrome
Fuchs corneal dystrophy
Monocular patients
Neurotrophic corneas
Patients who are pregnant or breastfeeding
Patients with unreasonable expectations
Patients younger than 18 years
Previous herpes simplex infection
Previous herpes zoster ophthalmicus
Thyroid eye disease
Uncontrolled systemic diabetes mellitus

hydrochloride were excluded from undergoing excimer laser procedures, although there is little evidence that these drugs adversely affect laser keratorefractive outcomes.

Patients with epithelial basement membrane dystrophy (EBMD) are better candidates for surface ablation than for LASIK because surface ablation may be therapeutic, reducing epithelial irregularity and improving postoperative quality of vision while enhancing epithelial adhesion. In contrast, LASIK may cause a frank epithelial defect in eyes with EBMD, especially when performed with a mechanical microkeratome.

Any patient undergoing excimer laser photoablation should have a pachymetric and topographic evaluation (see Chapter 2). Younger patients and patients with thin corneas, low predicted residual stromal bed (RSB) thickness, or irregular topography may be at increased risk for the development of ectasia with LASIK. As such, these patients may be better candidates for surface ablation. Patients with subtle topographic pattern abnormalities need to be evaluated on a case-by-case basis. In some circumstances, patients who are stable may be offered surface ablation but with a clear acknowledgment, as well as a signed informed consent form, that they understand there may still be a risk of progression to corneal ectasia.

Smith RJ, Maloney RK. Laser in situ keratomileusis in patients with autoimmune diseases. *J Cataract Refract Surg.* 2006;32(8):1292–1295.

Special Considerations for LASIK

The preoperative evaluation of patients for LASIK is similar to that for surface ablation. A narrow palpebral fissure and a prominent brow with deep-set globes increase the difficulty of creating a successful corneal flap. The presence of either may lead a surgeon to consider surface ablation over LASIK.

Many reports indicate that postoperative dry eye due to corneal denervation is more common with LASIK than with surface ablation. This difference is important to remember when considering refractive surgery in a patient with known dry eye syndrome. Nevertheless, many patients undergoing PRK will also experience postoperative dry eye; however, it is believed that this occurs to a lesser extent than for LASIK patients.

Corneal topography must be performed to assess corneal cylinder and rule out the presence of forme fruste keratoconus, pellucid marginal degeneration, or contact lens–induced corneal warpage. Corneas steeper than 48.00 D are more likely to have thin flaps or frank buttonholes (central perforation of the flap) with procedures using mechanical microkeratomes. Corneas flatter than 40.00 D are more likely to have smaller-diameter flaps and are at increased risk for creation of a free cap due to transection of the hinge with mechanical microkeratomes. These problems may be reduced by using a smaller or larger suction ring, which changes the flap diameter; modifying the hinge length; slowing passage of the microkeratome to create a thicker flap or using a microkeratome head designed to create thicker flaps; applying higher suction levels and creating a higher intraocular pressure (IOP); or selecting a femtosecond laser to create the lamellar flap. If a patient is having both eyes treated in a single session, the surgeon must be aware that using the same microkeratome blade to create the flap in the second eye typically results in a flap that is 10–20 μm thinner than the flap in the first eye. In addition, there is some concern about transferring epithelium and/or infectious agents between eyes. These specific concerns are greatly minimized with the use of a femtosecond laser for flap creation.

Preoperative pachymetric measurement of corneal thickness is mandatory because an adequate stromal bed must remain to decrease the possibility of postoperative corneal ectasia, although the definition of what constitutes an adequate RSB remains controversial. The following formula is used to calculate the RSB:

RSB = Central Corneal Thickness – Thickness of Flap – Depth of Ablation

Although most practitioners use a minimum RSB of 250 μm as a guideline, this figure is clinically derived rather than based on any definitive laboratory investigations or controlled prospective studies. A thicker stromal bed after ablation does not guarantee that postoperative corneal ectasia will not develop. Moreover, the actual LASIK flap may be thicker than that noted on the label of the microkeratome head, making the stromal bed thinner than the calculated minimum of 250 μm. Consequently, many surgeons use intraoperative pachymetry—especially for high myopic corrections, enhancements, or thin corneas—to determine actual flap thickness.

Determining flap thickness and RSB via intraoperative pachymetry, rather than by estimating thickness based on the markings on the plate, provides the most accurate data. This is accomplished by measuring the central corneal thickness at the beginning of the procedure, creating the LASIK flap with the surgeon's instrument of choice, lifting the flap, measuring the untreated stromal bed, and subtracting the intended thickness of corneal ablation from the stromal bed to ascertain whether the RSB will be 250 μm or whatever safe threshold is desired following ablation. Flap thickness is then calculated by subtracting the untreated stromal bed measurement from the initial central corneal thickness. It is important to measure the corneal bed thickness quickly after making the flap in order to avoid corneal thinning from exposure to the air.

The surgeon should preoperatively inform patients with thinner corneas or higher corrections that future LASIK enhancement may not be possible because of an inadequate RSB. These patients may be better candidates for surface ablation enhancements if needed.

Many ophthalmologists believe that excessive corneal flattening or steepening after LASIK may reduce vision quality and increase aberrations. Thus, many of them avoid creating overly flat or overly steep corneas, although no established guidelines are available on the specific values to avoid. The surgeon can estimate the postoperative keratometry by calculating a flattening of 0.80 D for every diopter of myopia treated and a steepening of 1.00 D for every diopter of hyperopia treated (see Chapter 2).

If wavefront-guided laser ablation is planned, wavefront error is measured preoperatively, as discussed in Chapter 1. Although wavefront data are used to program the laser, the surgeon must still compare these data to the manifest refraction before surgery to prevent data-input errors. In general, substantial differences between the manifest refraction and the wavefront refraction should alert the surgeon to a potentially poor candidate for the procedure.

Flanagan G, Binder PS. Estimating residual stromal thickness before and after laser in situ keratomileusis. *J Cataract Refract Surg.* 2003;29(9):1674–1683.

Kim WS, Jo JM. Corneal hydration affects ablation during laser in situ keratomileusis surgery. *Cornea.* 2001;20(4):394–397.

Randleman JB, Hebson CB, Larson PM. Flap thickness in eyes with ectasia after laser in situ keratomileusis. *J Cataract Refract Surg.* 2012;38(5):752–757. Epub 2012 Mar 16.

Randleman JB, Woodward M, Lynn MJ, Stulting RD. Risk assessment for ectasia after corneal refractive surgery. *Ophthalmology.* 2008;115(1):37–50. Epub 2007 Jul 12.

Salib GM, McDonald MB, Smolek M. Safety and efficacy of cyclosporine 0.05% drops versus unpreserved artificial tears in dry-eye patients having laser in situ keratomileusis. *J Cataract Refract Surg.* 2006;32(5):772–778.

Williams LB, Dave SB, Moshirfar M. Correlation of visual outcome and patient satisfaction with preoperative keratometry after hyperopic laser in situ keratomileusis. *J Cataract Refract Surg.* 2008;34(7):1083–1088.

Surgical Technique for Photoablation

Many of the steps in keratorefractive surgery are identical for surface ablation and LASIK. These include calibration and programming of the laser and patient preparation. The major difference between surface ablation and LASIK is preparation for ablation, which is by exposure of the Bowman layer for surface ablation and the midstroma for LASIK. A list of FDA-approved lasers for refractive surgery can be found on the FDA website.

US Food & Drug Administration. List of FDA-approved lasers for LASIK. Medical Devices website. Published August 17, 2015. Available at https://goo.gl/WvNaRY. Accessed November 5, 2016.

Calibration of the Excimer Laser

At the start of each surgery day and between patients, the technician should check the laser for proper homogeneous beam profile, alignment, and power output, according to the instructions of the manufacturer. Ultimately, however, it is the surgeon's responsibility to ensure that the laser is functioning correctly before treating each patient.

Preoperative Planning and Laser Programming

An important part of preoperative planning is programming the laser with the appropriate refraction. Often, the patient's manifest and cycloplegic refractions differ, or the amount and axis of astigmatism differ between the topographic evaluation and refractive examination. Thus, it may be unclear which refractive data to enter into the laser. The surgeon's decision about whether to use the manifest or the cycloplegic refraction is based on his or her individual nomogram and technique. The manifest refraction is more accurate than the cycloplegic refraction in determining cylinder axis and amount. If the refractive cylinder is confirmed to differ from the topographic cylinder, lenticular astigmatism or posterior corneal curvature is assumed to be the cause. In this case, the laser is still programmed with the axis and amount of cylinder noted on refraction. The surgeon should take particular care to check the axis obtained on the refraction with the value programmed into the laser. Entering an incorrect value is a potential source of error, particularly when converting between plus and minus cylinder formats. Before each surgery, the surgeon and the technician should review a checklist of information, confirming the patient's name, the refraction, and the eye on which surgery is to be performed. In wavefront procedures, the treatment should correspond to the patient's refraction, and adjustments may be required to compensate for accommodation.

For many laser models, the surgeon also must enter the size of the optical zone and indicate whether a blend of the ablation zone should be performed. The *blend zone* is an area of peripheral asphericity designed to reduce the possible undesirable effects of an abrupt transition from the optical zone to the untreated cornea (see Fig 5-1B). A prolate blend zone reduces the risk of glare and halo after excimer laser photoablation.

Special considerations for wavefront-guided techniques

Several wavefront mapping systems and wavefront-guided lasers are available commercially. Wavefront mapping systems are unique to the specific wavefront-guided laser used. Calibration should be performed according to the manufacturer's specifications.

For wavefront-guided ablations, the wavefront maps are taken with the patient sitting up at an aberrometer under scotopic conditions; the mapping results are then applied to the cornea in the laser suite with the patient lying down under the operating microscope. Some systems require pupillary dilation to capture wavefront data. The wavefront refraction indicated on wavefront analysis is then compared with the manifest refraction. If the difference between them exceeds 0.75 D, the manifest refraction and the wavefront analysis may need to be repeated. The data are either electronically transferred to the laser or downloaded to a portable drive and then transferred to the laser. Unlike conventional or wavefront-optimized excimer laser treatment, in which the manifest or cycloplegic refraction is used to program the laser, wavefront-guided laser treatment uses programmed wavefront data to create a custom ablation pattern.

Preoperative Preparation of the Patient

Many surgeons administer topical antibiotic prophylaxis preoperatively. The patient's skin is prepared with povidone-iodine, 5%–10%, or alcohol wipes before or after the patient enters the laser suite, and povidone-iodine solution, 5%, is sometimes applied as drops to the ocular surface and then irrigated out for further antisepsis. There is no consensus about the utility of these measures. When preparing the patient, the surgeon should take care to avoid irritation of the conjunctiva, which could lead to swelling of the conjunctiva and difficulties with suction.

In addition, before laser treatment, patients should be informed about the sounds and smells they will experience during the laser treatment. They may receive an oral antianxiety medication, such as diazepam.

If substantial astigmatism is being treated, some surgeons mark the cornea at the horizontal or vertical axis while the patient is sitting up to ensure accurate alignment under the laser. This step is done to compensate for the cyclotorsion that commonly occurs when the patient changes from a sitting to a lying position. A 15° offset in the axis of treatment can decrease the effective cylinder change by 35% and can result in a significant axis shift. There are multiple methods for marking the cornea or limbus.

After the patient is positioned under the laser, a sterile drape may be placed over the skin and eyelashes according to the surgeon's preference. Before doing so, a "time-out" should be performed during which the correct patient is identified, and the treatment and eye(s) to which treatment will be performed are confirmed. Topical anesthetic drops are placed in the eye; for LASIK patients, care should be taken to ensure that the drops are not instilled too early, as doing so may loosen the epithelium substantially. An eyelid speculum is placed in the eye to be treated, and an opaque patch is placed over the fellow eye to avoid cross-fixation. A gauze pad may be taped over the temple between the eye to be treated and the ear to absorb any excess fluid. The patient is asked to fixate on the laser centration light while the surgeon reduces ambient illumination from the microscope, focuses on the cornea, and centers the laser. It is important for the plane of the eye to remain parallel to the plane of the laser, for the patient to maintain fixation, and for the surgeon to control centration even when using lasers with tracking systems. For most patients, voluntary fixation during photoablation produces more accurate centration than globe immobilization by the surgeon.

Preparation of the Bowman Layer or Stromal Bed for Excimer Ablation

The next surgical step for all excimer photoablation procedures is preparation of the cornea for ablation. With surface ablation procedures, such preparation consists of epithelial removal to expose the Bowman layer. With LASIK, preparation involves the creation of a lamellar flap with a mechanical microkeratome or a femtosecond laser to expose the central stroma.

Epithelial debridement techniques for surface ablation

The epithelium can be removed with

- a sharp blade
- a blunt spatula
- a rotary corneal brush
- application of 20% absolute alcohol to the corneal surface for 10–45 seconds to loosen the epithelium (Video 5-1)
- a mechanical microkeratome with an epi-LASIK blade
- transepithelial ablation from the excimer laser itself

Figure 5-2 shows de-epithelialization techniques. In both transepithelial ablation and epi-LASIK, the peripheral margin of de-epithelialization is defined by the laser or epi-keratome itself. For other epithelial debridement techniques, the surgeon often defines the outer limit of de-epithelialization with an optical zone marker and then debrides from the periphery toward the center. An ophthalmic surgical cellulose sponge can be brushed

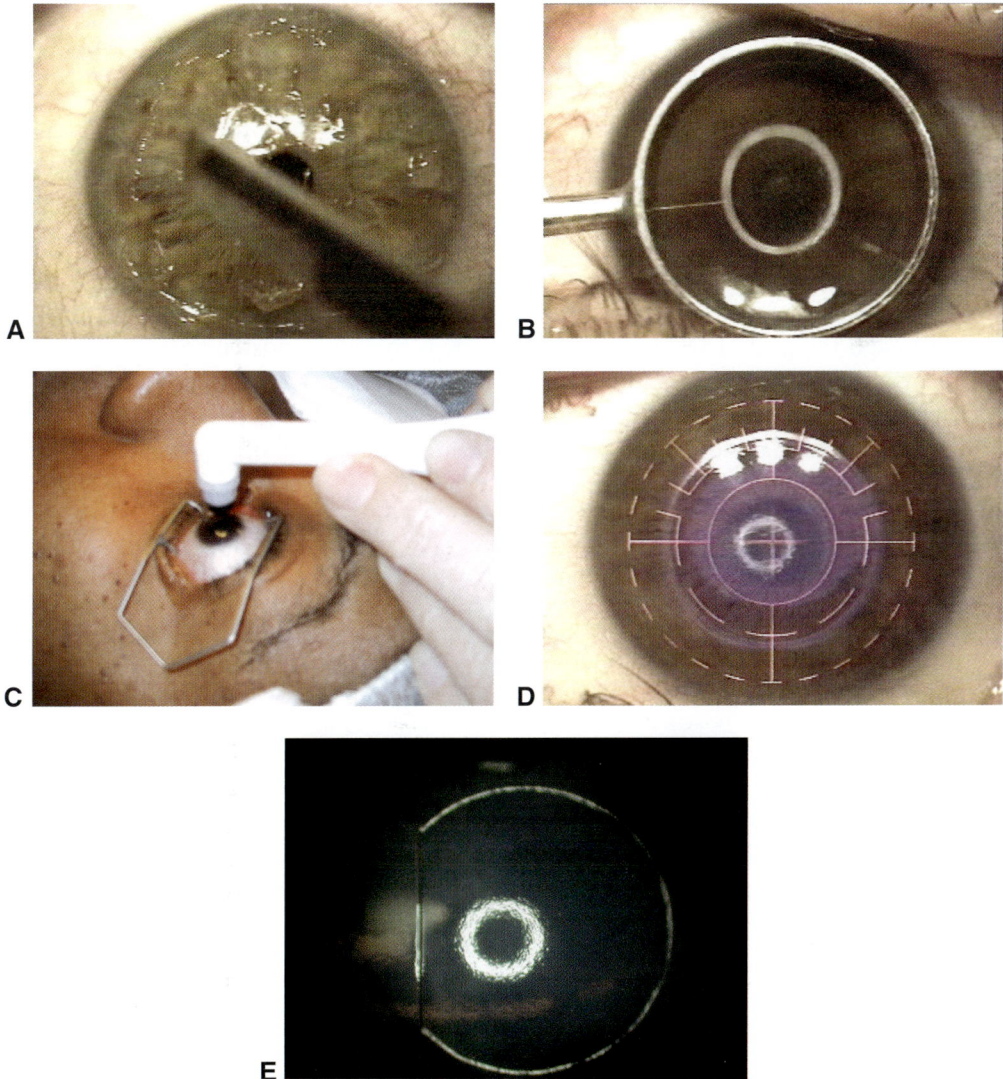

Figure 5-2 Techniques for de-epithelialization for surface ablation. **A,** Scraping with a blade. **B,** 20% dilution of absolute ethanol in an optical zone marker well. **C,** Rotary brush debridement. **D,** "Laser scrape," in which a broad-beam laser exposes the entire treatment zone to ablation pulses; these pulses remove most of the epithelium that is fluorescing brightly, after which the basal epithelial layer is removed by scraping with a blade. **E,** Epi-LASIK with a mechanical microkeratome (the epithelial flap may be removed or retained). *(Parts A, B, and D courtesy of Roger F. Steinert, MD; part C courtesy of Steven C. Schallhorn, MD; part E courtesy of Eric D. Donnenfeld, MD.)*

uniformly over the surface of the cornea to remove any residual epithelium and provide a smooth surface. The epithelium should be removed efficiently and consistently to prevent hydration changes in the stroma, because excessive corneal stromal dehydration may increase the amount of tissue removed and lead to overcorrection. The laser treatment zone must be free of epithelial cells, debris, and excess fluid before ablation.

VIDEO 5-1 Photorefractive keratectomy procedure.
Courtesy of George O. Waring IV, MD.
Access all Section 13 videos at www.aao.org/bcscvideo_section13.

Epithelial preservation techniques

LASEK In the LASEK variant of surface ablation, the goal is to preserve the patient's epithelium. Instead of debriding and discarding the epithelium or ablating the epithelium with the excimer laser, the surgeon loosens the epithelium with 20% alcohol for 20 seconds and folds back an intact sheet of epithelium.

Epi-LASIK In epi-LASIK, an epithelial flap is fashioned with a microkeratome fitted with a blunt epikeratome and a thin applanation plate that mechanically separates the epithelium.

Although the goal of LASEK and epi-LASIK is to reduce postoperative pain, speed the recovery of visual acuity, and decrease postoperative haze formation compared with PRK, controlled studies have had mixed results. In addition, the epithelial flap may not remain viable and may slough off, actually delaying healing and vision recovery. To date, epi-LASIK and LASEK have not proved to be superior to PRK in reducing corneal haze.

Ambrósio R Jr, Wilson S. LASIK vs LASEK vs PRK: advantages and indications. *Semin Ophthalmol.* 2003;18(1):2–10.
Matsumoto JC, Chu YS. Epi-LASIK update: overview of techniques and patient management. *Int Ophthalmol Clin.* 2006;46(3):105–115.
Stevens SX, Bowyer BL. Corneal modulators and their use in excimer laser phototherapeutic keratectomy. *Int Ophthalmol Clin.* 1996;36(4):119–125.

Flap creation for LASIK

Lamellar flap creation can be performed using a mechanical microkeratome or a femtosecond laser. Many surgeons make asymmetric sterile ink marks in the corneal periphery, away from the intended flap hinge, just before placement of the suction ring. These marks can aid in alignment of the flap at the end of surgery and in proper orientation in the rare event of a free cap.

Microkeratome Before each surgery, the microkeratome and vacuum unit are assembled, carefully inspected, and tested to ensure proper functioning. The importance of meticulously maintaining the microkeratome and carefully following the manufacturer's recommendations cannot be overemphasized.

The basic principles of the microkeratome and the role of the suction ring and cutting head are illustrated in Figure 5-3. The suction ring has 2 functions: (1) to adhere to the globe, providing a stable platform for the microkeratome cutting head, and (2) to raise the IOP to a high level, which stabilizes the cornea. The dimensions of the suction ring determine the diameter of the flap and the size of the stabilizing hinge. The thicker the vertical dimension of the suction ring and the smaller the diameter of the ring opening, the less

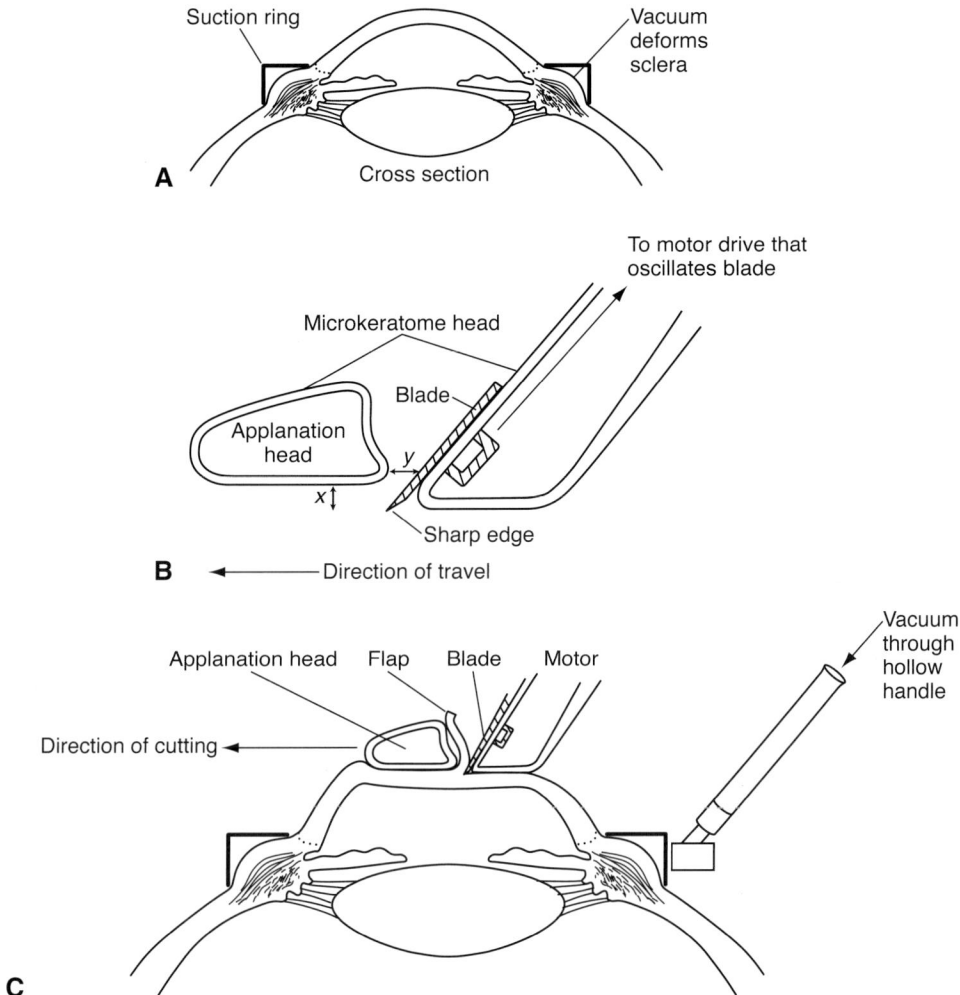

Figure 5-3 Schematic representation of the principles of a microkeratome. **A,** The suction ring serves as a platform for the microkeratome head, gripping the conjunctiva and sclera adjacent to the limbus. **B,** Simplified cross-section schematic of a typical microkeratome head. **C,** Creation of the flap. When the microkeratome head passes across the cornea, the applanating surface of the head flattens the cornea in advance of the blade. *(Illustration by Jeanne Koelling.)*

the cornea will protrude, and hence a smaller-diameter flap will be produced. The suction ring is connected to a vacuum pump, which typically is controlled by an on–off foot pedal.

The microkeratome cutting head has several key components. Its highly sharpened, disposable cutting blade is discarded after each patient, either after treatment of a single eye (if the patient is only having a single eye treated or if the surgeon chooses to discard the blade after the first eye) or after bilateral treatment. It is common practice to use the same blade on the second eye of the same patient.

The applanation head, or plate, serves to flatten the cornea in advance of the cutting blade. The length of the blade that extends beyond the applanation plate and the clearance between the blade and the applanation surface are the principal determinants of flap thickness. The motor, either electrical or gas-driven turbine, oscillates the blade rapidly, typically between 6000 and 15,000 cycles per minute. The same motor or a second motor is used to mechanically advance the cutting head, which is attached to the suction ring, across the cornea, although in some models the surgeon manually controls the advance of the cutting head. Smaller and thinner flap size and longer hinge cord length may be more important than hinge location in sparing the nerves and reducing the incidence and severity of dry eyes. Regardless of hinge type, patients generally recover most corneal sensation to preoperative levels within 6–12 months after surgery.

Once the ring is properly positioned, suction is activated (Fig 5-4). The patient should be notified prior to surgery that when the suction is applied, there may be some discomfort and vision may diminish temporarily. The IOP should be assessed at this point; low IOP can result in a poor-quality, thin, or incomplete flap. It is essential to have both excellent exposure of the eye, allowing free movement of the microkeratome, and proper suction ring fixation. Inadequate suction may result from blockage of the suction ports caused by eyelashes under the suction ring or redundant or scarred conjunctiva. To avoid the possibility of pseudosuction (occlusion of the suction port with conjunctiva but not sclera), the surgeon can confirm the presence of true suction by observing that the eye moves when the suction ring is gently moved, the pupil is mildly dilated, and the patient can no longer see the fixation light. Methods used to assess whether the IOP is adequately elevated include use of a handheld Barraquer plastic applanator or a pneumotonometer and palpation of the eye by the surgeon. Surgeons without extensive experience are advised to use an objective rather than a subjective method.

Before the lamellar cut is made, the surface of the cornea is moistened with proparacaine with glycerin or with nonpreserved artificial tears. Use of balanced salt solution should be avoided at this point because mineral deposits may develop within the microkeratome and interfere with its proper function. The surgeon places the microkeratome on the suction ring (if it is a 2-piece system) and checks that its path is free of obstacles such as the eyelid speculum, drape, or overhanging eyelid. The microkeratome is then

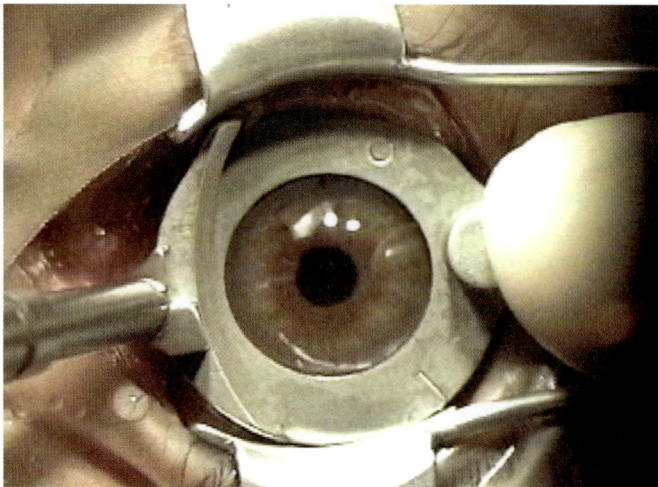

Figure 5-4 Placement of a suction ring. *(Courtesy of Roger F. Steinert, MD.)*

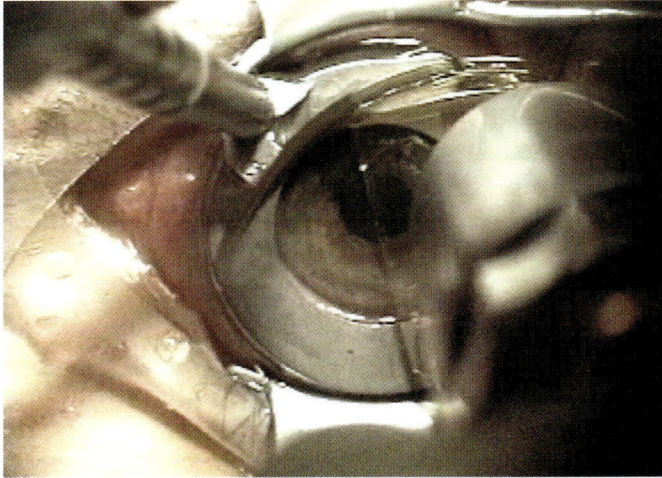

Figure 5-5 Movement of the microkeratome head across the cornea. *(Courtesy of Roger F. Steinert, MD.)*

activated, passed over the cornea (Fig 5-5) until it is halted by the hinge-creating stopper, and then reversed off the cornea.

In addition, the surgeon should be aware that, regardless of the label describing the flap thickness of a specific device, the actual flap thickness varies with the type of microkeratome, patient age, preoperative corneal thickness, preoperative keratometry reading, preoperative astigmatism, corneal diameter, and translation speed of the microkeratome pass. It is important to maintain a steady translation speed to avoid creating irregularities in the stromal bed.

Barequet IS, Hirsh A, Levinger S. Effect of thin femtosecond LASIK flaps on corneal sensitivity and tear function. *J Refract Surg.* 2008;24(9):897–902.

Calvillo MP, McLaren JW, Hodge DO, Bourne WM. Corneal reinnervation after LASIK: prospective 3-year longitudinal study. *Invest Ophthalmol Vis Sci.* 2004;45(11):3991–3996.

Donnenfeld ED, Ehrenhaus M, Solomon R, Mazurek J, Rozell JC, Perry HD. Effect of hinge width on corneal sensation and dry eye after laser in situ keratomileusis. *J Cataract Refract Surg.* 2004;30(4):790–797.

Hardten DR, Feder RS, Rosenfeld SI. Mechanical microkeratomes. In: Feder RS, ed. *The LASIK Handbook: A Case-Based Approach.* 2nd ed. Philadelphia: Lippincott Williams & Wilkins; 2013:chap 4.

Kumano Y, Matsui H, Zushi I, et al. Recovery of corneal sensation after myopic correction by laser in situ keratomileusis with a nasal or superior hinge. *J Cataract Refract Surg.* 2003; 29(4):757–761.

Solomon KD, Donnenfeld E, Sandoval HP, et al; Flap Thickness Study Group. Flap thickness accuracy: comparison of 6 microkeratome models. *J Cataract Refract Surg.* 2004;30(5): 964–977.

Femtosecond laser The femtosecond laser can also be used to create a lamellar dissection within the stroma. Each laser pulse creates a discrete area of photodisruption of the collagen. The greater the number of laser spots and the more the spots overlap, the more easily the tissue will separate when lifted. The femtosecond laser allows adjustments for several variables involved in making the flap, including flap thickness, flap diameter, hinge location, hinge angle, bed energy, and spot separation. Although the goal is to try to minimize the total energy used in flap creation, a certain level of power is necessary to ensure complete photodisruption. With the computer programmed for flap diameter, depth, and hinge location and size, thousands of adjacent pulses are scanned across the cornea in a controlled pattern that results in creation of a flap. Some potential advantages of the femtosecond laser include excellent depth control, reduction of complications such as buttonhole perforations, precise control of flap dimensions and location, and the ability to create pockets and channels within the cornea. Utilization of the femtosecond laser allows the geometry of the side cut to be modified in a manner that may reduce the incidence of epithelial ingrowth and flap slippage.

Femtosecond laser complications can occur, however. One study of 208 eyes showed that 1.9% had a loss of suction during femtosecond laser flap creation but that all had successful flap creation after reapplanation of the eye. Occasionally, an opaque bubble layer (OBL) may form from gas expansion into in the stroma adjacent to the flap interface and lead to improper flap creation. To prevent an OBL, most lasers now create a pocket deep within the cornea to disperse the gas away from the flap interface.

Although some variation exists between femtosecond lasers, all systems require centration and vacuum adherence to the patient's cornea. Complete applanation of the cornea must be achieved, or an incomplete flap or incomplete side cut may result. Figures 5-6, 5-7, and 5-8 illustrate some components of the femtosecond laser. Video 5-2 demonstrates the

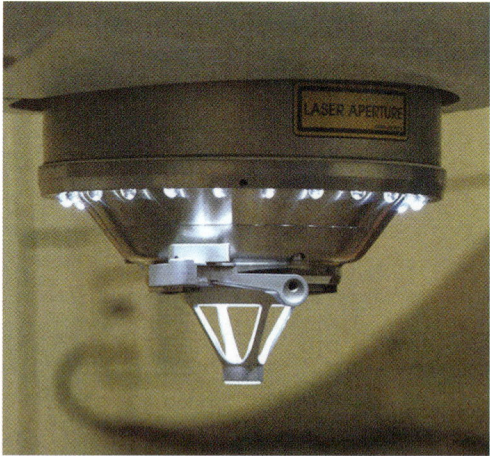

Figure 5-6 IntraLase femtosecond laser with cone attached. *(Reproduced with permission from Feder RS, Rapuano CJ. The LASIK Handbook: A Case-Based Approach. Philadelphia: Lippincott Williams & Wilkins; 2007:45, fig 2.7. Image courtesy of Robert Feder, MD.)*

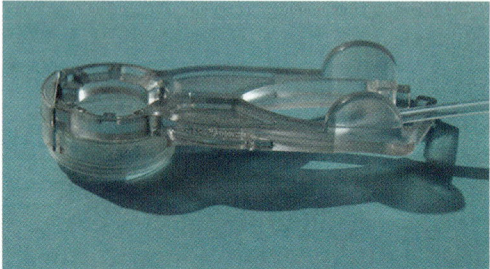

Figure 5-7 IntraLase suction ring. *(Reproduced with permission from Feder RS, Rapuano CJ. The LASIK Handbook: A Case-Based Approach. Philadelphia: Lippincott Williams & Wilkins; 2007:45, fig 2.8. Image courtesy of Robert Feder, MD.)*

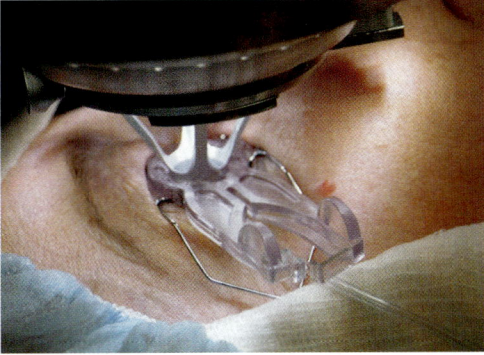

Figure 5-8 Docking of IntraLase cone with suction ring positioned on the eye. *(Reproduced with permission from Feder RS, Rapuano CJ. The LASIK Handbook: A Case-Based Approach. Philadelphia: Lippincott Williams & Wilkins; 2007:46, fig 2.9. Image courtesy of Robert Feder, MD.)*

use of a femtosecond laser for flap creation and the subsequent treatment with the excimer laser.

Once centration is confirmed on the laser, the surgeon administers the femtosecond laser treatment. The vacuum is then released, the suction ring is removed, and the patient is positioned under the excimer laser. A spatula with a semisharp edge is used to identify and score the flap edge near the hinge (Fig 5-9). The instrument is then passed across the

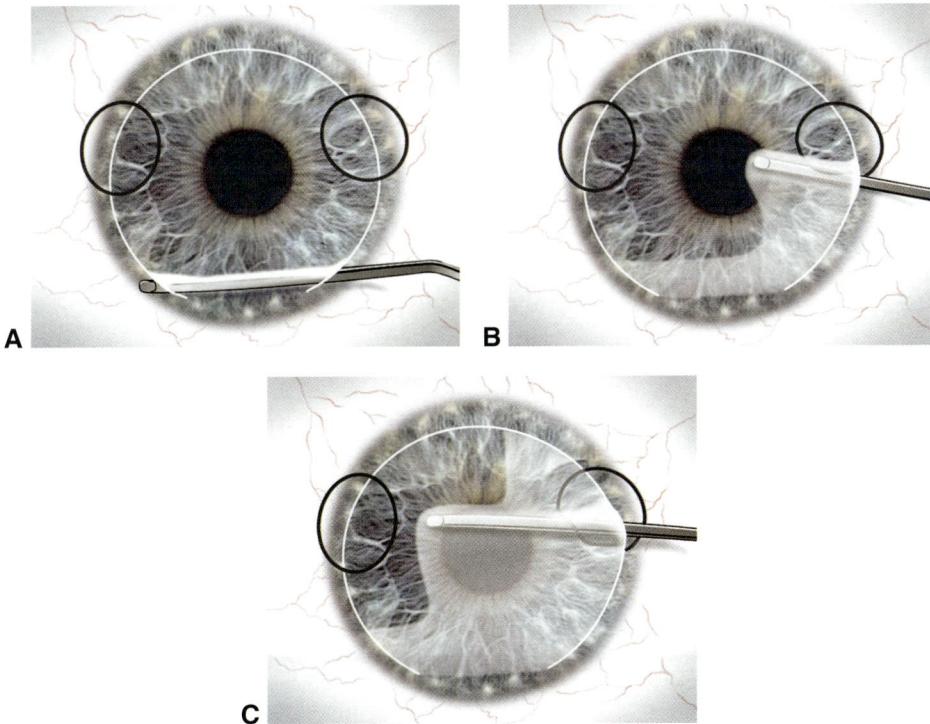

Figure 5-9 Flap lift technique following femtosecond laser application. **A,** After the flap edge is scored near the hinge on either side *(black ovals)*, a spatula is passed across the flap. **B,** The interface is separated by starting at the superior hinge and sweeping inferiorly. **C,** Dissecting one-third of the flap at a time reduces the risk of tearing the hinge. *(Reproduced with permission from Feder RS, Rapuano CJ. The LASIK Handbook: A Case-Based Approach. Philadelphia: Lippincott Williams & Wilkins; 2007:48, fig 2.12. Image courtesy of Robert Feder, MD.)*

flap along the base of the hinge, and the flap is lifted by sweeping inferiorly and separating the flap interface, dissecting one-third of the flap at a time and thus reducing the risk of tearing.

Several studies have compared the benefits of the mechanical microkeratome with those of femtosecond lasers for creating flaps. Minimal differences between the techniques have been found for most patients (Table 5-2).

VIDEO 5-2 Femtosecond laser procedure.
Courtesy of George O. Waring IV, MD.

Bryar PJ, Hardten DR, Vrabec M. Femtosecond laser flap creation. In: Feder RS, ed. *The LASIK Handbook: A Case-Based Approach.* 2nd ed. Philadelphia: Lippincott Williams & Wilkins; 2013:chap 5.

Chen S, Feng Y, Stojanovic A, Jankov MR II, Wang Q. IntraLase femtosecond laser vs mechanical microkeratomes in LASIK for myopia: a systematic review and meta-analysis. *J Refract Surg.* 2012;28(1):15–24.

Davison JA, Johnson SC. Intraoperative complications of LASIK flaps using the IntraLase femtosecond laser in 3009 cases. *J Refract Surg.* 2010;26(11):851–857.

Holzer MP, Rabsilber TM, Auffarth GU. Femtosecond laser–assisted corneal flap cuts: morphology, accuracy, and histopathology. *Invest Ophthalmol Vis Sci.* 2006;47(7): 2828–2831.

Slade SG, Durrie DS, Binder PS. A prospective, contralateral eye study comparing thin-flap LASIK (sub-Bowman keratomileusis) with photorefractive keratectomy. *Ophthalmology.* 2009;116(6):1075–1082.

Zhang ZH, Jin HY, Suo Y, et al. Femtosecond laser versus mechanical microkeratome laser in situ keratomileusis for myopia: metaanalysis of randomized controlled trials. *J Cataract Refract Surg.* 2011;37(12):2151–2159.

Table 5-2 Advantages and Disadvantages of the Femtosecond Laser

Advantages	Disadvantages
More customizable flap parameters	Longer suction time
	More flap manipulation
Size and thickness of flap less dependent on corneal contour	Opaque bubble layer may interfere with excimer ablation
Centration easier to control	Bubbles in the anterior chamber may interfere with tracking and registration
Epithelial defects on flap are rare	Increased overall treatment time
Less risk of free cap and buttonhole	Difficulty lifting flap after 6 months
	Increased risk of transient light sensitivity
More reliable flap thickness	Increased cost
Hemorrhage from limbal vessels less likely	Delayed photosensitivity or good acuity plus photosensitivity, which may require prolonged topical corticosteroid therapy
Ability to re-treat immediately if incomplete femtosecond laser ablation	

Modified with permission from Feder RS, Rapuano CJ. *The LASIK Handbook: A Case-Based Approach.* Philadelphia: Lippincott Williams & Wilkins; 2007.

Application of Laser Treatment

Tracking, centration, and ablation

For surface ablation, the exposed Bowman layer should be inspected and found to be smooth, uniformly dry, and free of debris and residual epithelial islands. For LASIK, the flap must be lifted and reflected, and the stromal bed must be uniformly dry before treatment. Fluid or blood accumulation on the stromal bed should be avoided, as it can lead to an irregular ablation.

Excimer lasers in current use employ open-loop tracking systems, which have improved clinical outcomes. The tracker uses video technology to monitor the location of an infrared image of the pupil and to shift the laser beam accordingly.

The laser is centered and focused according to the manufacturer's recommendations. Tracking systems, although effective, do not lessen the importance of keeping the reticule centered on the patient's entrance pupil. If the patient is unable to maintain fixation, the illumination of the operating microscope should be reduced. If decentration occurs and the ablation does not stop automatically, the surgeon should immediately stop the treatment until adequate refixation is achieved. It is still important for the surgeon to monitor for excessive eye movement, which can result in decentration despite the tracking device.

The change in illumination and in patient position (ie, from sitting to lying down) can cause pupil centroid shift and cyclotorsion. In most patients, the pupil moves nasally and superiorly when it is constricted. *Registration* is a technique in which a fixed landmark is used at the time of aberrometry and treatment to apply the ablation to the correct area of the cornea; it relies on iris landmarks and not on the pupil for laser centration (Fig 5-10). Once the patient confirms that the fixation light of the excimer laser is still visible and

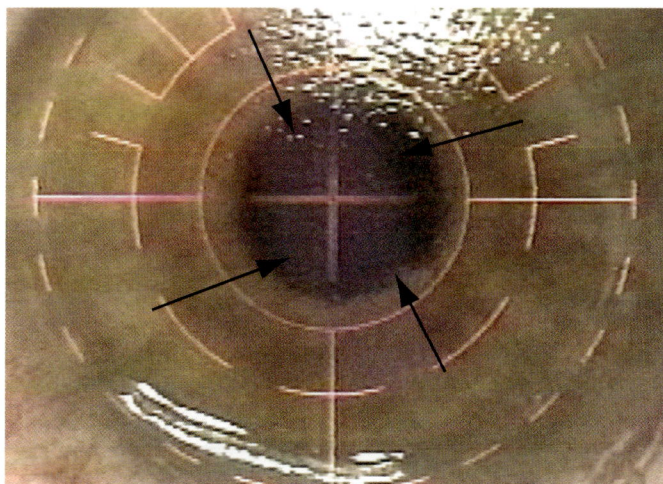

Figure 5-10 Excimer laser ablation of the stromal bed. Note the faint blue fluorescence of the stromal bed from the laser pulse *(arrows)*. The rectangular shape of the exposure by this broad-beam laser indicates that the laser is correcting the cylindrical portion of the treatment. (Photograph is enhanced to visualize fluorescence; the surgeon usually sees minimal or no fluorescence through the operating microscope.) *(Courtesy of Roger F. Steinert, MD.)*

that he or she is looking directly at it, ablation begins. Neither tracking nor iris registration is a substitute for accurate patient fixation. It is important to initiate stromal ablation promptly, before excessive stromal dehydration takes place. During larger-diameter ablations, a flap protector may be needed to shield the underside of the LASIK flap near the hinge from the laser pulses. In addition, it is important to remove the excessive fluid that can accumulate during treatment, especially in patients undergoing high corrections.

> Donnenfeld E. The pupil is a moving target: centration, repeatability, and registration. *J Refract Surg.* 2004;20(5):S593–S596.
> Moshirfar M, Chen MC, Espandar L, et al. Effect of iris registration on outcomes of LASIK for myopia with the VISX CustomVue platform. *J Refract Surg.* 2009;25(6):493–502.

Immediate Postablation Measures

Surface ablation

One of the major potential complications of surface ablation is corneal haze. To decrease the chance of post–surface ablation corneal haze, especially for eyes with previous corneal surgery such as PRK, LASIK, PKP, RK, or primary surface ablations for moderate to high treatments or deeper ablation depths, a pledget soaked in mitomycin C (usually 0.02% or 0.2 mg/mL) can be placed on the ablated surface for approximately 12 seconds to 2 minutes at the end of the laser exposure. The concentration and duration of mitomycin C application varies by diagnosis and surgeon preference; however, most surgeons tend toward shorter durations of mitomycin C exposure. Application of mitomycin C for 12 seconds appears to be as efficacious for prophylaxis as prolonged times. Some surgeons reduce the amount of treatment when applying mitomycin C in surface ablation due to reports of potential endothelial cell toxicity. The cornea is then copiously irrigated with balanced salt solution to remove excess mitomycin C. To avoid damage to limbal stem cells, care should be taken not to expose the limbus or conjunctiva to mitomycin C. Confocal microscopy studies of human eyes have shown a reduced keratocyte population and less haze in eyes that received mitomycin C.

Some surgeons apply sterile, chilled, balanced salt solution or a frozen cellulose sponge before and/or after the surface ablation procedure in the belief that cooling reduces pain and haze formation. However, the advantage of this practice has not been substantiated in a controlled study. Care should be taken to not expose the eye to tap water, which may result in infectious contamination.

If the LASEK or epi-LASIK variant has been performed, the surgeon carefully floats and moves the epithelial sheet back into position with balanced salt solution. Antibiotic, corticosteroid, and, sometimes, nonsteroidal anti-inflammatory drugs (NSAIDs) are then placed on the eye, followed by a bandage contact lens. Some NSAIDs and antibiotics can be placed directly on the corneal bed, whereas others should be placed only on the surface of the contact lens, as they have been associated with poor corneal healing. If the patient cannot tolerate a bandage contact lens, a pressure patch may be used. Of note, the American Society of Cataract and Refractive Surgery released a clinical alert on February 14, 2013, discussing the postoperative risks posed by certain medications used topically prior to or during LASIK or PRK. The medications listed in this statement have the potential to cause flap slippage and/or diffuse lamellar keratitis (DLK) following LASIK surgery and poor epithelial healing following PRK.

ASCRS Cornea and Refractive Surgery Clinical Committees. Medication alert for LASIK and PRK. [Eyeworld website.] March 2013. Available at www.eyeworld.org/article-medication -alert-for-lasik-and-prk. Accessed November 5, 2016.

Carones F, Vigo L, Scandola E, Vacchini L. Evaluation of the prophylactic use of mitomycin-C to inhibit haze formation after photorefractive keratectomy. *J Cataract Refract Surg.* 2002; 28(12):2088–2095.

Lee DH, Chung HS, Jeon YC, Boo SD, Yoon YD, Kim JG. Photorefractive keratectomy with intraoperative mitomycin-C application. *J Cataract Refract Surg.* 2005;31(12):2293–2298.

Virasch VV, Majmudar PA, Epstein RJ, Vaidya NS, Dennis RF. Reduced application time for prophylactic mitomycin C in photorefractive keratectomy. *Ophthalmology.* 2010;117(5): 885–889.

LASIK

After the ablation is completed, the flap is replaced onto the stromal bed. The interface is irrigated until all interface debris is eliminated (which is apparent more readily with oblique than with coaxial illumination). The surface of the flap is gently stroked using a smooth instrument, such as an irrigation cannula or a moistened microsurgical spear sponge, from the hinge, or center, to the periphery. This approach helps to ensure that wrinkles are eliminated and that the flap settles back into its original position, as indicated by realignment of the corneal marks made earlier. The peripheral gutters should be symmetric and even. The physiologic dehydration of the stroma by the endothelial pump will begin to secure the flap in position within several minutes. If a significant epithelial defect or a large, loose sheet of epithelium is present, a bandage contact lens should be put in place. Once the flap is adherent, the eyelid speculum is removed carefully so as not to disturb the flap. Most surgeons place varying combinations of antibiotic, NSAID, and corticosteroid drops on the eye at the conclusion of the procedure. The flap is usually rechecked at the slit lamp before the patient leaves to make sure it has remained in proper alignment. A clear shield or protective goggles are often placed to guard against accidental trauma that could displace the flap. Patients are instructed not to rub or squeeze their eyes.

Lui MM, Silas MA, Fugishima H. Complications of photorefractive keratectomy and laser in situ keratomileusis. *J Refract Surg.* 2003;19(Suppl 2):S247–S249.

Price FW Jr. LASIK. *Focal Points: Clinical Modules for Ophthalmologists.* San Francisco: American Academy of Ophthalmology; 2000, module 3.

Schallhorn SC, Amesbury EC, Tanzer DJ. Avoidance, recognition, and management of LASIK complications. *Am J Ophthalmol.* 2006;141(4):733–739.

Postoperative Care

Surface ablation

After surface ablation, patients may experience variable degrees of pain, from minimal to severe, and some may need oral NSAID, narcotic, or neuropathic pain medications. Studies have shown that topical NSAID drops reduce postoperative pain, although they may also slow the rate of re-epithelialization and promote sterile infiltrates (see Chapter 6). Corneal melting and stromal scarring have been described after the use of some topical NSAIDs. For patients who are not healing normally after surface ablation, use of any topical NSAID should be discontinued.

Patients should be monitored closely until the epithelium is completely healed, which usually occurs within 4–7 days. As long as the bandage contact lens is in place, patients are treated with topical broad-spectrum antibiotics and corticosteroids, usually 4 times daily. Once the epithelium is healed, the bandage contact lens, antibiotic drops, and NSAID drops (if used) may be discontinued. In addition, most clinicians recommend avoidance of swimming and the use of hot tubs for at least 2 weeks postoperatively to help lessen the risk of infection.

The use of topical corticosteroids to modulate postoperative wound healing, reduce anterior stromal haze, and decrease regression of the refractive effect remains controversial. Although some studies have demonstrated that corticosteroids have no significant long-term effect on corneal haze or visual outcome after PRK, other studies have shown that corticosteroids are effective in limiting haze and myopic regression after PRK, particularly after higher myopic corrections. Some surgeons who advocate use of topical corticosteroids after the removal of the bandage contact lens restrict their use to patients with higher levels of myopia (eg, myopia greater than –4.00 or –5.00 D). When used after removal of the bandage contact lens, corticosteroid drops are typically tapered over a 1- to 4-month period, depending on the patient's corneal haze and refractive outcome. Patients who received mitomycin C at the time of surgery have a reduced risk of haze formation and thus may have a shorter duration of corticosteroid use. Patients who had PRK for hyperopia may experience prolonged epithelial healing because of the larger epithelial defect resulting from the larger ablation zone, as well as a temporary reduction in best-corrected visual acuity (BCVA; also called *corrected distance visual acuity, CDVA*) in the first week to month, which usually improves with time. Many patients with hyperopia also experience a temporary myopic overcorrection, which regresses over several weeks to months. In the absence of complications, routine follow-up examinations are typically scheduled at approximately 2–4 weeks, 2–3 months, 6 months, and 12 months postoperatively and perhaps more frequently, depending on the steroid taper used.

LASIK

Many surgeons instruct their patients to use topical antibiotics and corticosteroids postoperatively for 3–7 days. With femtosecond laser procedures, some surgeons prescribe more frequent applications of corticosteroid eye drops or a longer period of use due to a tendency of older femtosecond lasers to create more intrastromal inflammation. LASIK flaps made with current generation femtosecond lasers have similar inflammation profiles to microkeratome cut flaps. In addition, it is very important for the surface of the flap to be kept well lubricated in the early postoperative period. Patients may be told to use the protective shield for 1–7 days when they shower or sleep and to avoid swimming and the use of hot tubs for 2 weeks. Patients are examined 1 day after surgery to ensure that the flap has remained in proper alignment and that there is no evidence of infection or excessive inflammation. In the absence of complications, the next examinations are typically scheduled at approximately 1 week, 1 month, 3 months, 6 months, and 12 months postoperatively.

Santhiago MR, Kara-Junior N, Waring GO IV. Microkeratome versus femtosecond flaps: accuracy and complications. *Curr Opin Ophthalmol.* 2014;25(4):270–274.

Santhiago MR, Wilson SE. Cellular effects after laser in situ keratomileusis flap formation with femtosecond lasers: a review. *Cornea.* 2012;31(2):198–205.

Solomon KD, Donnenfeld ED, Raizman M, et al; Ketorolac Reformulation Study Groups 1 and 2. Safety and efficacy of ketorolac tromethamine 0.4% ophthalmic solution in post–photorefractive keratectomy patients. *J Cataract Refract Surg.* 2004;30(8):1653–1660.

Refractive Outcomes

As the early broad-beam excimer laser systems improved and surgeons gained experience, the results achieved with surface ablation and LASIK improved markedly. The ablation zone diameter was enlarged because it was found that small ablation zones, originally selected to limit depth of tissue removal, produced more haze and regression in surface ablation treatments and concerns about subjective glare and halos for both surface ablation and LASIK. The larger treatment diameters currently used, including for optical zones and gradual aspheric peripheral blend zones, improve optical quality and refractive stability in both myopic and hyperopic treatments. Central island elevations have become less common with improvements in beam quality, vacuums to remove the ablation plume, and the development of scanning and variable-spot-size excimer lasers.

Solomon KD, Fernández de Castro LE, Sandoval HP, et al; Joint LASIK Study Task Force. LASIK world literature review: quality of life and patient satisfaction. *Ophthalmology.* 2009;116(4):691–701.

Outcomes for Myopia

Initial FDA clinical trials of conventional excimer laser treatments limited to myopia of 6.00 D or less revealed that 56%–86% of eyes treated with either PRK or LASIK achieved uncorrected visual acuity (UCVA; also called *uncorrected distance visual acuity, UDVA*) of at least 20/20, 88%–100% achieved UCVA of at least 20/40, and 82%–100% were within 1.00 D of emmetropia. Up to 2.1% of eyes lost 2 or more lines of BCVA. Reports since 2000 have demonstrated significantly improved outcomes and safety profiles, with fewer than 0.6% of eyes losing 2 or more lines of BCVA.

el Danasoury MA, el Maghraby A, Klyce SD, Mehrez K. Comparison of photorefractive keratectomy with excimer laser in situ keratomileusis in correcting low myopia (from –2.00 to –5.50 diopters): a randomized study. *Ophthalmology.* 1999;106(2):411–420.

Kanellopoulos AJ, Asimellis G. Long-term bladeless LASIK outcomes with the FS200 femtosecond and EX500 excimer laser workstation: the refractive suite. *Clin Ophthalmol.* 2013;7:261–269.

Kulkarni SV, AlMahmoud T, Priest D, Taylor SE, Mintsioulis G, Jackson WB. Long-term visual and refractive outcomes following surface ablation techniques in a large population for myopia correction. *Invest Ophthalmol Vis Sci.* 2013;54(1):609–619.

Luger MH, Ewering T, Arba-Mosquera S. Influence of patient age on high myopic correction in corneal laser refractive surgery. *J Cataract Refract Surg.* 2013;39(2):204–210.

Sugar A, Rapuano CJ, Culbertson WW, et al. Laser in situ keratomileusis for myopia and astigmatism: safety and efficacy: a report by the American Academy of Ophthalmology. *Ophthalmology.* 2002;109(1):175–187.

Tole DM, McCarty DJ, Couper T, Taylor HR. Comparison of laser in situ keratomileusis and photorefractive keratectomy for the correction of myopia of −6.00 diopters or less. Melbourne Excimer Laser Group. *J Refract Surg.* 2001;17(1):46–54.

Watson SL, Bunce C, Alan BD. Improved safety in contemporary LASIK. *Ophthalmology.* 2005;112(8):1375–1380.

Outcomes for Hyperopia

In myopic ablations, the central cornea is flattened, whereas in hyperopic ablations, more tissue is removed from the midperiphery than from the central cornea, resulting in an effective steepening (see Fig 5-1B). To ensure that the size of the central hyperopic treatment zone is adequate, a large ablation area is required for hyperopic treatments. Most studies have employed hyperopic treatment zones with transition zones out to 9.0–9.5 mm. FDA clinical trials of PRK and LASIK for hyperopia up to +6.00 D reported that 46%–59% of eyes had postoperative UCVA of 20/20 or better, 92%–96% had UCVA of 20/40 or better, and 84%–91% were within 1.00 D of emmetropia; loss of more than 2 lines of BCVA occurred in 1%–3.5%. The VISX FDA clinical trial of hyperopic astigmatic PRK up to +6.00 D sphere and +4.00 D cylinder reported an approximate postoperative UCVA of 20/20 or better in 50% of eyes, UCVA of 20/40 or better in 97%, and 87% within ±1.00 D of emmetropia, with loss of more than 2 lines of BCVA in 1.5%. For the same amount of correction, the period from surgery to postoperative stabilization is longer for hyperopic than for myopic corrections. Overall, studies with larger ablation zones have demonstrated good results for refractive errors up to +4.00 D for conventional treatments, but predictability and stability are markedly reduced with LASIK treatments for hyperopia above this level. Consequently, most refractive surgeons do not treat up to the highest levels of hyperopia that have been approved by the FDA for conventional treatments.

Gil-Cazorla R, Teus MA, de Benito-Llopis L, Mikropoulos DG. Femtosecond laser vs mechanical microkeratome for hyperopic laser in situ keratomileusis. *Am J Ophthalmol.* 2011;152(1): 16–21.

Llovet F, Galal A, Benitez-del-Castillo JM, Ortega J, Martin C, Baviera J. One-year results of excimer laser in situ keratomileusis for hyperopia. *J Cataract Refract Surg.* 2009;35(7): 1156–1165.

Salz JJ, Stevens CA; LADARVision LASIK Hyperopia Study Group. LASIK correction of spherical hyperopia, hyperopic astigmatism, and mixed astigmatism with the LADARVision excimer laser system. *Ophthalmology.* 2002;109(9):1647–1656.

Tabbara KF, El-Sheikh HF, Islam SM. Laser in situ keratomileusis for the correction of hyperopia from +0.50 to +11.50 diopters with the Keracor 117C laser. *J Refract Surg.* 2001;17(2): 123–128.

Varley GA, Huang D, Rapuano CJ, Schallhorn S, Boxer Wachler BS, Sugar A; Ophthalmic Technology Assessment Committee Refractive Surgery Panel. LASIK for hyperopia, hyperopic astigmatism, and mixed astigmatism: a report by the American Academy of Ophthalmology. *Ophthalmology.* 2004;111(8):1604–1617.

Williams L, Moshirfar M, Dave S. Preoperative keratometry and visual outcomes after hyperopic LASIK. *J Refract Surg.* 2009;25(12):1052.

Wavefront-Guided, Wavefront-Optimized, and Topography-Guided Treatment Outcomes for Myopia and Hyperopia

Wavefront-guided or wavefront-optimized LASIK coupled with sophisticated eye-tracking systems has greatly improved the accuracy and reproducibility of results, allowing even higher percentages of patients to obtain UCVA of 20/20 and 20/40. In wavefront-guided LASIK for myopic astigmatism, for example, up to about –10.00 to –12.00 D, 79%–95% of patients obtained 20/20 UCVA, and 96%–100% obtained 20/40 UCVA. In wavefront-guided LASIK for hyperopic astigmatism up to +6.00 D, 55%–59% of patients obtained 20/20 UCVA, and 93%–97% obtained 20/40 UCVA. In wavefront-guided LASIK for mixed astigmatism with up to +5.00 D of cylinder, 56%–61% of patients obtained 20/20 UCVA, and 95% obtained 20/40 UCVA. A recent study found that the visual acuity results for the vast majority of patients were equivalent between wavefront-guided and wavefront-optimized LASIK.

Recent clinical trial data on topography-guided ablations demonstrated that for corrections up to –9.00 D of spherical equivalent myopia with up to –8.00 D spherical and –3.00 D astigmatic components, 93% of eyes had UCVA of 20/20 or better. The data also demonstrated that 32% of eyes achieved 20/12.5 or better and 69% achieved 20/16 or better. In 30% of patients, postoperative UCVA improved 1 line or more compared to preoperative BCVA.

Fares U, Otri AM, Al-Aqaba MA, Faraj L, Dua HS. Wavefront-optimized excimer laser in situ keratomileusis for myopia and myopic astigmatism: refractive outcomes and corneal densitometry. *J Cataract Refract Surg*. 2012;38(12):2131–2138.

Keir NJ, Simpson T, Jones LW, Fonn D. Wavefront-guided LASIK for myopia: effect on visual acuity, contrast sensitivity, and higher order aberrations. *J Refract Surg*. 2009;25(6): 524–533.

Randleman JB, Perez-Straziota CE, Hu MH, White AJ, Loft ES, Stulting RD. Higher-order aberrations after wavefront-optimized photorefractive keratectomy and laser in situ keratomileusis. *J Cataract Refract Surg*. 2009;35(2):260–264.

Schallhorn SC, Farjo AA, Huang D, et al; American Academy of Ophthalmology. Wavefront-guided LASIK for the correction of primary myopia and astigmatism: a report by the American Academy of Ophthalmology. *Ophthalmology*. 2008;115(7):1249–1261.

Tan J, Simon D, Mrochen M, Por YM. Clinical results of topography-based customized ablations for myopia and myopic astigmatism. *J Refract Surg*. 2012;28(Suppl 11):S829–S836.

Re-treatment (Enhancements)

Although excimer laser ablation reduces refractive error and improves UCVA in almost all cases, some patients have residual refractive errors and would benefit from re-treatment. The degree of refractive error that warrants re-treatment varies depending on the patient's lifestyle and expectations. Re-treatment rates also vary, depending on the degree of refractive error being treated, the laser and nomograms used, and the expectations of the patient. One advantage of LASIK over surface ablation is that refractive stability generally occurs earlier, allowing earlier enhancements, typically within the first 3 months after

LASIK. With surface ablation, the ongoing activation of keratocytes and the risk of haze after enhancement usually require a wait of 3–6 months before an enhancement surface ablation is undertaken. Typically, re-treatment rates are higher for hyperopia and for high astigmatism than for other indications.

Studies showed that rates of re-treatment are higher for higher initial correction, residual astigmatism, and patients older than 40 years. One should be careful when enhancing a myopic shift in a patient older than 50 years, as this may be due to a lens-induced myopic shift rather than post–refractive surgery regression. Re-treatment rates vary from 1% to 11%, based on surgeon experience, patient demands, and the other factors just described. Surface ablation re-treatment is nearly identical to primary surface ablation treatment, whereas LASIK re-treatment can be performed either by lifting the preexisting lamellar flap and applying additional ablation to the stromal bed or by performing surface ablation on the LASIK flap. In most cases, the flap can be lifted many years after the original procedure. However, because of the safety of surface ablation after LASIK and the increased risk of epithelial ingrowth with flap lifts, many surgeons now prefer to perform surface ablation re-treatment if the primary LASIK was performed more than 2–3 years earlier. Creating a new flap with a mechanical microkeratome should be avoided because free slivers of tissue, irregular stromal beds, and irregular astigmatism may be produced. Using the femtosecond laser to create a new side cut within the boundaries of the previous flap may facilitate flap-lift enhancements; however, it is important to have an adequate exposed diameter for ablation, and tissues slivers can result if the old and new side cuts overlap. When attempting to lift or manipulate a femtosecond laser–created flap, the surgeon must take care to avoid tearing it, because the femtosecond laser usually creates a thinner flap than traditional microkeratomes.

When a preexisting flap is lifted, it is important to minimize epithelial disruption. A jeweler's forceps, Sinskey hook, or 27-gauge needle can be used to localize the edge of the previous flap. Because the edge of the flap can be seen more easily with the slit lamp than with the diffuse illumination of the operating microscope of the laser, some surgeons find it easier to begin a flap lift at the slit lamp and complete it at the excimer laser. Alternatively, the surgeon can often visualize the edge of the flap under the diffuse illumination of the operating microscope by applying pressure with a small Sinskey hook or similar device; the edge of the flap will dimple and disrupt the light reflex (Fig 5-11). A careful circumferential epithelial dissection is performed so that the flap can then be lifted without tearing the epithelial edges. Smooth forceps, iris spatulas, and several instruments specifically designed for dissecting the flap edge can be used to lift the original flap.

Once the ablation has been performed, the flap is repositioned and the interface is irrigated, as in the initial LASIK procedure. Special care must be taken to ensure that no loose epithelium is trapped beneath the edge of the flap that could lead to epithelial ingrowth; the risk of epithelial ingrowth is greater after re-treatment than after primary treatment.

Surface ablation may be considered to enhance a previous primary LASIK treatment. Surface ablation performed on a LASIK flap carries an increased risk of haze formation and irregular astigmatism, but it is an appealing alternative when the RSB is insufficient for further ablation; when the LASIK was performed by another surgeon and the flap

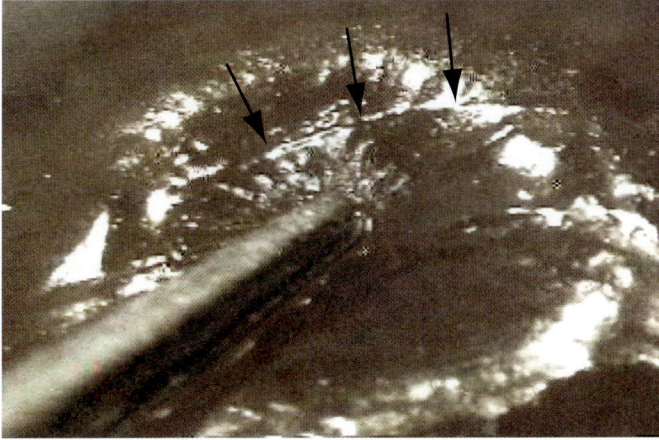

Figure 5-11 Indenting the cornea with forceps to visualize the edge of the flap *(arrows)* through an operating microscope prior to an enhancement procedure. *(Courtesy of Roger F. Steinert, MD.)*

thickness, or RSB, is not known; or with conditions such as a buttonhole or incomplete flap. Care must be taken when removing the epithelium over a flap to avoid inadvertently lifting or dislocating the flap. Applying 20% ethanol for 20–30 seconds inside a corneal well will loosen the epithelium, after which scraping motions are applied that extend from the hinge toward the periphery. A rotating brush should not be used to remove the epithelium from a LASIK flap. The risk of postoperative haze due to surface ablation over a previous LASIK flap may be avoided or reduced by administering intraoperative topical mitomycin C, 0.02%, and postoperative topical corticosteroids.

The appropriate choice between conventional and wavefront-guided treatment for enhancing the vision of patients who have previously undergone conventional LASIK is not yet established. Some studies report better results in both safety and efficacy with conventional LASIK re-treatment. With wavefront-guided re-treatments, particularly in patients with high spherical aberrations, the risk of overcorrection may be greater. Caution should be exercised in evaluating the degree of higher-order aberrations and the planned depth of the ablation when deciding between conventional and wavefront-guided treatments.

Carones F, Vigo L, Carones AV, Brancato R. Evaluation of photorefractive keratectomy retreatments after regressed myopic laser in situ keratomileusis. *Ophthalmology.* 2001; 108(10):1732–1737.

Caster AI, Friess DW, Schwendeman FJ. Incidence of epithelial ingrowth in primary and retreatment laser in situ keratomileusis. *J Cataract Refract Surg.* 2010;36(1):97–101.

Davis EA, Hardten DR, Lindstrom M, Samuelson TW, Lindstrom RL. LASIK enhancements: a comparison of lifting to recutting the flap. *Ophthalmology.* 2002;109(12):2308–2313.

Hersh PS, Fry KL, Bishop DS. Incidence and associations of retreatment after LASIK. *Ophthalmology.* 2003;110(4):748–754.

Hiatt JA, Grant CN, Boxer Wachler BS. Complex wavefront-guided retreatments with the Alcon CustomCornea platform after prior LASIK. *J Refract Surg.* 2006;22(1):48–53.

Jin GJ, Merkley KH. Conventional and wavefront-guided myopic LASIK retreatment. *Am J Ophthalmol.* 2006;141(4):660–668.

Randleman JB, White AJ Jr, Lynn MJ, Hu MH, Stulting RD. Incidence, outcomes, and risk factors for retreatment after wavefront-optimized ablations with PRK and LASIK. *J Refract Surg.* 2009;25(3):273–276.

Rubinfeld RS, Hardten DR, Donnenfeld ED, et al. To lift or recut: changing trends in LASIK enhancement. *J Cataract Refract Surg.* 2003;29(12):2306–2317.

Santhiago MR, Smadja D, Zaleski K, Espana EM, Armstrong BK, Wilson SE. Flap relift for retreatment after femtosecond laser–assisted LASIK. *J Refract Surg.* 2012;28(7):482–487.

Vaddavalli PK, Diakonis VF, Canto AP, Culbertson WW, Wang J, Kankariya VP, Yoo SH. Complications of femtosecond laser-assisted re-treatment for residual refractive errors after LASIK. *J Refract Surg.* 2013;29(8):577–580.

Weisenthal RW, Salz J, Sugar A, et al. Photorefractive keratectomy for treatment of flap complications in laser in situ keratomileusis. *Cornea.* 2003;22(5):399–404.

Photoablation: Complications and Adverse Effects

Photorefractive keratectomy (PRK) and laser in situ keratomileusis (LASIK), 2 of the most common kinds of refractive surgeries, are relatively safe and effective procedures. As with all types of surgery, there are potential risks and complications, and thus it is important to understand how to avoid, diagnose, and treat the complications of refractive surgery. Comprehensive ophthalmologists, as well as refractive surgeons, should be knowledgeable about these postoperative problems, given the increasing number of patients who undergo refractive surgery each year.

General Complications Related to Laser Ablation

Overcorrection

Overcorrection may occur if significant stromal dehydration develops prior to initiation of the excimer treatment, as more stromal tissue will be ablated per pulse. This overcorrection may occur if there is a long delay prior to beginning the ablation, following either removal of the epithelium in surface ablation or lifting the flap in LASIK. Controlling the humidity and temperature in the laser suite within the recommended excimer laser guidelines may decrease variability and ideally improve refractive outcomes. Overcorrection tends to occur more often in older individuals, as their wound-healing response is less vigorous and their corneas ablate more rapidly for reasons not fully understood.

Myopic or hyperopic surface ablation typically undergoes some degree of refractive regression for at least 3–6 months. In general, patients with higher degrees of myopia and any degree of hyperopia require more time to attain refractive stability, which must be achieved before any decision is made regarding possible re-treatment of the overcorrection.

Various modalities are available for treating small amounts of overcorrection. Myopic regression can be induced after surface ablation by abrupt discontinuation of corticosteroids. Patients with consecutive hyperopia (ie, hypcropia due to overcorrection of myopia) or consecutive myopia (ie, myopia due to overcorrection of hyperopia) require less treatment to achieve emmetropia compared with previously untreated eyes, as both are considered to have over-responded to the initial treatment. When re-treating such patients, the surgeon should take care not to overcorrect a second time. With conventional ablation, most surgeons will reduce the ablation by 20%–25% for consecutive treatments. For wavefront procedures, review of the depth of the ablation and the amount of higher-order aberration helps titrate the re-treatment.

Undercorrection

Undercorrection occurs much more commonly with treatment of higher degrees of ametropia. Patients with regression after treatment of their first eye have an increased likelihood of regression in their second eye. Topical mitomycin C, administered at the time of initial surface ablation, can be used to modulate the response, especially in patients with higher levels of ametropia. Sometimes the regression may be reversed with aggressive administration of topical corticosteroids. The patient may undergo a re-treatment generally no sooner than 3 months postoperatively, once the refraction has stabilized. A patient with significant corneal haze and regression after surface ablation is at higher risk after re-treatment for further regression, recurrence, or worsening of the corneal haze, as well as loss of best-corrected visual acuity (BCVA; also called *corrected distance visual acuity, CDVA*). It is recommended that the surgeon wait at least 6–12 months for the haze to improve spontaneously before repeating surface ablation. In patients with significant haze and myopic regression, removal of the haze with adjunctive use of mitomycin C should not be coupled with a refractive treatment, as the resolution of the haze will commonly improve the refractive outcome. Undercorrection after LASIK typically requires flap lift and laser treatment of the residual refractive error after the refraction has remained stable for at least 3 months. Cases of delayed and progressive regression, especially with concomitant development of irregular astigmatism, may suggest ectasia, or, in an older patient, refractive shift due to the development of cataract.

Optical Aberrations

After undergoing surface ablation or LASIK, some patients report symptoms related to optical aberrations, including glare, ghost images, and halos. These symptoms are most prevalent after treatment with smaller ablation zones (<6.0 mm in diameter), after attempted higher spherical and cylindrical correction, and in patients with symptoms prior to refractive surgery. These vision problems seem to be exacerbated in dim-light conditions when mydriasis occurs. Wavefront mapping can reveal higher-order aberrations associated with these subjective concerns. In general, a larger, more uniform, and well-centered optical zone provides a better quality of vision, especially at night.

Night-vision concerns are often the result of spherical aberration, although other higher-order aberrations also contribute. The cornea and lens have inherent spherical aberration. In addition, excimer laser ablation increases positive spherical aberration in the midperipheral cornea. Wavefront-guided and optimized corneal treatment patterns are designed to reduce existing aberrations and to help prevent the creation of new aberrations, with the goal of achieving a better quality of vision after laser ablation.

Although the excimer laser photoablation causes most of the post-LASIK changes in lower- and higher-order aberrations, several studies have demonstrated that the creation of the flap itself can also result in aberrations (Fig 6-1). Some studies have demonstrated that femtosecond lasers cause little or no change in higher-order aberrations, in contrast to mechanical microkeratomes. Pallikaris showed that LASIK flap creation alone, without

OS   -1.28 DS -0.62 DC x 4° @12.5 mm (4.00 Rx Calc)
20-Oct-2008 10:18:46   W.F. Diam (mm): 5.25   High Order: 13.4 %
Eff. Blur (D): 1.72   Rms Err.(µ): 1.71   Quality: ✓ ✓ ✓ ✓

Eye Image   Limbus Diam:12.6 mm   Pupil: 5.5 x 5.2 mm @86° (avg 5.4)

High Order Aberrations - Log 50%   Eff. Blur (D): 0.23

Range: -8.0 to +8.0 minutes of arc

Wavefront High Order Aberrations   Rms Error (µ): 0.23
Range: -0.7 to +1.0 microns   Grid spacing: 1 mm.

Normalized Polar Zernike Coefficients (µ)   High Order Aberrations Graph

	Value	Name	0.0 0.19506	Axis
Z	1.61040	Defocus		
Z	0.52059 @ 94°	Astigmatism		
Z	0.08501 @ 216°	Coma		
Z	0.19506 @ 91°	Trefoil		
Z	0.04095	Sph. Aberration		
Z	0.00615 @ 149°			
Z	0.06444 @ 27°			
Z	0.01122 @ 66°			
Z	0.00456 @ 96°			
Z	0.02383 @ 8°			
Z	0.00130			
Z	0.03598 @ 9°			
Z	0.02033 @ 65°			
Z	0.01591 @ 4°			

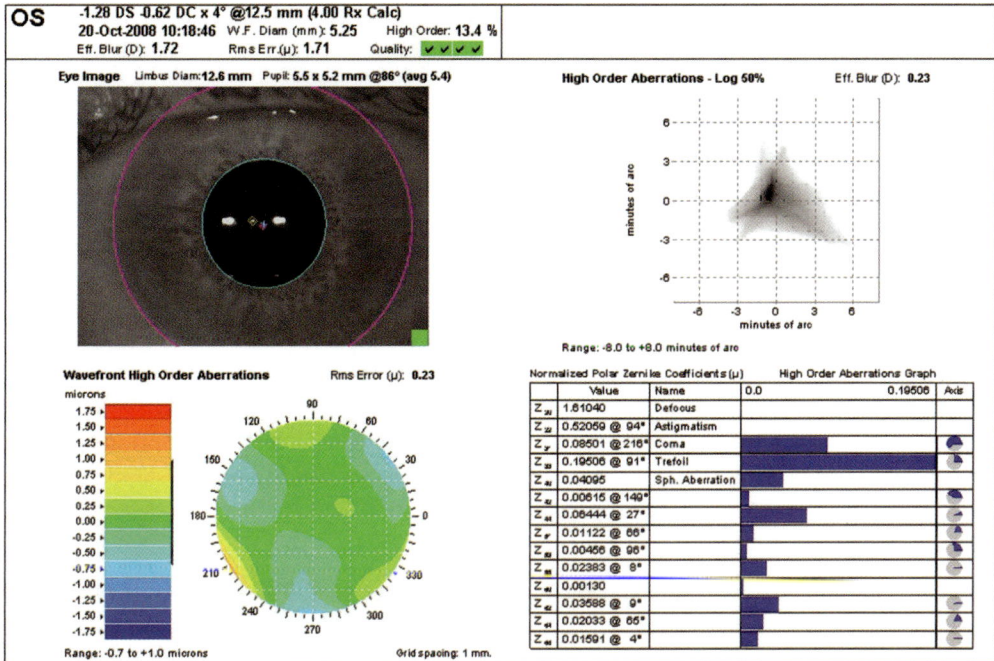

Figure 6-1 Wavefront analysis depicting higher-order aberrations after laser in situ kerato-mileusis (LASIK), including coma and trefoil. *(Courtesy of Steven I. Rosenfeld, MD.)*

lifting, caused no significant change in refractive error or visual acuity but did cause a significant increase in total higher-order wavefront aberrations.

Pallikaris IG, Kymionis GD, Panagopoulou SI, Siganos CS, Theodorakis MA, Pellikaris AI. Induced optical aberrations following formation of a laser in situ keratomileusis flap. *J Cataract Refract Surg.* 2002;28(10):1737–1741.

Tran DB, Sarayba MA, Bor Z, et al. Randomized prospective clinical study comparing induced aberrations with IntraLase and Hansatome flap creation in fellow eyes: potential impact on wavefront-guided laser in situ keratomileusis. *J Cataract Refract Surg.* 2005; 31(1):97–105.

Waheed S, Chalita MR, Xu M, Krueger RR. Flap-induced and laser-induced ocular aberrations in a two-step LASIK procedure. *J Refract Surg.* 2005;21(3):346–352.

Central Islands

A central island is defined as a steepening of at least 1.00 D with a diameter of less than 1 mm compared with the paracentral flattened area. A central island appears on computerized corneal topography as an area of central corneal steepening surrounded by an area of flattening that corresponds to the myopic treatment zone in the paracentral region (Fig 6-2). Central islands may be associated with decreased visual acuity, monocular diplopia and multiplopia, ghost images, and decreased contrast sensitivity.

The occurrence of central islands has been reduced significantly through the use of scanning and variable-spot-size lasers and is now rarely encountered with modern laser technology. Fortunately, most central islands diminish over time, especially after

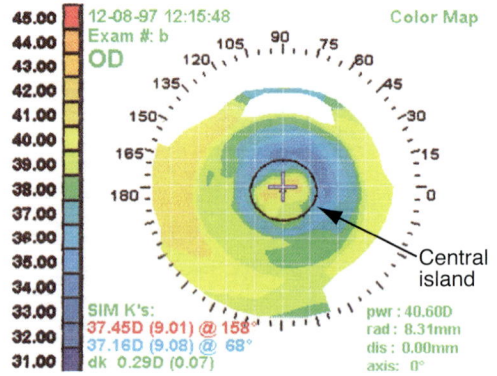

Figure 6-2 Corneal topography findings of a myopic ablation *(blue)* with a central island *(yellow)* in the visual axis. *(Courtesy of Roger F. Steinert, MD.)*

surface ablation, although resolution may take 6–12 months. Treatment options such as topography-guided ablations may be helpful in treating persistent central islands.

Decentered Ablations

Accurate centration during the excimer laser procedure is important in optimizing the visual results. Centration is even more crucial for hyperopic than myopic treatments. A decentered ablation may occur if the patient's eye slowly begins to drift and loses fixation, if the surgeon initially positions the patient's head improperly, or if the patient's eye is not perpendicular to the laser treatment (Fig 6-3). The incidence of decentration increases with surgeon inexperience, hyperopic ablations, and higher refractive correction, due to longer ablation times. Decentration may be reduced by ensuring that the patient's head remains in the correct plane throughout the treatment—that is, perpendicular to the laser (parallel to the ground)—and that there is no head tilt. Treatment of decentration with topography-guided technology, and/or with the use of masking agents may be effective.

Corticosteroid-Induced Complications

The incidence of increased intraocular pressure (IOP) after surface ablation has been reported to range from 11% to 25%. Occasionally, the IOP may be quite high. In 1 study, 2% of patients had a postoperative IOP greater than 40 mm Hg. Most cases of elevated IOP are associated with prolonged topical corticosteroid therapy. Accordingly, postoperative

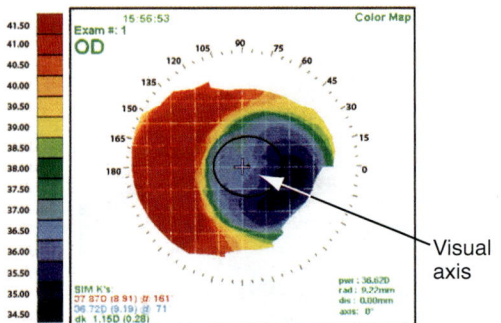

Figure 6-3 Corneal topography findings indicating a decentered ablation. *(Courtesy of Roger F. Steinert, MD.)*

corticosteroid-associated IOP elevations are more likely to occur after surface ablation (after which corticosteroid therapy may be used for 2–4 months to prevent postoperative corneal haze) or after complicated LASIK cases. Corticosteroid-induced elevated IOP occurs in 1.5%–3.0% of patients using fluorometholone but in up to 25% of patients using dexamethasone. The increase in IOP is usually controlled with topical IOP-lowering medications and typically normalizes after the corticosteroids are decreased or discontinued. Because of the changes in corneal curvature and/or corneal thickness, Goldmann tonometry readings after myopic surface ablation and LASIK are artifactually reduced (see Glaucoma After Refractive Surgery in Chapter 11). Several alternative techniques of measuring IOP have been suggested, but dynamic contour tonometry is the only technique shown to have sufficient reproducible accuracy in eyes after refractive ablation. In addition, with high IOP, fluid can collect in the flap interface and mask dangerously high IOPs, as applanation devices will artifactually measure the pressure of the fluid chamber created between the stroma and the LASIK flap. Other corticosteroid-associated complications that have been reported after surface ablation are reactivation of herpes simplex virus keratitis, ptosis, and cataracts.

Central Toxic Keratopathy

Central toxic keratopathy is a rare, acute, noninflammatory central corneal opacification that can occur within days after uneventful LASIK or PRK (Fig 6-4). The etiology is unknown but may be related to enzymatic degradation of keratocytes.

Confocal microscopy has demonstrated activated keratocytes without inflammatory cells, with initial keratocyte loss from the stromal bed and gradual repopulation over time. Central toxic keratopathy has been reported to result in anterior curvature flattening without alteration of posterior curvature in anterior segment tomography; however,

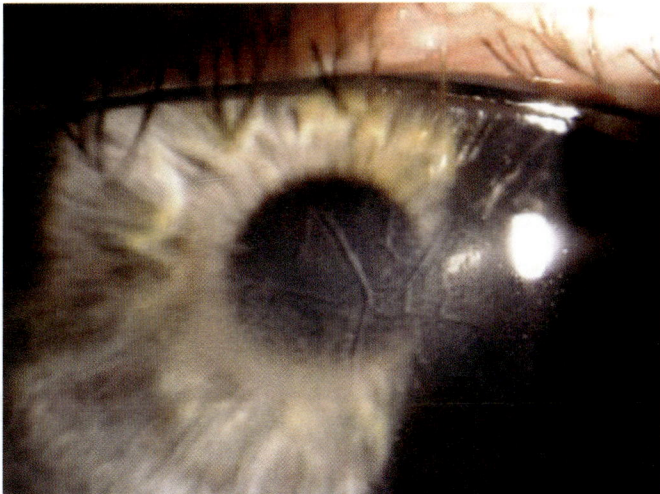

Figure 6-4 Clinical photograph of central toxic keratopathy, a rare, acute, noninflammatory central corneal opacification that can occur within days after uneventful LASIK or photorefractive keratectomy. *(Courtesy of Parag Majmudar, MD.)*

some cases do appear to alter all tomographic findings, likely as measurement artifact. The onset is acute without worsening over time, unlike in most other interface entities.

Marked hyperopic shift is often observed and tends to resolve over time. Enhancement can be deferred in these cases until refractive stability is achieved and the clinical findings have resolved. The use of topical hypertonic solutions for the treatment of central toxic keratopathy has been proposed in anecdotal reports.

Moshirfar M, Hazin R, Khalifa YM. Central toxic keratopathy. *Curr Opin Ophthalmol.* 2010;
 21(4):274–279.
Thornton IL, Foulks GN, Eiferman RA. Confocal microscopy of central toxic keratopathy.
 Cornea. 2012;31(8):934–936.

Infectious Keratitis

Infectious keratitis may occur after surface ablation procedures or LASIK, as both types of surgery involve disturbance of the ocular surface (Fig 6-5). As a result, eyelid preparation and proper draping are recommended. The risk of infection varies depending on the specific technique, with surface ablation more commonly at risk of postoperative infection compared to LASIK. The most common etiologic agents for these infections are gram-positive organisms, including *Staphylococcus aureus,* methicillin-resistant *Staphylococcus aureus (MRSA), Streptococcus pneumoniae,* and *Streptococcus viridans.* Although health care workers and others exposed in hospital and nursing home settings may be at greatest risk for MRSA infection, MRSA infections have been diagnosed in increasing numbers of cases without known risk factors. Atypical mycobacteria, *Nocardia asteroides,* and fungi have also been reported to cause infectious keratitis after surface ablation and LASIK.

PRK and other surface ablation techniques involve creation of an iatrogenic corneal epithelial defect that may take 3–5 days to heal. During this time, the risk of postoperative infectious keratitis is greatest because of exposure of the stroma, use of a bandage contact lens, and administration of topical corticosteroid drops, all of which increase the opportunity for eyelid and conjunctival bacterial flora to gain access to the stroma. Treatment of postoperative infectious keratitis consists of culture and sensitivity testing of contact lens and corneal scrapings and institution of appropriate intensive, topical, broad-spectrum antibiotic coverage, being cognizant of the higher prevalence of keratitis secondary to gram-positive organisms. Treatment may require a combination of antimicrobial agents. Fungal keratitis can also occur, especially with concomitant corticosteroid use. With that

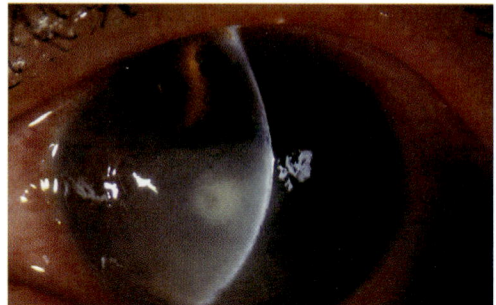

Figure 6-5 Infectious keratitis 1 month postoperatively after LASIK. *(Courtesy of M. Bowes Hamill, MD.)*

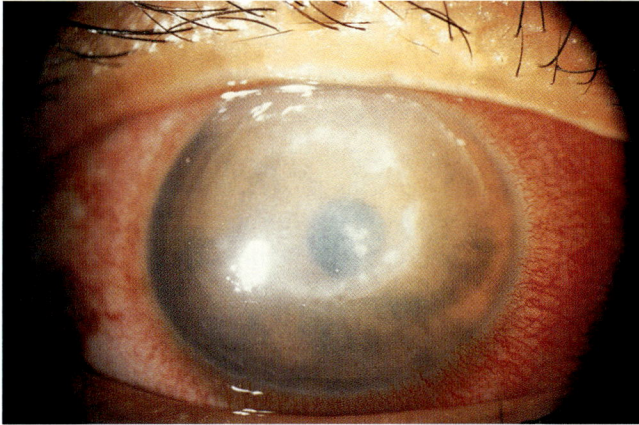

Figure 6-6 Infectious keratitis in a LASIK flap after recurrent epithelial abrasion. *(Courtesy of Jayne S. Weiss, MD.)*

in mind, cultures should include fungal assays, and treatment for keratitis should include antifungal agents in suspected cases (see BCSC Section 8, *External Disease and Cornea*).

During or shortly after LASIK, which involves creation of a corneal flap, eyelid and conjunctival flora may enter and remain sequestered under the flap. The antimicrobial components in the tears and in topically applied antibiotic drops have difficulty penetrating into the deep stroma to reach the organisms (Fig 6-6). If a post-LASIK infection is suspected, the surgeon can lift the flap, scrape the stromal bed for culture and sensitivity testing, and irrigate with antibiotics prior to flap repositioning. Intensive treatment with topical antibiotic drops, as described previously, can be started pending culture results. If there is lack of clinical progress, additional scrapings and irrigation may be necessary, the flap may be amputated, and the antibiotic regimen may be altered.

Llovet F, de Rojas V, Interlandi E, et al. Infectious keratitis in 204,586 LASIK procedures. *Ophthalmology.* 2010;117(3):232–238.

Mozayan A, Madu A, Channa P. Laser in-situ keratomileusis infection: review and update of current practices. *Curr Opin Ophthalmol.* 2011;22(4):233–237.

Solomon R, Donnenfeld ED, Perry HD, et al. Methicillin-resistant *Staphylococcus aureus* infectious keratitis following refractive surgery. *Am J Ophthalmol.* 2007;143(4):629–634.

Wroblewski KJ, Pasternak JF, Bower KS, et al. Infectious keratitis after photorefractive keratectomy in the United States Army and Navy. *Ophthalmology.* 2006;113(4):520–525.

Complications Unique to Surface Ablation

Persistent Epithelial Defects

Usually, the epithelial defect created during surface ablation heals within 3 or 4 days with the aid of a bandage contact lens. A frequent cause of delayed reepithelialization is keratoconjunctivitis sicca or other tear film abnormalities. Proper diagnosis and targeted treatment are critical. Treatment options include aggressive nonpreserved lubrication, topical cyclosporine, temporary punctal occlusion, amniotic membrane grafting, and autologous serum drops. Patients who have autoimmune connective tissue disease or diabetes mellitus or who smoke may also have poor epithelial healing and may require a more aggressive approach. Topical nonsteroidal anti-inflammatory drugs (NSAIDs) should be discontinued in patients with delayed reepithelialization. Nonpreserved drops are preferable. Oral tetracycline-family antibiotics may be beneficial for persistent epithelial defects because they inhibit collagenase activity and in turn improve wound healing. In some cases, epithelial healing may be impaired by the presence of necrotic epithelium on the corneal surface. Gentle debridement of the necrotic epithelial border can promote reepithelialization. The importance of closely monitoring patients until re-epithelialization occurs cannot be overemphasized, as a persistent epithelial defect increases the risk of corneal haze, irregular astigmatism, refractive instability, delayed recovery of vision, and infectious keratitis.

Sterile Infiltrates

The use of bandage contact lenses to aid epithelial healing is associated with sterile infiltrates, which may occur more frequently in patients using topical NSAIDs for longer than 24 hours without concomitant topical corticosteroids. The infiltrates, which have been reported in approximately 1 in 300 cases, are secondary to an immune reaction (Fig 6-7). They are treated with institution of topical corticosteroids, tapering and discontinuation of topical NSAIDs, and close follow-up. Any infiltrate may be infectious and should be monitored and managed appropriately. If infectious keratitis is suspected, the cornea is typically scraped and cultured for suspected organisms.

Corneal Haze

The presentation of wound healing after surface ablation is important in determining postoperative topical corticosteroid management. Eyes that have haze and are undercorrected may benefit from increased corticosteroid use. After surface ablation, eyes with clear

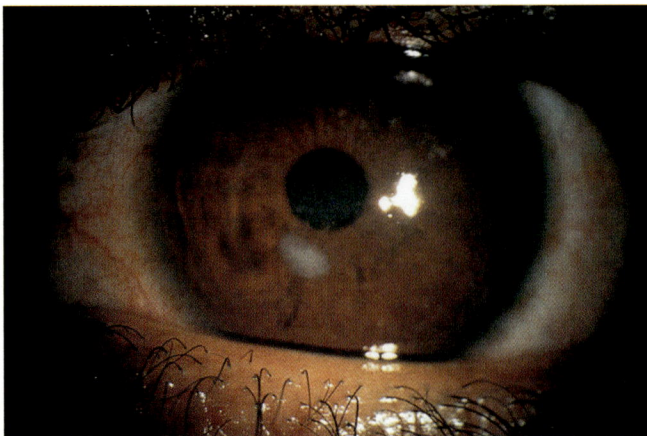

Figure 6-7 Stromal infiltrates after use of a bandage contact lens following photorefractive keratectomy. *(Courtesy of Jayne S. Weiss, MD.)*

corneas that are overcorrected may benefit from a reduction in topical corticosteroids, which may lead to regression of the overcorrection.

When present, subepithelial corneal haze typically appears several weeks after surface ablation, peaks in intensity at 1–2 months, and gradually diminishes or disappears over the following 6–12 months (Fig 6-8). *Late-onset corneal haze* may occur several months or even a year or more postoperatively after a period in which the patient had a relatively clear cornea. Histologic studies in animals with corneal haze after PRK demonstrate abnormal glycosaminoglycans and/or nonlamellar collagen deposited in the anterior stroma as a consequence of epithelial–stromal wound healing. Most histologic studies from animals and humans show an increase in the number and activity of stromal keratocytes, which suggests that increased keratocyte activity may be the source of the extracellular deposits.

Persistent severe haze is usually associated with greater amounts of correction or smaller ablation zones. Animal studies have demonstrated that ultraviolet B exposure after PRK prolongs the stromal healing process, with an increase in subepithelial haze. Clinical cases of haze after high ultraviolet exposure (such as at high altitude) corroborate these studies.

If clinically unacceptable haze persists, a superficial keratectomy or phototherapeutic keratectomy (PTK) may be performed. In addition, topical mitomycin C (0.02%), with PTK or debridement, may be used to prevent recurrence of subepithelial fibrosis. Because haze is known to resolve spontaneously with normal wound remodeling, re-ablation should be delayed for at least 6–12 months. The clinician should be aware that, in the presence of haze, refraction is often inaccurate, typically with an overestimation of the amount of myopia.

Ayres BD, Hammersmith KM, Laibson PR, Rapuano CJ. Phototherapeutic keratectomy with intraoperative mitomycin C to prevent recurrent anterior corneal pathology. *Am J Ophthalmol.* 2006;142:490–492.

Donnenfeld ED, O'Brien TP, Solomon R, Perry HD, Speaker MG, Wittpenn J. Infectious keratitis after photorefractive keratectomy. *Ophthalmology.* 2003;110(4):743–747.

Hofmeister EM, Bishop FM, Kaupp SE, Schallhorn SC. Randomized dose-response analysis of mitomycin-C to prevent haze after photorefractive keratectomy for high myopia. *J Cataract Refract Surg.* 2013;39(9):1358–1365.

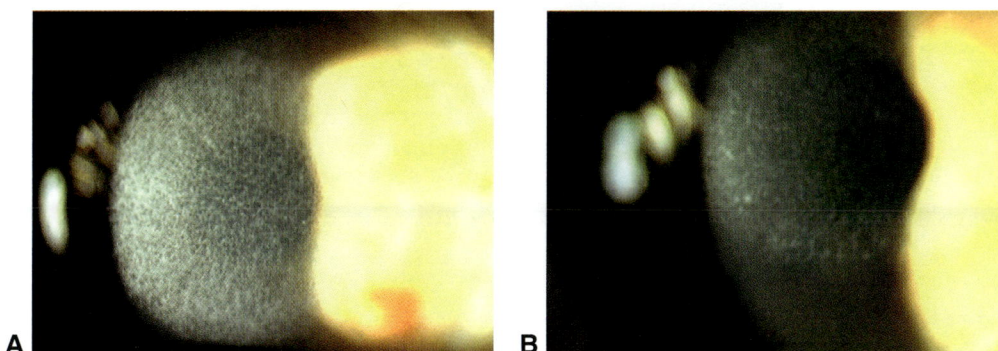

Figure 6-8 Corneal haze after photorefractive keratectomy (PRK). **A,** Severe haze 5 months after PRK. The reticular pattern is characteristic of PRK-induced haze. **B,** Haze has improved to a moderate level by 13 months postoperatively. *(Courtesy of Roger F. Steinert, MD.)*

Krueger RR, Saedy NF, McDonnell PJ. Clinical analysis of steep central islands after excimer laser photorefractive keratectomy. *Arch Ophthalmol.* 1996;114(4):377–381.

Moller-Pedersen T, Cavanagh HD, Petroll WM, Jester JV. Stromal wound healing explains refractive instability and haze development after photorefractive keratectomy: a 1-year confocal microscopic study. *Ophthalmology.* 2000;107(7):1235–1245.

Complications Unique to LASIK

The complications associated with LASIK are primarily related to flap creation, postoperative flap positioning, or interface problems.

Microkeratome Complications

In the past, the more severe complications associated with LASIK were related to problems with the manual microkeratome, which caused the planned LASIK procedure to be abandoned in an estimated 0.6%–1.6% of cases. In current practice, advances in microkeratome technology and the advent of femtosecond laser–created flaps have substantially reduced the incidence of severe, sight-threatening complications.

When a manual microkeratome is used, meticulous care must be taken in the cleaning and assembly of the instrument to ensure a smooth, uninterrupted keratectomy. Defects in the blade, poor suction, or uneven progression of the microkeratome across the cornea can produce an irregular, thin, or buttonhole flap (Fig 6-9), which can result in irregular astigmatism with loss of BCVA. Steep corneal curvature can result in a nonuniform fit of the keratome suction device, exposing additional corneal surface area to the cutting blade,

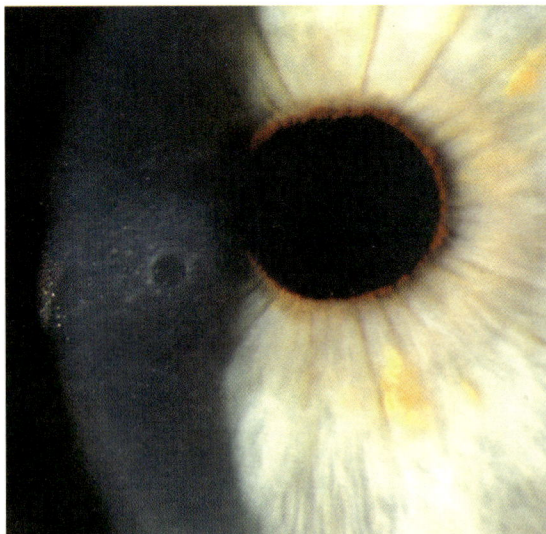

Figure 6-9 LASIK flap with buttonhole. *(Reproduced with permission from Feder RS, Rapuano CJ. The LASIK Handbook: A Case-Based Approach. Philadelphia: Lippincott Williams & Wilkins; 2007:95, fig 5.1. Image courtesy of Christopher J. Rapuano, MD.)*

leading to the risk of thin, irregular, or buttonhole flaps. If a thin or buttonhole flap is created, or if an incomplete flap does not provide a sufficiently large corneal stromal surface to perform the laser ablation, the flap should be replaced and the ablation should not be performed. Substantial loss of vision can be prevented if, under such circumstances, the ablation is not performed and the flap is allowed to heal before another refractive procedure is attempted, typically 3–6 months later. In such cases, a bandage contact lens is applied to stabilize the flap, typically for several days to a week. Although a new flap can usually be cut safely using a deeper cut after at least 3 months of healing, most surgeons prefer to use a surface ablation technique.

Occasionally, a free cap is created instead of a hinged flap (Fig 6-10). In these cases, if the stromal bed is large enough to accommodate the laser treatment, the corneal cap is placed in a moist chamber while the ablation is performed. It is important to replace the cap with the epithelial side up and to position it properly on a dried stromal bed, using the previously placed radial marks. A temporary 10-0 nylon suture can be placed to create an artificial hinge, but the physiologic dehydration of the stroma by the endothelial pump will generally keep the cap secured in proper position. A bandage contact lens can help protect the cap. A flat corneal curvature (<40.00 D) is a risk factor for creating a free cap because the flap diameter is often smaller than average in flat corneas.

Corneal perforation is a rare but devastating intraoperative complication that can occur if the microkeratome is not properly assembled or if the depth plate in an older-model microkeratome is not properly placed. It is imperative for the surgeon to double-check that the microkeratome has been properly assembled before beginning the procedure. Modern microkeratomes are constructed with a prefixed depth plate, which eliminates this source of error. Corneal perforation can also occur when LASIK is performed on an excessively thin cornea. Corneal thickness must be measured with pachymetry prior to the LASIK procedure, especially in patients who are undergoing re-treatment.

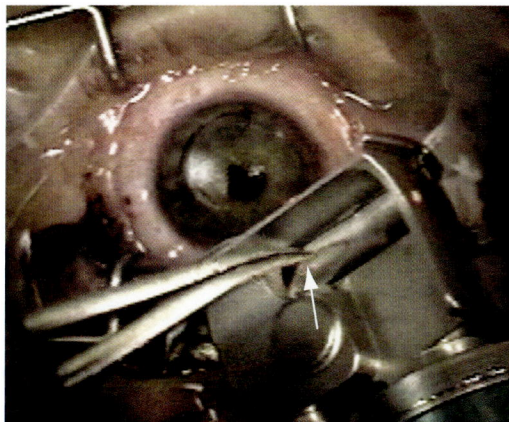

Figure 6-10 A free cap resulting from transection of the hinge. The cap is being lifted from the microkeratome with forceps *(arrow)*, and care is being taken to maintain the orientation of the epithelial external layer to prevent accidental inversion of the cap when it is replaced. *(Courtesy of Roger F. Steinert, MD.)*

Jacobs JM, Taravella MJ. Incidence of intraoperative flap complications in laser in situ keratomileusis. *J Cataract Refract Surg.* 2002;28(1):23–28.

Lee JK, Nkyekyer EW, Chuck RS. Microkeratome complications. *Curr Opin Ophthalmol.* 2009; 20(4):260–263.

Nakano K, Nakano E, Oliveira M, Portellinha W, Alvarenga L. Intraoperative microkeratome complications in 47,094 laser in situ keratomileusis surgeries. *J Refract Surg.* 2004;20 (Suppl 5):S723–726.

Epithelial Sloughing or Defects

The friction of microkeratome passage across the pressurized cornea may loosen a sheet of epithelium (termed *epithelial slough*) or cause a frank epithelial defect. Although patients with epithelial basement membrane dystrophy are at particular risk—in which case surface ablation rather than LASIK is advisable—other patients show no preoperative epithelial abnormalities. The risk of epithelial abnormality during LASIK correlates with older age. Also, in bilateral LASIK procedures with mechanical microkeratomes, the second eye has a greater likelihood of sustaining an epithelial defect (57%) if an intraoperative epithelial defect developed in the first eye. Techniques suggested to decrease the rate of epithelial defects include limiting medications to avoid toxicity, using chilled proparacaine, minimizing use of topical anesthetic, using nonpreserved drops until just before performing the skin prep or starting the procedure, having patients keep their eyes closed after topical anesthetic is administered, frequent use of corneal lubricating drops, meticulous microkeratome maintenance, and shutting off suction on the microkeratome reverse pass. The femtosecond laser is associated with a reduced incidence of epithelial defects because there is no microkeratome movement across the epithelium.

In cases of significant epithelial defects, a bandage contact lens is often applied immediately postoperatively and retained until stable reepithelialization occurs, with subsequent use of intensive lubricants and, occasionally, punctal occlusion. Persistent abnormal epithelium with recurrent erosions or loss of BCVA may require debridement and even superficial PTK using the technique employed for treatment of recurrent erosions (see BCSC Section 8, *External Disease and Cornea*). Epithelial defects are associated with an increased incidence of postoperative diffuse lamellar keratitis, infectious keratitis, flap striae, and epithelial ingrowth, and surgeons should watch closely for these conditions.

Chen S, Feng Y, Stojanovic A, Jankov MR II, Wang Q. IntraLase femtosecond laser vs mechanical microkeratomes in LASIK for myopia: a systematic review and meta-analysis. *J Refract Surg.* 2012;28(1):15–24.

Tekwani NH, Huang D. Risk factors for intraoperative epithelial defect in laser in-situ keratomileusis. *Am J Ophthalmol.* 2002;134(3):311–316.

Flap Striae

Flap folds, or striae, are a potential cause of decreased visual quality or acuity after LASIK. When present, most (56%) flap folds are noted on the first postoperative day, and 95% are noted within the first week. Risk factors for development of folds include excessive irrigation under the flap during LASIK, thin flaps, and deep ablations with mismatch of the flap to the new bed. Recognition of visually significant folds is important. Early intervention is often crucial in treating folds that cause loss of BCVA or visual distortion.

The first step in evaluating a patient with corneal folds is determining the BCVA. Folds are not treated if the BCVA and the subjective visual acuity are good. Folds are examined with a slit lamp using direct illumination, retroillumination, and fluorescein staining. Circumferential folds may be associated with high myopia and typically resolve with time. Folds that are parallel and emanate from the flap hinge grouped in the same direction indicate flap slippage, which requires prompt intervention. Corneal topography is usually not helpful in diagnosing folds.

Folds are often categorized as either macrostriae or microstriae, although there is significant overlap between these types (Table 6-1). *Macrostriae* represent full-thickness, undulating stromal folds. These folds invariably occur because of initial flap malposition or postoperative flap slippage (Fig 6-11A). Current approaches to smoothing the flap and avoiding striae at the end of the LASIK procedure vary widely. No matter which technique is used, however, the surgeon must carefully examine for the presence of striae once the flap is repositioned. The surgeon can apply momentary medical grade compressed air and instruct the patient to not overly squeeze the eyelids upon removal of the speculum. Coaxial and oblique illumination should be used at the operating microscope to examine for striae. Macrostriae may occur as patients attempt to squeeze their eyelids shut when the speculum and drape are removed. Accordingly, before removing the speculum, the surgeon should instruct the patient to actively suppress the otherwise natural reflex to squeeze the eyelids at this stage. Checking the patient in the early postoperative period is important to detect flap slippage. A protective plastic shield is often used for the first 24 hours to discourage the patient from touching the eyelids and inadvertently disrupting the flap.

Flap dislocation has been reported to occur in up to 1.4% of eyes. Careful examination will disclose a wider gutter on the side where the folds are most prominent. Flap slippage should be rectified as soon as it is recognized because the folds rapidly become fixed. Under the operating microscope or at the slit lamp, an eyelid speculum is placed, the flap is lifted and repositioned, copious irrigation with sterile balanced salt solution is used in the interface, and the flap is repeatedly stroked perpendicular to the fold until the striae resolve or improve. Using hypotonic saline or sterile distilled water as the interface-irrigating solution swells the flap and may initially reduce the striae, but swelling also reduces the flap diameter, which widens the gutter, delays flap adhesion because of prolonged endothelial dehydration time, and may worsen the striae after the flap dehydrates. If the macrostriae have been present for more than 24 hours, reactive epithelial hyperplasia in the valleys and hypoplasia over the elevations of the macrostriae tend to fix the folds into position. In such a case, in addition to refloating of the flap, the central 6 mm of the flap over the macrostriae may be de-epithelialized to remove this impediment to smoothing the wrinkles. A bandage contact lens should be used to stabilize the flap and to protect the surface until full reepithelialization occurs. In cases of intractable macrostriae, a tight 360° antitorque running suture or multiple interrupted sutures using 10-0 nylon may be placed and retained for several weeks, but irregular astigmatism may still be present after suture removal.

Table 6-1 Differentiation Between Macrostriae and Microstriae in LASIK Flaps

Characteristic		Macrostriae	Microstriae
Pathology		Large folds involving entire flap thickness	Fine folds, principally in Bowman layer
Cause		Flap slippage	Mismatch of flap to new bed; contracture of flap
Slit-lamp appearance	Direct illumination	Broad undulations as parallel or radial converging lines; widened flap gutter may be present	Fine folds, principally in Bowman layer; gutter usually symmetric
	Retroillumination	Same as above	Folds more obvious on retroillumination
	Fluorescein	Same as above, with negative staining pattern	Often has normal fluorescein pattern
Analogy		Wrinkles in skewed carpet	Dried, cracked mud
Topography		Possible disruption over striae	Color map may be normal or slightly disrupted; Placido disk mires show fine irregularity
Vision		Decreased BCVA and/or multiplopia if central	Subtle decreased BCVA or multiplopia if clinically significant; microstriae masked by epithelium are universal and asymptomatic
Treatment options	Acute	Refloat/reposition flap immediately	Observe; support surface with aggressive lubrication
	Established	Refloat, de-epithelialize over striae, hydrate and stroke, apply traction, or suture	If visually significant, refloat; try hydration, stroking, suturing
		Phototherapeutic keratectomy	Phototherapeutic keratectomy

BCVA = best-corrected visual acuity; LASIK = laser in situ keratomileusis.

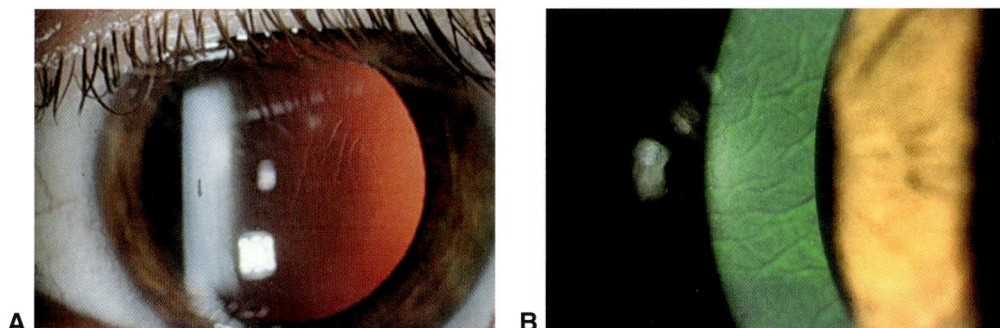

Figure 6-11 Post-LASIK striae. **A,** Retroillumination of multiple horizontal parallel macrostriae in the visual axis from mild flap dislocation. **B,** Numerous randomly directed microstriae on fluorescein staining. These striae resemble dried, cracked mud, are apparent on the first postoperative day after LASIK, and usually resolve without intervention. *(Part A courtesy of Parag Majmudar, MD; part B courtesy of Steven C. Schallhorn, MD.)*

Microstriae are fine, hairlike optical irregularities that are best viewed on red reflex illumination or by light reflected off the iris (Fig 6-11). They are very small folds in the Bowman layer, and this anterior location accounts for the disruption of BCVA in some eyes. Computer topographic color maps do not usually show these subtle irregularities. However, disruption of the surface contour may result in irregularity of the Placido disk image. In addition, application of dilute fluorescein often reveals so-called *negative staining,* in which the elevated striae disrupt the tear film and fluorescence is lost over them.

If optically significant microstriae persist, the flap may be sutured in an attempt to reduce the striae by means of tension. As with macrostriae, however, suturing has the potential to induce new irregular astigmatism. An alternative procedure is PTK. Pulses from a broad-beam laser, set to a maximal diameter of 6.5 mm, are initially applied to penetrate the epithelium in about 200 pulses. The epithelium acts as a masking agent, exposing the elevated striae before the valleys between the striae. After the transepithelial ablation, additional pulses are applied, and a thin film of medium-viscosity artificial tears is administered every 5–10 pulses, up to a maximum of 100 additional pulses. If these suggestions are followed, little to no haze results, and an average hyperopic shift of less than +1.00 D occurs as a result of the minimal tissue removal.

Ashrafzadeh A, Steinert RF. Results of phototherapeutic keratectomy in the management of flap striae after LASIK before and after developing a standardized protocol: long-term follow-up of an expanded patient population. *Ophthalmology.* 2007;114(6):1118–1123.

Jackson DW, Hamill MB, Koch DD. Laser in situ keratomileusis flap suturing to treat recalcitrant flap striae. *J Cataract Refract Surg.* 2003;29(2):264–269.

Traumatic Flap Dislocation

Flap dislocation has been reported to occur in up to 1.4% of eyes. Dislocation of the LASIK flap is not uncommon on the first postoperative day, when dryness and adhesion of the flap to the upper tarsal conjunctiva are sufficient to cause the flap to slip. After the first day, however, the reepithelialization of the gutter begins the process of increasing flap stability. Within several weeks, keratocytes begin to lay down new collagen at the cut edge of the Bowman layer, and eventually a fine scar is established at the edge of the flap. However, minimal healing occurs across the stromal interface. Late dislocation from blunt trauma has been reported many years after LASIK. This can occur if the shearing force exceeds the strength of the peripheral Bowman layer–level healing. Flap dislocation requires urgent treatment to replace the flap in its proper anatomical position. The surgeon should make sure that there is no epithelium on the underside of the flap or in the interface, a situation that significantly increases the chances of epithelial ingrowth.

LASIK-Interface Complications

Diffuse lamellar keratitis

The presentation of diffuse lamellar keratitis (DLK) (Fig 6-12) can range from asymptomatic interface haze near the edge of the flap to marked diffuse haze under the center of the flap with decreased BCVA. The condition represents a nonspecific sterile inflammatory response to a variety of mechanical and toxic insults. The interface under the flap is a potential space; any cause of anterior stromal inflammation may trigger the accumulation of white blood cells therein. DLK has been reported in association with epithelial defects that occur during primary LASIK or during enhancement, or even months after

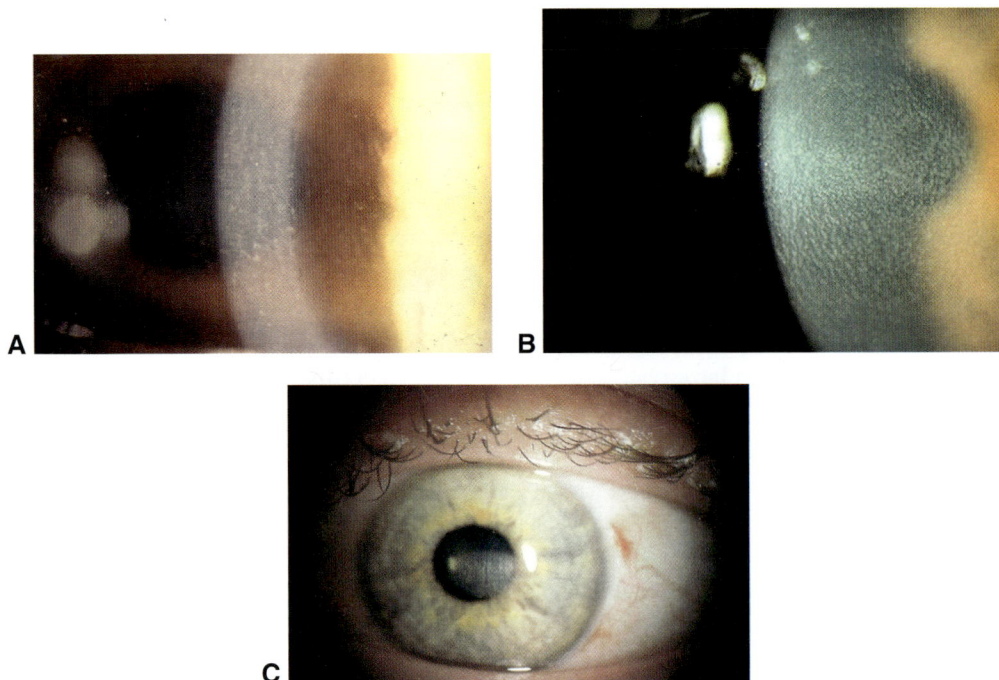

Figure 6-12 Diffuse lamellar keratitis (DLK). **A,** High magnification image of stage 2 DLK. Note accumulation of inflammatory cells in the fine ridges created by the oscillating microkeratome blade. **B,** Stage 3 DLK showing dense accumulation of inflammatory cells centrally. **C,** Stage 4 DLK with central scar and folds. *(Parts A and B courtesy of Roger F. Steinert, MD; part C courtesy of Jayne S. Weiss, MD.)*

Table 6-2 Staging of Diffuse Lamellar Keratitis

Stage	Findings
1	Peripheral faint white blood cells; granular appearance
2	Central scattered white blood cells; granular appearance
3	Central dense white blood cells in visual axis
4	Permanent scarring or stromal melting

the LASIK procedure from corneal abrasions or infectious keratitis. Other reported inciting factors include foreign material on the surface of the microkeratome blade or motor, trapped meibomian gland secretions, povidone-iodine solution (from the preoperative skin preparation), marking ink, substances produced by laser ablation, contamination of the sterilizer with gram-negative endotoxin, and red blood cells in the interface. The inflammation generally resolves with topical corticosteroid treatment alone without sequelae, but severe cases can lead to scarring or flap melting; therefore, early detection and management is important.

DLK is typically classified by the stages described in Table 6-2. Although stages 1 and 2 usually respond to frequent topical corticosteroid application, stages 3 and 4 usually require lifting the flap and irrigating, followed by intensive topical corticosteroid treatment. Oral corticosteroids may be used adjunctively in severe cases. Some surgeons use topical and systemic corticosteroids in stage 3 DLK instead of, or in addition to, lifting the flap. Recovery of vision in DLK is usually excellent if the condition is detected and treated promptly.

A surgeon should have a low threshold for lifting or irrigating underneath the flap in suspected cases of severe DLK. Lifting the flap allows removal of inflammatory mediators from the interface and direct placement of corticosteroids and NSAIDs to suppress inflammation and necrosis. If there is any suspicion that the inflammation is due to infection, lifting the flap and obtaining samples for corneal cultures of the interface should be considered. Topical antibiotics can also be placed in the flap interface at the same time. In cases of suspected DLK not responsive to corticosteroids within 7–10 days of initiation, the diagnosis should be reconsidered, as infectious keratitis or pressure-induced stromal keratopathy (PISK, discussed later) can mimic DLK and require corticosteroid cessation.

Haft P, Yoo SH, Kymionis GD, Ide T, O'Brien TP, Culbertson WW. Complications of LASIK flaps made by the IntraLase 15- and 30-kHz femtosecond lasers. *J Refract Surg.* 2009; 25(11):979–984.

Holland SP, Mathias RG, Morck DW, Chiu J, Slade SG. Diffuse lamellar keratitis related to endotoxins released from sterilizer reservoir biofilms. *Ophthalmology.* 2000;107(7): 1227–1233.

Randleman JB, Shah RD. LASIK interface complications: etiology, management, and outcomes. *J Refract Surg.* 2012;28(8):575–586.

LASIK infectious keratitis

It is important to differentiate sterile interface inflammation from potentially devastating infectious inflammation. Increased pain and decreased vision are the primary indicators of infection. However, postoperative discomfort is common, so it is difficult for patients to distinguish between normal and abnormal eye pain. Moreover, because corneal nerves are severed during flap creation, corneal sensation may be reduced, along with the subjective symptom of pain that usually accompanies infection. Infection after LASIK is usually associated with redness, photophobia, and decreased vision. Several distinct features can help distinguish between DLK and infectious keratitis (Table 6-3). DLK is usually visible with slit lamp biomicroscopy within 24 hours of surgery and typically begins at the periphery of the flap. There is usually a gradient of inflammation, with the inflammation being most intense at the periphery and diminishing toward the center of the cornea. In general, the inflammatory reaction in DLK is diffusely distributed but localized and confined to the area of the flap interface; it does not extend far beyond the edge of the flap (Fig 6-13). In contrast, post-LASIK infectious keratitis usually begins 2 or 3 days after surgery and involves a more focal inflammatory reaction that is not confined to the lamellar interface. An anterior chamber reaction may further help differentiate between an infectious and a sterile process. The inflammatory reaction can extend up into the flap, deeper into the stromal bed, and even beyond the confines of the flap.

Infection within the interface can lead to flap melting, severe irregular astigmatism, and corneal scarring that may require corneal transplantation. If infection is suspected, the flap should be lifted and the interface cultured and irrigated with antibiotics. The most common infections are from gram-positive organisms, followed in frequency by those

Table 6-3 Diffuse Lamellar Keratitis vs Infectious Keratitis After LASIK

Diffuse Lamellar Keratitis	Infectious Keratitis
Usually visible within first 24 hours	Usual onset at least 2–3 days postoperatively
Typically begins at flap periphery	Can occur anywhere under flap
More intense inflammation at periphery decreasing toward center	
Inflammation primarily confined to interface	Inflammation extends above and below interface, and beyond flap edge
Diffuse inflammation	Focal inflammation around infection
Minimal to no anterior chamber reaction	Mild to moderate anterior chamber reaction
Flap melts can occur	Flap melts can occur

Modified with permission from Culbertson WW. Surface ablation and LASIK patients share similar infection potential. *Refractive Eyecare.* September 2006:12.

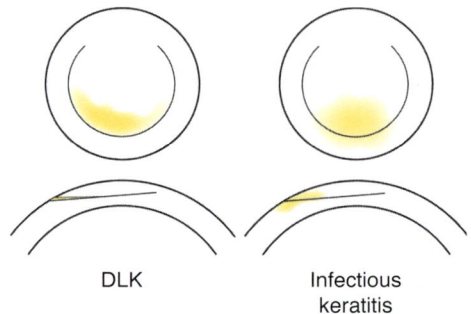

Figure 6-13 DLK is differentiated from infectious keratitis by the confinement of the infiltrate to the interface alone in DLK. *(Reproduced with permission from Culbertson WW. Surface ablation and LASIK patients share similar infection potential. Refractive Eyecare. September 2006:12.)*

caused by atypical mycobacteria. Mycobacterial infection can be diagnosed more rapidly by using acid-fast and fluorochrome stains rather than by waiting for culture results (see Fig 6-5).

In general, the timing of the onset of symptoms provides a clue as to the etiology of the infection. Infections occurring within 10 days of surgery are typically bacterial, with the preponderance being from gram-positive organisms (see BCSC Section 8, *External Disease and Cornea*). If the infection does not respond to treatment, amputation of the flap may be necessary to improve antimicrobial penetration. The fourth-generation fluoroquinolones gatifloxacin and moxifloxacin have excellent efficacy against the more common bacteria that cause post-LASIK infections, including some atypical mycobacteria; however, monotherapy with these drugs may not be sufficient. A LASIK flap infection may occur after a recurrent erosion (see Fig 6-6).

Freitas D, Alvarenga L, Sampaio J, et al. An outbreak of *Mycobacterium chelonae* infection after LASIK. *Ophthalmology.* 2003;110(2):276–285.

Llovet F, de Rojas V, Interlandi E, Martín C, Cobo-Soriano R, Ortega-Usobiaga J, Baviera J. Infectious keratitis in 204,586 LASIK procedures. *Ophthalmology.* 2010;117(2):232–238.

Moshirfar M, Welling JD, Feiz V, Holz H, Clinch TE. Infectious and noninfectious keratitis after laser in situ keratomileusis: occurrence, management, and visual outcomes. *J Cataract Refract Surg.* 2007;33(3):474–483.

Pressure-induced stromal keratopathy

A diffuse stromal and interface opacity termed *pressure-induced stromal keratopathy (PISK)* has been reported as a result of elevated IOP; it can be mistaken for DLK and is sometimes associated with a visible fluid cleft in the interface (Fig 6-14). The surgeon must be aware of this rare condition in order to properly diagnose and treat it. The pressure-induced haze from PISK is associated with prolonged corticosteroid treatment and usually presents after 10 days to 2 weeks. Key differentiators between DLK and PISK are that with DLK, the onset is earlier and the IOP is not elevated. IOP should be measured both centrally and peripherally in suspected cases, possibly with a pneumotonometer or Tono-Pen (Reichert Technologies, Depew, NY), because applanation pressure may be falsely lowered centrally in PISK by fluid accumulation in the lamellar interface. Several alternative techniques of measuring IOP have been suggested, but dynamic contour tonometry is the only technique shown to have sufficient reproducible accuracy in eyes that have undergone refractive ablation. Treatment of PISK involves rapid cessation of corticosteroid drops and the use of glaucoma medications to lower IOP. Severe glaucomatous vision loss has been reported in cases with delayed diagnosis.

Belin MW, Hannush SB, Yau CW, Schultze RL. Elevated intraocular pressure–induced interlamellar stromal keratitis. *Ophthalmology.* 2002;109(10):1929–1933.

Dawson DG, Schmack I, Holley GP, Waring GO III, Grossniklaus HE, Edelhauser HF. Interface fluid syndrome in human eye bank corneas after LASIK: causes and pathogenesis. *Ophthalmology.* 2007;114(10):1848–1859.

Hamilton DR, Manche EE, Rich LF, Maloney RK. Steroid-induced glaucoma after laser in situ keratomileusis associated with interface fluid. *Ophthalmology.* 2002;109(4):659–665.

Moya Calleja T, Iribarne Ferrer Y, Sanz Jorge A, Sedó Fernandez S. Steroid-induced interface fluid syndrome after LASIK. *J Refract Surg.* 2009;25(2):235–239.

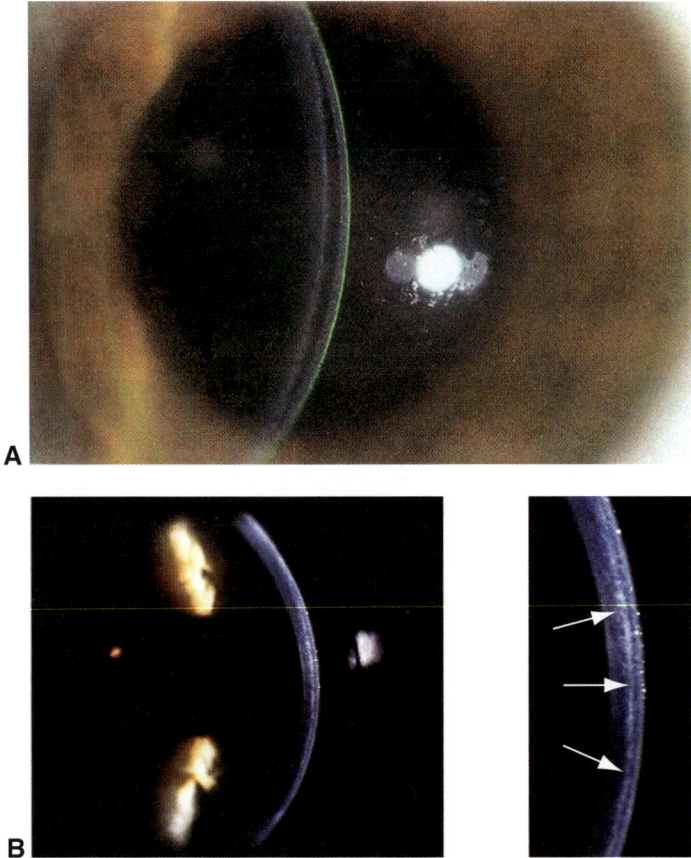

Figure 6-14 Pressure-induced stromal keratopathy (PISK) after LASIK. **A,** An optically clear, fluid-filled space between the flap and stromal bed. This condition is hypothesized to be caused by transudation of fluid across the endothelium as a result of corticosteroid-induced elevation of intraocular pressure (IOP). **B,** PISK without interface gap. A diffuse stromal and interface opacity without an interface fluid cleft can also result from elevated IOP with prolonged corticosteroid use *(left panel)*. Close-up *(right panel, arrows)* further demonstrates the opacification of the stroma and interface. *(Part A reproduced with permission from Hamilton DR, Manche EE, Rich LF, Maloney RK. Steroid-induced glaucoma after laser in situ keratomileusis associated with interface fluid. Ophthalmology. 2002;109(4):659–665; part B reprinted with permission from Randleman JB, Shah RD. Lasik interface complications: etiology, management, and outcomes. J Refract Surg. 2012;28(8):575–586.)*

Epithelial ingrowth

Epithelial ingrowth occurs in less than 3% of eyes (Fig 6-15). There is no need to treat isolated nests of epithelial cells in the peripheral lamellar interface that are not advancing and are not affecting vision. However, if the epithelium is advancing toward the visual axis, is associated with decreased vision from irregular astigmatism (Fig 6-16), or triggers overlying flap melting, it should be removed by lifting the flap, scraping the epithelium from both the underside of the flap and the stromal bed, and then repositioning the flap. After scraping the under-flap surface and stromal bed, some surgeons also remove epithelium

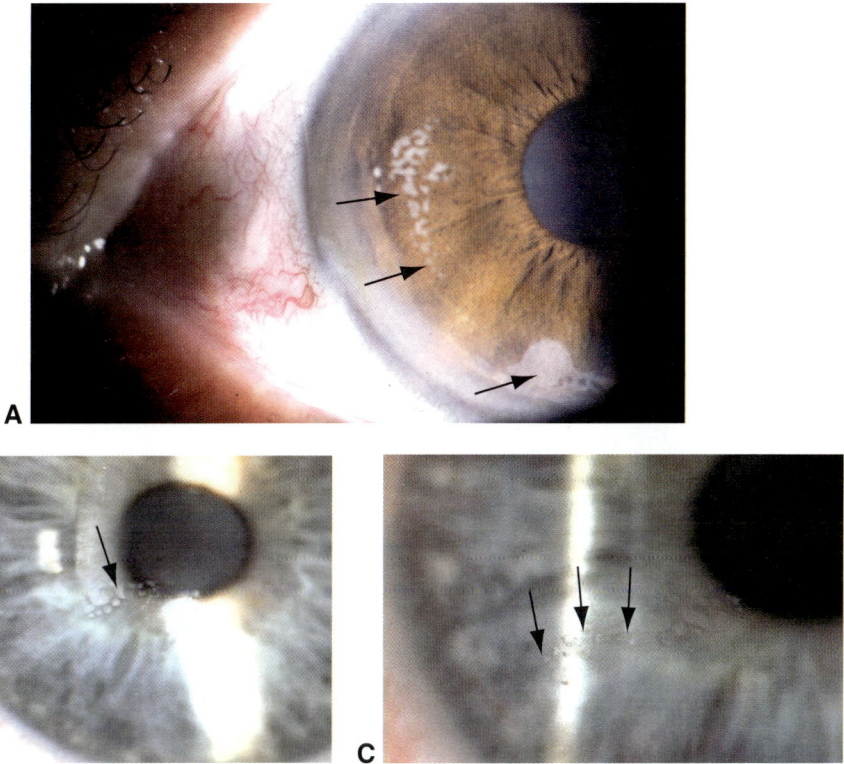

Figure 6-15 Epithelial ingrowth in the interface under a LASIK flap. **A,** Peripheral ingrowth of 1–2 mm *(arrows)* is common and inconsequential and does not require intervention unless it induces melting of the overlying flap. **B,** Central nests of epithelial cells *(arrow)* disrupt the patient's vision by elevating and distorting the flap. The flap must be lifted and the epithelium debrided. **C,** Inspection of the midperiphery shows the track followed by the invading epithelium from the periphery toward the center *(arrows). (Courtesy of Roger F. Steinert, MD.)*

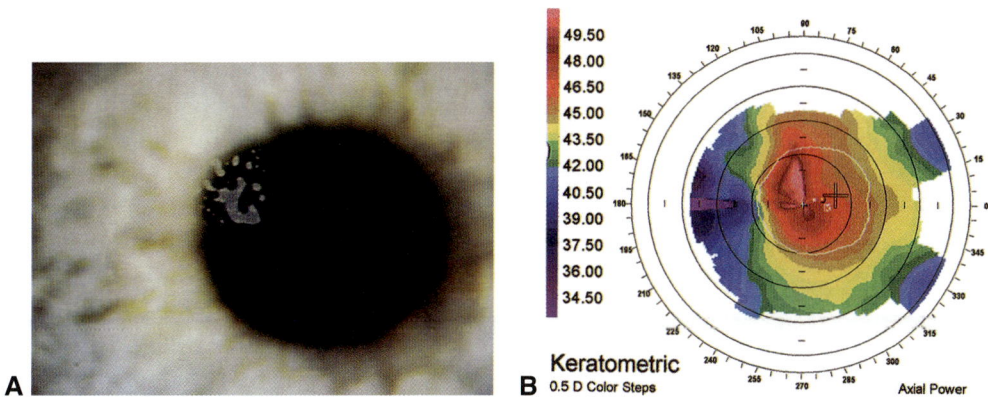

Figure 6-16 **A,** Epithelial ingrowth in visual axis. **B,** Corresponding topographic steepening and irregularity. *(Courtesy of J. Bradley Randleman, MD.)*

from both the periphery of the flap and the bed to allow for flap adherence before the epithelial edge advances to the flap edge. Recurrent epithelial ingrowth can be treated with repeated lifting and scraping, with or without flap suturing or using fibrin glue at the flap edge. Some surgeons treat the undersurface of the flap with absolute alcohol to identify and treat any residual epithelium. Nd:YAG laser has also been described to treat early epithelial ingrowth.

The incidence of epithelial ingrowth is greater in eyes that develop an epithelial defect at the time of the procedure, undergo a re-treatment with lifting of a preexisting flap, or have traumatic flap dehiscence. In such cases, special care should be taken to ensure that no epithelium is caught under the edge of the flap when it is repositioned. Placement of a bandage contact lens at the conclusion of the procedure may also decrease the incidence of epithelial ingrowth for patients at higher risk of developing this complication.

Ayala MJ, Alió JL, Mulet ME, De La Hoz F. Treatment of laser in situ keratomileusis interface epithelial ingrowth with neodymium:yytrium-aluminum-garnet laser. *Am J Ophthalmol.* 2008;145(4):630–634.

Caster AI, Friess DW, Schwendeman FJ. Incidence of epithelial ingrowth in primary and retreatment laser in situ keratomileusis. *J Cataract Refract Surg.* 2010;36(1):97–101.

Henry CR, Canto AP, Galor A, Vaddavalli PK, Culbertson WW, Yoo SH. Epithelial ingrowth after LASIK: clinical characteristics, risk factors, and visual outcomes in patients requiring flap lift. *J Refract Surg.* 2012;28(7):488–492.

Rapuano CJ. Management of epithelial ingrowth after laser in situ keratomileusis in a tertiary care cornea service. *Cornea.* 2010;29(3):307–313.

Interface debris

Debris in the interface is occasionally observed postoperatively. The principal indication for intervention by flap lifting, irrigation, and manual removal of debris is an inflammatory reaction elicited by the foreign material. Small amounts of lint, nondescript particles, or tiny metal particles from stainless steel surgical instruments are usually well tolerated. A small amount of blood that may have oozed into the interface from transected peripheral vessels may also be tolerated and typically resolves spontaneously with time; however, a significant amount of blood usually elicits an inflammatory cell response and should be irrigated from the interface at the time of the LASIK procedure (Fig 6-17). Use of a topical vasoconstrictor such as epinephrine applied with a fiber-free sponge to facilitate constriction when the flap is being replaced helps minimize this problem. The surgeon should be aware that applying epinephrine prior to laser ablation can result in pupillary dilation, difficulty for the patient to fixate on a fixation light, and thus treatment decentration.

Complications Related to Femtosecond Laser LASIK Flaps

Opaque bubble layer and possible sequelae

One of the most common adverse effects of the intrastromal photo-disruption procedure is the generation of opaque bubble layer (OBL). This bubble layer, created as a result of tissue disruption by the femtosecond laser, is composed of carbon dioxide and water. Laser tracking systems can be significantly impaired by the OBL. Time and/or mechanical

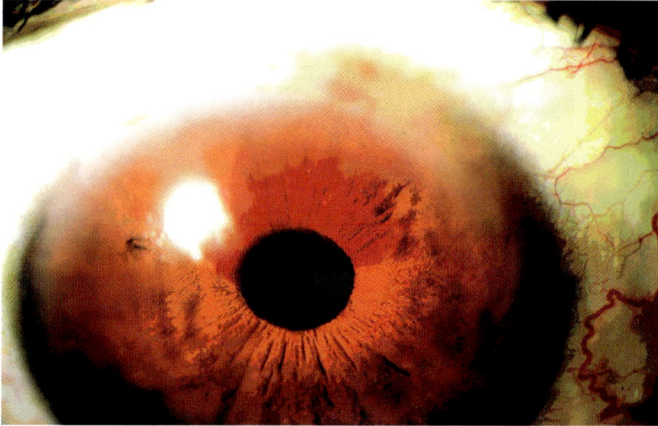

Figure 6-17 Blood in the LASIK interface. *(Courtesy of Jayne S. Weiss, MD.)*

massage will allow for OBL to dissipate. Newer-generation femtosecond lasers with higher repetition rates tend to create fewer OBLs.

Epithelial gas breakthrough is a rare but serious complication of OBL production. Similar to a buttonhole from a mechanical keratome, the breakthrough should be allowed to heal and stabilize generally for at least 3 months, at which time surface ablation may be considered.

In rare cases, the gas liberated from the plasma cavitations can travel into the anterior chamber, potentially interfering with the laser tracking systems. If this occurs, the surgeon can allow a few hours for the bubbles to resolve. In addition, instillation of a mydriatic drop may allow the pupil to begin to dilate around the bubbles, which can allow laser recognition and capture.

Kaiserman I, Maresky HS, Bahar I, Rootman DS. Incidence, possible risk factors, and potential effects of an opaque bubble layer created by a femtosecond laser. *J Cataract Refract Surg.* 2008;34(3):417–423.

Transient light sensitivity

Several weeks to months after LASIK with femtosecond laser flaps, some patients experience acute onset of pain and light sensitivity in an otherwise white and quiet eye with excellent uncorrected visual acuity (UCVA; also called *uncorrected distance visual acuity, UDVA*). The cornea and flap interface appear normal. It has been speculated that an acute onset of ocular inflammation or dry eyes is somehow related to use of the femtosecond laser. Treatment consists of frequent administration of topical corticosteroids (eg, prednisolone acetate, 1%, every 2 hours) and topical cyclosporine A, titrated to the clinical condition. Almost all cases respond to treatment and resolve in weeks to months.

Rainbow glare

Rainbow glare, an optical adverse effect of treatment with the femtosecond laser, is described as bands of color around white lights at night. This complication seems to be related to higher raster energy levels and increased length of time between service calls for the laser.

Farjo AA, Sugar A, Schallhorn SC, et al. Femtosecond lasers for LASIK flap creation: a report by the American Academy of Ophthalmology. *Ophthalmology.* 2013;120(3):e5–e20.

Krueger RR, Thornton IL, Xu M, Bor Z, van den Berg TJ. Rainbow glare as an optical side effect of IntraLASIK. *Ophthalmology.* 2008;115(7):1187–1195.

Ectasia

Corneal ectasia develops after excimer laser ablation when the corneal biomechanical integrity is reduced beyond its functional threshold; this complication results from performing surgery in patients who either are otherwise predisposed to developing corneal ectatic disorders or have a significantly reduced postablation residual stromal bed (RSB). The importance of an adequate RSB to prevent structural instability and postoperative corneal ectasia is discussed in Chapter 2. Ectasia has been reported far more frequently after LASIK than after surface ablation. Cumulative analysis of more than 200 eyes with postoperative ectasia found that ectasia is usually associated with LASIK performed in patients with preoperative topographic abnormalities. Other risk factors include younger patient age, thinner corneas, higher myopic corrections, and patients who have undergone several laser ablations. However, cases of ectasia without any demonstrable factors have also been reported.

For postoperative ectasia, corneal crosslinking (CCL) is becoming the first-line treatment worldwide. In 2016 its use was approved by the US Food and Drug Administration. Often, functional visual acuity can be restored with rigid gas-permeable or hybrid contact lens wear. The implantation of symmetric or asymmetric intrastromal ring segments to reduce the irregular astigmatism has been successful in select cases. In extreme cases, corneal transplantation may be required.

In 2005, a joint statement was issued by the American Academy of Ophthalmology, the International Society for Refractive Surgery, and the American Society of Cataract and Refractive Surgery summarizing current knowledge of corneal ectatic disorders and ectasia after LASIK. Their 8 conclusions at the time were

1. No specific test or measurement is diagnostic of a corneal ectatic disorder.
2. A decision to perform LASIK should take into account the entire clinical picture, not just the corneal topography.
3. Although some risk factors have been suggested for ectasia after LASIK, none is an absolute predictor of its occurrence.
4. Because keratoconus may develop in the absence of refractive surgery, the occurrence of ectasia after LASIK does not necessarily mean that LASIK was a causative or contributing factor for its development.
5. Risk factors for ectasia after LASIK may not also predict ectasia after surface ablation.
6. Ectasia is a known risk of laser vision correction.
7. Forme fruste keratoconus is a topographic diagnosis rather than a clinical one. It is not a variant of keratoconus. Rather, forme fruste implies subclinical disease with the potential for progression to clinically evident keratoconus.

8. Although to date no formal guidelines exist and good scientific data for future guidelines are presently lacking, in order to reduce some of the risks of ectasia after LASIK, the groups recommended that surgeons review topographic findings prior to surgery. Intraoperative pachymetry should be used to measure flap thickness and calculate the RSB after ablation to ascertain if the RSB is near the safe lower limits for the procedure, for that patient.

Current screening strategies that include a combination of these risk factors in a weighted fashion have been found to improve screening sensitivity and specificity. In addition, see the Preferred Practice Pattern on corneal ectasia published by the American Academy of Ophthalmology.

American Academy of Ophthalmology Cornea/External Disease Panel. Preferred Practice Pattern Guidelines. *Corneal Ectasia.* San Francisco, CA: American Academy of Ophthalmology; 2013. Available at www.aao.org/ppp.

Ambrósio R Jr, Randleman JB. Screening for ectasia risk: what are we screening for and how should we screen for it? *J Refract Surg.* 2013:29(4):230–232.

Binder PS, Lindstrom RL, Stulting RD, et al. Keratoconus and corneal ectasia after LASIK. *J Cataract Refract Surg.* 2005;31(11):2035–2038.

Ou RJ, Shaw EL, Glasgow BJ. Keratectasia after laser in situ keratomileusis (LASIK): evaluation of the calculated residual stromal bed thickness. *Am J Ophthalmol.* 2002;134(5): 771–773.

Randleman JB, Woodward M, Lynn MJ, Stulting RD. Risk assessment of ectasia after corneal refractive surgery. *Ophthalmology.* 2008;115(1):37–50.

Richoz O, Mavrakanas N, Pajic B, Hafezi F. Corneal collagen cross-linking for ectasia after LASIK and photorefractive keratectomy: long-term results. *Ophthalmology.* 2013;120(7): 1354–1359.

Rare Complications

Rare, sometimes coincidental, complications of LASIK include optic nerve ischemia, premacular subhyaloid hemorrhage, macular hemorrhage associated with preexisting lacquer cracks or choroidal neovascularization, choroidal infarcts, postoperative corneal edema associated with preoperative cornea guttata, and ring scotoma. Diplopia is another rare complication that may occur in patients whose refractive error has been corrected and who have iatrogenic monovision, improper control of accommodation (in patients with strabismus), or decompensated phorias.

Gimbel HV, Penno EE, van Westenbrugge JA, Ferensowicz M, Furlong MT. Incidence and management of intraoperative and early postoperative complications in 1000 consecutive laser in situ keratomileusis cases. *Ophthalmology.* 1998;105(10):1839–1848.

Gunton KB, Armstrong B. Diplopia in adult patients following cataract extraction and refractive surgery. *Curr Opin Ophthalmol.* 2010;21(5):341–344.

Moshirfar M, Feiz V, Feilmeier MR, Kang PC. Laser in situ keratomileusis in patients with corneal guttata and family history of Fuchs' endothelial dystrophy. *J Cataract Refract Surg.* 2005;31(12):2281–2296.

Netto MV, Dupps W Jr, Wilson SE. Wavefront-guided ablation: evidence for efficacy compared to traditional ablation. *Am J Ophthalmol.* 2006;141(2):360–368.

Stulting RD, Carr JD, Thompson KP, Waring GO III, Wiley WM, Walker JG. Complications of laser in situ keratomileusis for the correction of myopia. *Ophthalmology.* 1999;106(1): 13–20.

Sugar A, Rapuano CJ, Culbertson WW, et al. Laser in situ keratomileusis for myopia and astigmatism: safety and efficacy: a report by the American Academy of Ophthalmology. *Ophthalmology.* 2002;109(1):175–187.

CHAPTER 7

Collagen Shrinkage and Crosslinking Procedures

Keratorefractive surgical procedures aim to alter the refractive power of the cornea by changing its shape. Various methods are used to alter corneal curvature, including incising or removing corneal tissue or implanting artificial material into the cornea. Procedures that change the character of the corneal collagen have also been developed. This chapter focuses on 2 such procedures: corneal collagen shrinkage and corneal crosslinking (CLL).

Collagen Shrinkage

The idea of using heat to alter the shape of the cornea was first proposed by Lans, a Dutch medical student, in 1898. When Lans used electrocautery to heat the corneal stroma, he noticed astigmatic changes in the cornea. In 1975, Gasset and Kaufman proposed a modified technique known as *thermokeratoplasty* to treat keratoconus. In 1984, Fyodorov introduced a technique of radial thermokeratoplasty that used a handheld, heated Nichrome inoculating needle designed for deeper thermokeratoplasty. The handheld probe contained a retractable 34-gauge wire heated to 600°C. For a duration of 0.3 second, a motor advanced the wire to a preset depth of 95% of the corneal thickness. Fyodorov used different patterns to treat hyperopia and astigmatism. However, excessive heating of the cornea resulted in necrosis, scarring, and variable corneal remodeling; regression and unpredictability of treatment limited the success of this technique. It is now known that the optimal temperature for avoiding stromal necrosis while still obtaining corneal collagen shrinkage is approximately 58°–76°C.

Neumann AC, Fyodorov S, Sanders DR. Radial thermokeratoplasty for the correction of hyperopia. *Refract Corneal Surg.* 1990;6(6):404–412.

Laser Thermokeratoplasty

In the 1990s, numerous lasers were tested for use in laser thermokeratoplasty (LTK) but only the holmium:yttrium-aluminum-garnet (Ho:YAG) laser reached commercial production. The Ho:YAG laser produces light in the infrared region at a wavelength of 2100 nm and has corneal tissue penetration to approximately 480–530 μm. A noncontact system slit-lamp delivery system was used to apply 8 simultaneous spots at a frequency of 5 Hz and a pulse duration of 250 μsec. The system was approved for the temporary correction of 0.75–2.50 D of hyperopia with less than 1.00 D of astigmatism. Interest in LTK waned, primarily because of the significant refractive regression that frequently occurred. Few LTK units remain in clinical use.

Conductive Keratoplasty

In 2004, conductive keratoplasty (CK) received US Food and Drug Administration (FDA) approval for treatment of presbyopia in the nondominant eye of a patient with an endpoint of –1.00 to –2.00 D. The nonablative, collagen-shrinking effect of CK is based on the delivery of radiofrequency energy through a fine conducting tip that is inserted into the peripheral corneal stroma (Fig 7-1). As the current flows through the tissue surrounding the tip, resistance to the current creates localized heat. Collagen lamellae in the area surrounding the tip shrink in a controlled fashion and form a column of denatured collagen. The shortening of the collagen fibrils creates a band of tightening and flattening in the periphery that increases the relative curvature of the central cornea.

For the treatment of hyperopia, the surgeon inserts the tip into the stroma in a ring pattern around the peripheral cornea. The number and location of spots determine the amount of refractive change, with an increasing number of spots and rings used for higher amounts of hyperopia. The CK procedure is performed using topical anesthesia and typically takes less than 5 minutes. The collagen shrinkage leads to visible striae between the treated spots, which fade with time (Fig 7-2). The treatment is not advised for use in patients who have undergone radial keratotomy, and it is not FDA approved for such use.

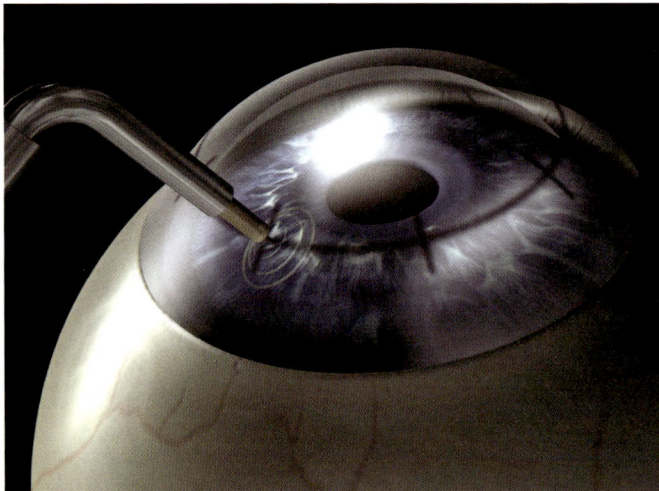

Figure 7-1 Schematic representation of an eye undergoing conductive keratoplasty, which delivers radiofrequency energy to the cornea through a handheld probe inserted into the peripheral cornea. *(Courtesy of Refractec, Inc.)*

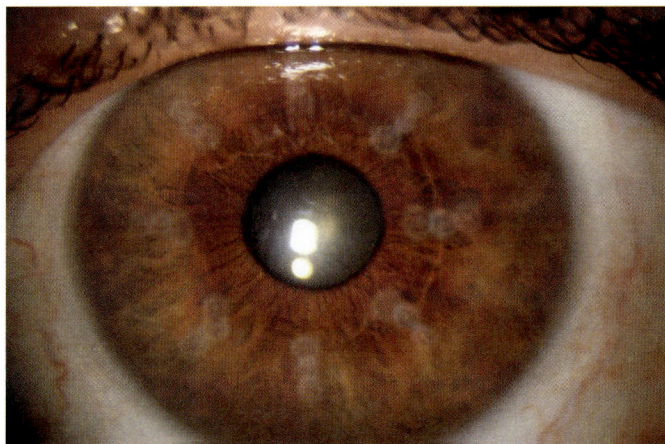

Figure 7-2 One month after a 24-spot conductive keratoplasty treatment in a patient with +2.00 D hyperopia, the spots are beginning to fade. Three sets of 8 spots each were applied at a 6.0-, 7.0-, and 8.0-mm optical zones. *(Courtesy of Refractec, Inc.)*

Despite initial reports of refractive stability, long-term follow-up has revealed regression and/or lack of adequate effect with CK. In a long-term (mean, 73.1 months; range, 44–90 months) follow-up of patients enrolled in the phase 3 multicenter trial of CK, Ehrlich and Manche found nearly complete regression of treatment effect in the 16 eyes (of the original 25 eyes) available for follow-up.

Ehrlich JS, Manche EE. Regression of effect over long-term follow-up of conductive keratoplasty to correct mild to moderate hyperopia. *J Cataract Refract Surg.* 2009;35(9):1591–1596.

Kymionis GD, Kontadakis GA, Naoumidi TL, Kazakos DC, Giapitzakis I, Pallikaris IG. Conductive keratoplasty followed by collagen cross-linking with riboflavin-UV-A in patients with keratoconus. *Cornea.* 2010;29(2):239–243.

McDonald MB. Conductive keratoplasty: a radiofrequency-based technique for the correction of hyperopia. *Trans Am Ophthalmol Soc.* 2005;103:512–536.

Other applications

Other potential off-label uses exist for CK. In cases of overcorrected myopic LASIK and myopic photorefractive keratectomy (PRK), CK can be used to correct hyperopia. In these procedures, CK obviates the need to lift or cut another flap. CK may also be used to treat keratoconus and post-LASIK ectasia. Although in 1 report corneal irregularities improved immediately, with some improvement in visual acuity, some cases showed regression of effect at 1 month.

Combination therapy with CK plus CCL may be effective in achieving a change in corneal curvature that does not regress with time.

Alió JL, Ramzy MI, Galal A, Claramonte PJ. Conductive keratoplasty for the correction of residual hyperopia after LASIK. *J Refract Surg.* 2005;21(6):698–704.

Claramonte PJ, Alió JL, Ramzy MI. Conductive keratoplasty to correct residual hyperopia after cataract surgery. *J Cataract Refract Surg.* 2006;32(9):1445–1451.

Corneal Crosslinking

Corneal crosslinking (CCL) was first described by Seiler, Spörl, and colleagues in 1997 as the "Dresden protocol." CCL involves the use of a riboflavin (vitamin B_2) solution plus exposure to ultraviolet A (UVA) light. The activated riboflavin causes collagen fibrils in tissue to form strong chemical bonds with adjacent fibrils. In the cornea, as in the skin, crosslinking of collagen can occur naturally, due to oxidative deamination within the end chains of the collagen molecule. In addition, other pathways can lead to crosslinking of collagen.

Most systems of corneal crosslinking employ oxidation through the release of oxygen free radicals. Riboflavin serves as a source for the generation of singlet oxygen and superoxide anion free radicals, which are split from its ring structure after excitation by UVA irradiation. It is this interaction of oxygen free radicals generated by the combination of riboflavin and exposure to UVA light that allows for crosslinking of collagen and increase corneal rigidity. In the presence of riboflavin, approximately 95% of the UVA light irradiance is absorbed in the anterior 300 μm of the corneal stroma. Therefore, a minimal corneal thickness of 400 μm after epithelial removal is recommended so as to avoid corneal endothelial damage by UVA irradiation. Thinner corneas may be thickened temporarily with application of a hypotonic riboflavin formulation prior to UVA treatment.

Although there may also be a slight flattening of the cornea, the most important effect of CCL is to stabilize the corneal curvature and prevent further steepening and bulging of the cornea in patients with ectatic conditions. There is no significant change in the refractive index or the clarity of the cornea. The primary clinical application of CCL is to prevent the progression of keratoconus and post–corneal refractive surgery ectasia.

In the Dresden protocol, riboflavin solution is continually applied to the de-epithelialized cornea for 30 minutes (in most studies), and the riboflavin is then activated by illumination of the cornea with UVA light for 30 minutes, during which time application of the riboflavin solution continues. The resultant corneas were shown to be nearly 300% stiffer and more resistant to enzymatic digestion. Investigation also proved that the treated corneas contained higher molecular weight polymers of collagen due to fibril crosslinking. Safety studies showed that the endothelium was not damaged by the treatment if proper UV irradiance was maintained and if the corneal thickness exceeded 400 μm. This type of cross-linking is commonly referred to as "epithelium-off" or "epi-off" CCL. Alternative riboflavin formulations and crosslinking techniques that avoid epithelial removal are being evaluated and seem promising.

CCL has rapidly become a first-line treatment for keratoconus throughout the world and was approved by the FDA in April 2016 for the treatment of progressive keratoconus and ectasia. Human studies of UV-induced CCL began in 2003 in Dresden, and early results were promising. The initial pilot study enrolled 16 patients with rapidly progressing keratoconus and all patients stopped progressing after treatment. In addition, 70% had flattening of their steep anterior corneal curvatures (decreases in average and maximum keratometric values), and 65% had an improvement in visual acuity. There were no reported complications.

In a clinical trial in the United States, all patients with keratoconus or post-LASIK ectasia had their corneal epithelium removed. This was followed by a 30-minute application of riboflavin (0.1% diluted in 20% dextran) every 2 minutes, and a subsequent 30-minute

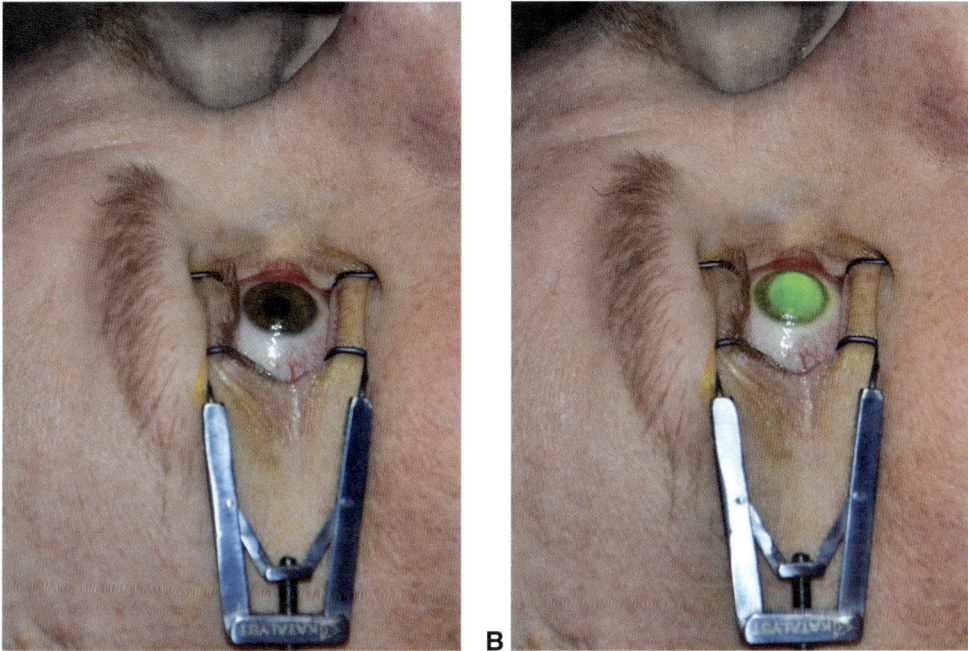

Figure 7-3 Patient undergoing corneal crosslinking. **A,** Patient preparing to undergo crosslinking of the cornea immediately prior to riboflavin application. **B,** After topical administration, the riboflavin fluoresces during application of ultraviolet irradiation to the cornea. *(Courtesy of Gregg J. Berdy, MD.)*

UVA treatment (365 nm; 3 mW/cm^2 irradiation), with concomitant administration of topical riboflavin as a photosensitizer (Fig 7-3). Two control groups—sham and fellow eye—were included in the study, and all patients were monitored for 1 year. Treated eyes initially showed a slight steepening of the cornea with a decrease in best-corrected visual acuity (BCVA; also called *corrected distance visual acuity, CDVA*), followed by corneal flattening of approximately 1.00–2.00 D, which peaked at between 1 and 3 months after crosslinking. In addition to a reduction in corneal cylinder, a transient compaction of the cornea and an increase in BCVA were observed. There appears to be stabilization in most treated eyes. Some eyes may require re-treatment, and there have been rare cases of loss of 2 or more lines of BCVA in these studies, however.

Spörl E, Huhle M, Kasper M, Seiler T. [Increased rigidity of the cornea caused by intrastromal cross-linking]. *Ophthalmologe.* 1997;94(12):902–906. German.

Wollensak G, Spoerl E, Seiler T. Riboflavin/ultraviolet-a-induced collagen crosslinking for the treatment of keratoconus. *Am J Ophthalmol.* 2003;135(5):620–627.

Patient Selection

Indications

The primary purpose of crosslinking is to stabilize the progression of ectasia. The most common indication for CCL is keratoconus. Other possible indications include pellucid marginal degeneration and ectasia resulting from refractive surgery.

Contraindications

Corneal crosslinking is relatively contraindicated in the following situations:

- corneal thickness of less than 400 μm (although some protocols may allow for treatment of corneas thicker than 300 μm)
- prior herpetic infection (due to concern of viral reactivation)
- severe corneal scarring or opacification
- history of poor epithelial wound healing
- severe ocular surface disease (eg, dry eye)
- autoimmune disorders

Surgical Technique

Variations of CCL procedures include the original Dresden protocol procedure, transepithelial CCL, accelerated CCL, and combined techniques. All have several prerequisites in common. The primary goal of the first stage of therapy is to allow sufficient riboflavin to diffuse into the cornea. In the initial studies, riboflavin was not able to penetrate an intact epithelium, and so the standard Dresden protocol required epithelial removal in order to allow riboflavin to rapidly penetrate into the stroma. However, newer formulations of riboflavin have been shown to penetrate intact epithelium and may have the additional advantage of faster healing, faster visual recovery, less pain, and lower incidence of complications. Studies are investigating the use of iontophoresis via an electrical charge gradient to allow for more complete penetration of riboflavin through the epithelium.

Once riboflavin has adequately diffused into the cornea, the second component of the CCL procedure is exposure to UVA light. The standard Dresden Protocol calls for 30-minute exposure to 370 nm UVA with an irradiance of 3 mWcm^{-2} for a total of 5.4 J/cm^2. Newer accelerated protocols attempt to decrease the duration of UVA exposure, while maintaining the same exposure (ie, 30 min at 3 mWcm^{-2} is equivalent to 3 min at 30 mWcm^{-2} or 10 min at 9 mWcm^{-2}). Table 7-1 reviews steps in the Dresden protocol.

Transepithelial corneal crosslinking

Postoperative discomfort, possible delayed epithelial healing, infection, stromal haze, and corneal melting represent the disadvantages of epithelial debridement that have led surgeons to explore transepithelial CCL. The reported clinical outcomes are promising. Experimental studies, however, have shown a significantly lower efficacy of transepithelial CCL compared to the standard epithelium-off approach due to the low epithelial permeability of riboflavin. Chemical agents such as benzalkonium chloride, trometamol, and ethylenediaminetetraacetic acid, as well as the use of hypotonic riboflavin solution without dextran, may to enhance riboflavin's penetration. The use of iontophoresis and partial disruption of the superficial epithelial layers also enhance riboflavin's penetration through the epithelium.

No matter which approach is used, stromal saturation with riboflavin is crucial and should always be visualized (Fig 7-4) before the UVA irradiation. Some researchers claim that, even with a sufficient stromal concentration of riboflavin, the effect of the

Table 7-1 Dresden Protocol

1. Prior to the procedure, the ultraviolet (UV) A light source is calibrated with the use of a light meter so that irradiance of 3 mWcm^{-2} is generated at the appropriate working distance (typically 3 or 4 inches from the apex of the cornea).
2. Topical anesthetic (typically proparacaine or tetracaine drops) is applied 3 times, once every 5 minutes.
3. An eyelid speculum is placed.
4. The central 8–10 mm of the epithelium are removed using a blunt spatula or a No. 64 blade. Alternately, dilute ethanol or an epithelial scrubber may be used.
5. Riboflavin drops (0.1% riboflavin-5-phosphate and 20% dextran T-500) are administered to the corneal surface every minute for 30 minutes. It is important to ensure adequate riboflavin penetration into the cornea. This is accomplished by visualizing the fluorescent riboflavin solution throughout the layers of the cornea or in the anterior chamber of the eye by use of the blue filter on slit-lamp examination.
6. Ultraviolet A irradiation is applied 5.4 J/cm^2 (3 mW/cm^2) for 30 minutes. Modern UV lamps use either a top hat instead of Gaussian beam profile or the spatially adjusted distribution of UV energy from the multiple UV diodes to compensate for the midperipheral loss of energy in the dome-shaped cornea.
7. Miosis may be induced with pilocarpine to protect the retroiridal structures and a cellulose-free ring may be used to shield the limbal area.
8. A bandage contact lens is placed.
9. Patients are prescribed topical antibiotic and corticosteroid, and oral analgesics.

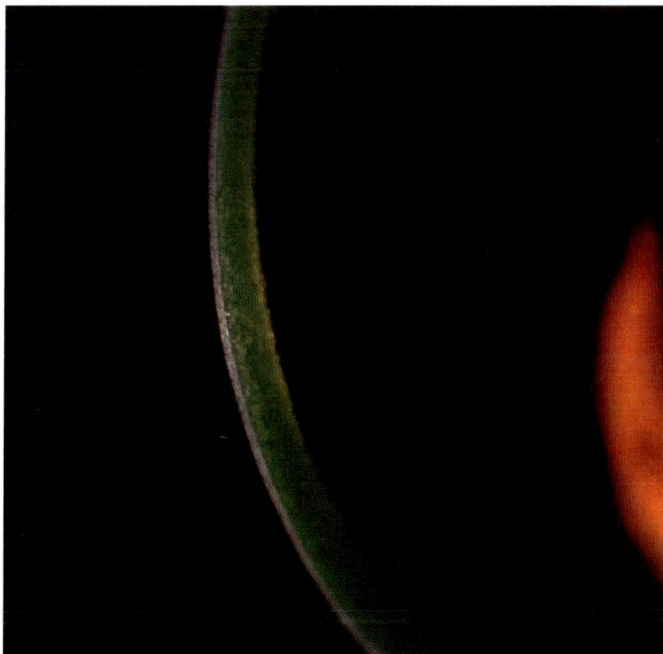

Figure 7-4 Full-thickness, homogeneous stromal penetration of riboflavin during epithelium-on (Epi-On) corneal crosslinking. Adequate riboflavin penetration is of paramount clinical importance prior to ultraviolet A light application. *(Courtesy of Roy S. Rubinfeld, MD, MA.)*

transepithelial CCL may be decreased due to the attenuation of UVA radiation by the epithelium. That would imply that UVA energy may need to be increased or otherwise modulated beyond the current level of 5.4 J/cm^2 when the epithelium is kept intact.

Baiocchi S, Mazzotta C, Cerretani D, et al. Corneal crosslinking: riboflavin concentration in corneal stroma exposed with and without epithelium. *J Cataract Refract Surg.* 2009;35(5): 893–899.

Bottos KM, Schor P, Dreyfuss JL, Nader HB, Chamon W. Effect of corneal epithelium on ultraviolet-A and riboflavin absorption. *Arq Bras Oftalmol.* 2011;74(5):348–351.

Filippello M, Stagni E, O'Brart D. Transepithelial corneal collagen crosslinking: bilateral study. *J Cataract Refract Surg.* 2012;38(2):283–291.

Kanellopoulos AJ. Long term results of a prospective randomized bilateral eye comparison trial of higher fluence, shorter duration ultraviolet A radiation, and riboflavin collagen cross linking for progressive keratoconus. *Clin Ophthalmol.* 2012;6:97–101.

Kissner A, Spoerl E, Jung R, Spekl K, Pillunat LE, Raiskup F. Pharmacological modification of the epithelial permeability by benzalkonium chloride in UVA/Riboflavin corneal collagen cross-linking. *Curr Eye Res.* 2010;35(8):715–721.

Stojanovic A, Zhou W, Utheim TP. Corneal collagen cross-linking with and without epithelial removal: a contralateral study with 0.5% hypotonic riboflavin solution. *Biomed Res Int.* 2014; 2014:619398. Epub 2014 Jun 22.

Accelerated corneal crosslinking

New-generation lamps have been developed to shorten the duration of UVA irradiation. Some offer fixed treatment times of 10 and 5 minutes with the use of a power of 10 and 18 mW/cm^2. Other systems allow a wide range of adjustable times (1–30 minutes) with a UV power of 3 to 45 mW and increased maximum irradiance to 10 J/cm^2. Kanellopoulos reported that the use of higher-fluence UVA for a shorter time (7 mW/cm^2 for 15 minutes) is safe and effective. He found that this approach achieves similar clinical results to the Dresden protocol in terms of stabilizing ectasia.

Kanellopoulos AJ. Collagen cross-linking in early keratoconus with riboflavin in a femtosecond laser–created pocket: initial clinical results. *J Refract Surg.* 2009;25(11):1034–1037.

Combined techniques

In some cases, patients do not achieve visual acuity improvement sufficient to provide functional vision after CCL treatment. Ophthalmologists, therefore, have attempted to combine CCL with various refractive surgical techniques (see Chapter 12). The implantation of intracorneal ring segments with sequential or subsequent CCL treatment has proven effective. The limited use of topography-guided transepithelial PRK followed by CCL has also been shown to improve visual acuity and stabilize keratoconus. Same-day PRK followed by CCL appears to be superior to sequential PRK after CCL, and the former has been widely used as the Athens protocol. Combining CCL with the implantation of a phakic toric intraocular lens safely and effectively corrects myopic astigmatism in eyes with mild to moderate keratoconus. The triple procedure of CCL combined with topography-guided PRK to regularize the corneal shape and the implantation of a phakic intraocular to optimize the refraction may rehabilitate the patient's vision with a higher predictability of the refractive outcome compared with CCL combined with topography-guided PRK alone.

Güell JL, Morral M, Malecaze F, Gris O, Elies D, Manero F. Collagen crosslinking and toric iris-claw phakic intraocular lens for myopic astigmatism in progressive mild to moderate keratoconus. *J Cataract Refract Surg.* 2012;38(3):473–484.

Kamburoglu G, Ertan A. Intacs implantation with sequential collagen cross-linking treatment in postoperative LASIK ectasia. *J Refract Surg.* 2008;24(7):S726–729.

Kanellopoulos AJ. Comparison of sequential vs same-day simultaneous collagen cross-linking and topography-guided PRK for treatment of keratoconus. *J Refract Surg.* 2009;25(9): S812–818.

Stojanovic A, Zhang J, Chen X, Nitter TA, Chen S, Wang Q. Topography-guided transepithelial surface ablation followed by corneal collagen cross-linking performed in a single combined procedure for the treatment of keratoconus and pellucid marginal degeneration. *J Refract Surg.* 2010;26(2):145–152.

Complications

Complications of CCL may include delayed epithelial healing, corneal haze (which may be visually significant), decreased corneal sensitivity, infectious keratitis, persistent corneal edema, and endothelial cell damage.

Summary

Corneal crosslinking is a very promising treatment modality, and studies are evaluating its place among the options for corneal therapy. In addition to conducting studies employing denuded epithelium for crosslinking, investigators are examining riboflavin penetration across intact epithelium for crosslinking. In addition, there have been reports of CCL employed successfully to treat fungal and bacterial infections of the cornea. This use may represent a potential new application of this technology.

Papaioannou L, Miligkos M, Papathanassiou M. Corneal collagen cross-linking for infectious keratitis: a systematic review and meta-analysis. *Cornea.* 2016;35(1):62–71.

CHAPTER 8

Intraocular Refractive Surgery

▶ *This chapter includes related videos, which can be accessed by scanning the QR codes provided in the text or going to www.aao.org/bcscvideo_section13.*

In its early history, *refractive surgery* was synonymous with *corneal refractive (keratorefractive)* surgery. In recent years, the scope of refractive surgery has expanded to include lens-based intraocular surgical techniques for achieving refractive outcomes.

In crystalline lens–sparing procedures, termed *phakic intraocular lens implantation,* the implantation of a phakic intraocular lens (PIOL) allows treatment of more extreme refractive errors, especially high myopia. Available PIOLs in the United States include iris-fixated and posterior chamber (sulcus) lenses for myopia. Outside the United States, angle-supported, iris-fixated, and posterior chamber lenses are available for hyperopia and myopia, and some phakic toric intraocular lenses (IOLs) are available to correct both myopic and hyperopic and astigmatism.

In crystalline lens–extraction procedures, termed *refractive lens exchange (RLE),* the patient's lens is removed and replaced with a prosthetic lens to address refractive errors of the eye. Advances in cataract surgical technique (small, predictable wounds, precision biometry, and improved IOL power calculation formulas) and expanded choices of intraocular lenses have afforded more accurate and predictable refractive outcomes allowing the elective correction of spherical, astigmatic, and presbyopic refractive errors.

The combination of corneal and intraocular refractive surgery, termed *bioptics,* allows patients at the extremes of refractive error, both spherical (myopia, hyperopia) and cylindrical (astigmatism), to attain good, predictable outcomes by combining the advantages of the intraocular refractive surgery in treating large corrections with the adjustability of keratorefractive techniques. In addition, the optical quality may be improved by dividing the refractive correction between the 2 surgical procedures.

This chapter discusses the intraocular surgical techniques that are now, or are soon expected to be, available to the refractive surgeon.

Phakic Intraocular Lenses

Background

The history of the PIOL in correcting refractive error began in Europe in the 1950s, but manufacturing-quality limitations precluded these IOLs from achieving widespread use until the 1990s. Refinements in IOL design have reduced the incidence of complications and, consequently, increased the popularity of these PIOLs both inside and outside the United States. Within the United States, 3 PIOLs are currently approved by the US Food and Drug Administration (FDA) for myopia: 2 nonfoldable polymethyl methacrylate (PMMA) iris-fixated PIOLs, and 1 foldable collamer posterior chamber PIOL. The 2 nonfoldable PMMA lenses are identical in design but have different dioptric ranges. Outside the United States, available models include foldable versions of the PIOLs, hyperopic and toric versions of all of these PIOLs, and an angle-fixated PIOL. Representative lenses in each category (Table 8-1) are discussed in the following sections.

> Huang D, Schallhorn SC, Sugar A, et al. Phakic intraocular lens implantation for the correction of myopia: a report by the American Academy of Ophthalmology. *Ophthalmology.* 2009;116(11):2244–2258.

Advantages

Phakic intraocular lenses have the advantage of treating a much larger range of refractive errors than can be treated safely and effectively with corneal refractive surgery. The skills required for insertion are, with a few exceptions, similar to those used in cataract surgery. The equipment needed for IOL implantation is substantially less expensive than an excimer laser and is similar to that used for cataract surgery. In addition, the PIOL is removable; therefore, the refractive effect should theoretically be reversible. However, any intervening change caused by the PIOL implantation is often permanent. Compared with refractive lens exchange (discussed later in this chapter), PIOL implantation has the advantage of preserving natural accommodation; it also has a lower risk of endophthalmitis and postoperative retinal detachment because the crystalline lens barrier is preserved and there is minimal vitreous destabilization.

Disadvantages

Phakic intraocular lens insertion is an intraocular procedure, with all the potential risks associated with intraocular surgery. In addition, each PIOL style has its own set of associated risks. Lenses currently available in the United States with PMMA optics are not foldable, so their insertion requires a relatively large wound, which may result in postoperative astigmatism. Posterior chamber PIOLs have a higher incidence of cataract formation. For patients with PIOLs in whom a visually significant cataract eventually develops, the PIOL will have to be explanted at the time of cataract surgery, possibly through a larger-than-usual wound. Although PIOLs to correct hyperopia are available outside the United States, indications for their implantation are narrower because the anterior chamber tends to be

Table 8-1 Phakic Intraocular Lenses

Position	Model	Available Power (D)	Optic Size/ Effective Diameter (mm)	Length (mm)	Material	Manufacturer	FDA Approval
Angle-supported	AcrySof Cachet	−6.00 to −16.50	6.0	12.5, 13.0, 13.5, 14.0	Acrylic	Alcon Laboratories	
	Kelman Duet	−6.00 to −20.00	6.3	12.0, 12.5, 13.0, 13.5	Silicone optic PMMA haptics	Tekia (Irvine, CA)	
Iris-supported	Verisyse model[a] VRSM5US	−5.00 to −20.00	5.0	8.5	PMMA	Abbott Medical Optics (Santa Ana, CA)	Approved
	Verisyse model[a] VRSM6US	−5.00 to −15.00	6.0	8.5	PMMA	Abbott Medical Optics	Approved
	Artisan model 203	+3.00 to +12.00	5.0 or 6.0	8.5	PMMA	Ophtec (Groningen, The Netherlands; USA, Boca Raton, FL)	
	Artisan toric IOL	Custom	5.0 or 6.0	8.5	PMMA	Ophtec	
	Artiflex/ Veriflex	−3.00 to −23.50	5.0 or 6.0	8.5	Polysiloxane	Ophtec	
Sulcus-supported	Visian ICL[b]	−3.00 to −20.00	4.9–5.8	12.1, 12.6, 13.2, 13.7	Collamer	STAAR (Monrovia, CA)	Approved
	Visian ICL Visian Toric ICL	+3.00 to +12.00 Up to +2.50 Custom to +4.00	4.75–5.50	11.5–13.2 11.5–13.2	Collamer Collamer	STAAR STAAR	

FDA = US Food and Drug Administration; ICL = implantable collamer lens; IOL = intraocular lens; PMMA = polymethyl methacrylate.

[a] The Artisan lens (Ophtec), marketed as the Verisyse lens (Abbott Medical Optics), has been FDA approved for use in the lens power range of −5.00 to −20.00 D.

[b] The Visian ICL (STAAR) posterior chamber phakic IOL has received FDA approval to correct myopia in the range of −3.00 to −20.00 D.

shallower than in patients with myopia, causing the IOL to sit too close to the corneal endothelium and resulting in increased endothelial cell loss.

Patient Selection

Indications

Phakic intraocular lenses can be offered as the primary surgical option for anyone who has refractive errors within the available treatment range and meets other screening criteria (discussed later). However, most surgeons reserve PIOL use for patients whose refractive limits are near or beyond the FDA-approved limits for laser vision correction, or who are otherwise not good candidates for keratorefractive surgery. Although excimer lasers can be used to treat high degrees of myopia, many surgeons have reduced the upper limits for laser in situ keratomileusis (LASIK) and surface ablation in their refractive practices because of the decreased predictability, high rate of regression, large amount of stromal tissue removed, increased incidence of microstriae, and night-vision problems that can occur with treatment of a patient with high myopia. Similarly, LASIK and surface ablation for correction of hyperopia greater than +4.00 D and astigmatism greater than 4.00 D of cylinder are less accurate than they are for lower corrections. If surgeons become comfortable with the use of PIOLs, they may also choose to implant them for refractive powers significantly lower than the maximal limits for programmable excimer laser treatments. In addition, due to the rapid visual recovery and low complication rate of currently available PIOLs, increasing numbers of surgeons are implanting these lenses bilaterally on the same day, providing a patient experience similar to bilateral same-day LASIK. The Ophthalmic Mutual Insurance Company (OMIC) has evaluated this practice.

PIOLs are available in powers between –3.00 D and –20.00 D in the United States (see Table 8-1). Outside the United States, PIOLs are available for correcting hyperopia up to +10.00 D. PIOLs may be considered off-label treatment for eyes with irregular topographies from forme fruste or frank keratoconus.

> Ophthalmic Mutual Insurance Company (OMIC). Am I covered for performing bilateral same-day RLE or bilateral same-day phakic implant procedures? OMIC website. Updated June 5, 2014. Available at https://goo.gl/bb9IcI. Accessed November 6, 2016.

Contraindications

Phakic intraocular lenses have specific contraindications. These include preexisting intraocular disease such as a compromised corneal endothelium, iritis, significant iris abnormality, rubeosis iridis, cataract, or glaucoma. The anterior chamber diameter, anterior chamber depth, and pupil size must be appropriate for the specific PIOL being considered.

Patient evaluation

A thorough preoperative evaluation is necessary, as detailed in Chapter 2. PIOLs are not approved in the United States for patients younger than 21 years.

Informed consent

As with any refractive procedure, an informed consent specifically for this procedure should be obtained before surgery. The patient should be informed of the potential short-term and long-term risks of the procedure and of available alternatives; he or she should also be counseled about the importance of long-term follow-up because of the potential for endothelial cell loss over time. The surgeon must also ensure that the patient has realistic expectations about the visual outcomes of the procedure.

Ancillary tests

Specular microscopy or confocal microscopy should be performed to evaluate endothelial cell count and morphology. Anterior chamber depth must also be assessed because adequate depth is required for safe implantation of a PIOL. If the anterior chamber depth is less than 3.2 mm, the risk of endothelial and iris or angle trauma from placement of an anterior chamber, iris-fixated, or posterior chamber PIOL is increased. Anterior chamber depth can be measured by ultrasound biomicroscopy, anterior segment optical coherence tomography (OCT), partial coherence interferometry, slit-beam topography, or Scheimpflug imaging. In the United States, PIOL implantation is contraindicated in individuals who do not meet the minimum endothelial cell count specified for each PIOL and who do not have a minimum anterior chamber depth of 3.2 mm. Methods for IOL power selection are specific to each PIOL and manufacturer, and some manufacturers provide software for use in IOL power calculation.

Surgical Technique

Topical anesthesia with an intracameral supplement is appropriate if the patient is able to cooperate and the PIOL can be inserted through a small incision. If the patient cannot cooperate for the use of topical anesthesia or if a large incision is required, peribulbar or general anesthesia is preferable. Retrobulbar anesthesia should be used with caution in patients whose eyes have a high axial length because of the increased risk of globe perforation.

A peripheral iridotomy is recommended for all currently FDA-approved PIOLs to reduce the risk of pupillary block and angle closure; however, this recommendation may soon change, and iridotomy is not required for angle-supported PIOLs. One or more laser iridotomies can be performed before the PIOL surgery, or an iridectomy can be performed as part of the implant procedure. Viscoelastic material should be meticulously removed at the conclusion of surgery to prevent postoperative elevation of IOP.

Iris-fixated phakic intraocular lens

Most surgeons induce pupillary miosis before they initiate iris-fixated PIOL implantation, both to protect the crystalline lens and to make the iris easier to manipulate. The lens is generally inserted through a superior limbal incision but can be implanted with the wound placed at the steep meridian to minimize postoperative astigmatism. The long axis of the PIOL is ultimately oriented perpendicular to the axis of the incision. A side port incision is made approximately 2–3 clock-hours on either side of the center of the incision; thus, a 12 o'clock incision requires side port incisions near the 10 and 2 o'clock meridians. The "claw" haptics are fixated to the iris in a process called *enclavation*. After the PIOL has been carefully centered over the pupil, it is stabilized with forceps while a specially designed enclavation needle is introduced through one of the side port incisions, and a small amount of iris is brought up into the claw haptic. This procedure is repeated on the other side. If adjustment of the PIOL position becomes necessary after fixation, the iris must be released before the PIOL is moved. Careful wound closure helps minimize surgically induced astigmatism. PMMA PIOLs require a 6-mm wound and thus generally require sutures for proper closure, whereas iris-fixated PIOLs made of flexible materials can be inserted through a small, self-sealing wound of approximately 3 mm. Video 8-1 demonstrates implantation of an iris-fixated IOL.

VIDEO 8-1 Implantation of an iris-fixated phakic IOL.
Courtesy of David R. Hardten, MD.
Access all Section 13 videos at www.aao.org/bcscvideo_section13.

Sizing the iris-fixated phakic intraocular lens Because this PIOL is fixated to the midperipheral iris, not the angle or sulcus, it has the advantage of having a "one-size-fits-all" length. It is 8.5 mm in length, with a 5.0- or 6.0-mm PMMA optic (Fig 8-1).

Posterior chamber phakic intraocular lens

Posterior chamber PIOLs require pupillary dilation prior to implantation. These PIOLs are made of a flexible collamer material and are implanted through a small wound approximately 3 mm in length (Fig 8-2). The optic of the PIOL is vaulted to avoid contact with the crystalline lens and to allow aqueous to flow over the crystalline lens. This vaulting can be viewed at the slit lamp as well as with ultrasound biomicroscopy or Scheimpflug imaging (Fig 8-3). The lens manufacturers suggest that an acceptable amount of vaulting of the lens optic over the crystalline lens is 1.0 ± 0.5 corneal thicknesses. Using the appropriate vault is crucial for reducing complications (discussed later in the chapter).

For lens implantation, following pupil dilation, a 3.0- to 3.2-mm temporal clear corneal incision is made, and 1–2 additional paracentesis incisions are created, usually

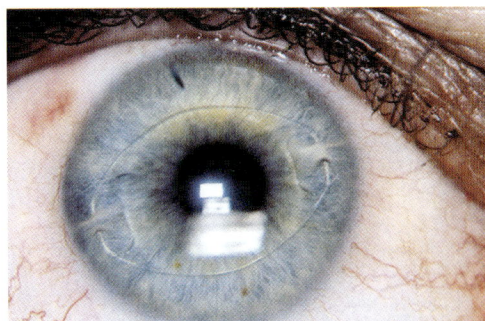

Figure 8-1 An iris-fixated phakic intraocular lens (PIOL) for myopic correction. *(Courtesy of Abbott Medical Optics.)*

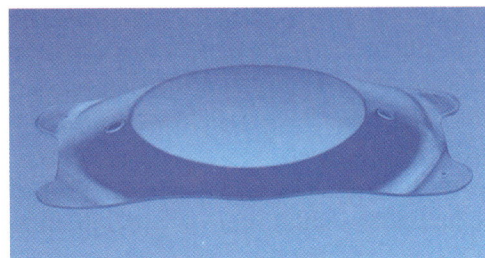

Figure 8-2 Side view of an implantable collamer posterior chamber PIOL. *(Courtesy of STAAR Surgical Company.)*

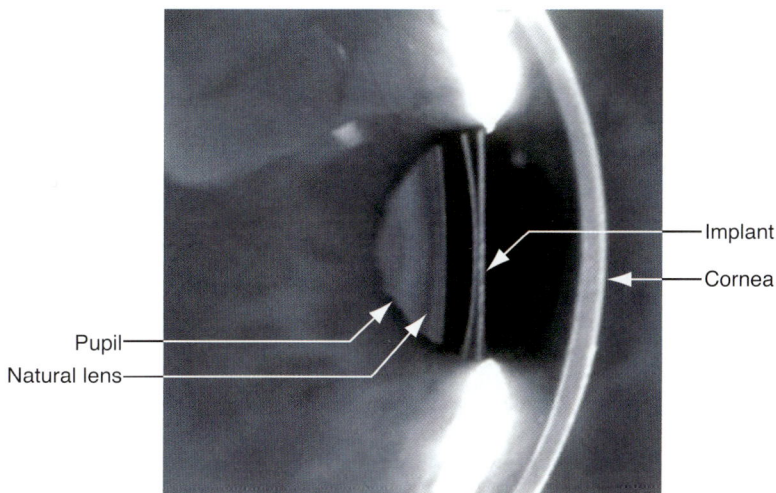

Figure 8-3 Scheimpflug image of a posterior chamber PIOL in place within the ciliary sulcus. *(Courtesy of STAAR Surgical Company.)*

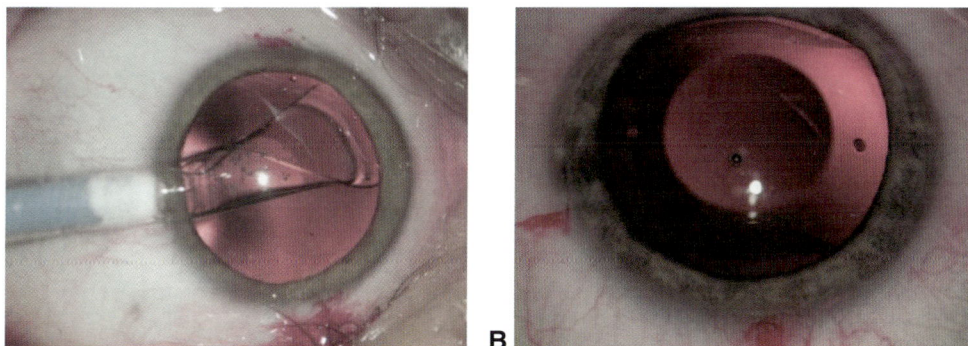

Figure 8-4 **A,** After placement with an IOL inserter, the posterior chamber PIOL unfolds in the anterior chamber. **B,** A posterior chamber PIOL shown unfolded and in position anterior to the crystalline lens in the posterior chamber. *(Courtesy of STAAR Surgical Company.)*

superiorly and inferiorly, to facilitate lens positioning. The lens is inserted using a cohesive viscoelastic material; after the lens unfolds, the footplates are positioned under the iris (Fig 8-4). The leading footplate is marked for identification and must be confirmed to be in the correct location once the lens exits the injector in order to ensure the lens is oriented with the correct side facing anteriorly. The surgeon should avoid contact with the central 6.0 mm of the lens, as any contact might damage the thin lens optic. Care should be taken to avoid touching the crystalline lens with the PIOL to minimize the risk of cataract formation. Positioning instruments should be inserted through the paracenteses and should be kept peripheral to this central area. The pupil is then constricted. It is crucial to remove all viscoelastic material at the conclusion of the procedure to reduce the risk of a postoperative spike in intraocular pressure (IOP). Video 8-2 demonstrates implantation of a posterior chamber PIOL.

VIDEO 8-2 Implantation of a posterior chamber phakic IOL.
Courtesy of George O. Waring IV, MD.

Sizing the posterior chamber phakic intraocular lens The correct IOL length is selected by using the white-to-white measurement between the 3 and 9 o'clock meridians or by direct sulcus measurements made by a variety of techniques, including high-frequency ultrasound, anterior segment OCT, slit-beam or Scheimpflug imaging, and laser interferometry. Although the FDA-approved technique for measurement remains white-to-white measurement, there is growing evidence that direct sulcus measurement using any of these methods is superior and minimizes the risk of incorrect PIOL sizing. For more information on PIOLs, please refer to the FDA website.

US Food and Drug Administration. Phakic intraocular lenses. Medical devices website. Available at https://goo.gl/aRyPgK. Updated June 24, 2014. Accessed November 6, 2016.

Angle-supported phakic intraocular lens

No angle-supported PIOLs are currently approved by the FDA. Outside the United States, several commercial angle-supported PIOLs are available. The most widely used lens is made of flexible acrylic material and can be inserted through a small incision without the need for pupil dilation.

Outcomes

With better methods for determining PIOL power, outcomes have steadily improved. The significant postoperative gains in lines of best-corrected visual acuity (BCVA), also referred to as *corrected distance visual acuity (CDVA),* over preoperative values are likely the result of a reduction in the image minification present with spectacle correction of high myopia. Loss of BCVA is rare. Moreover, the loss of contrast sensitivity noted after LASIK for high myopia does not occur after PIOL surgery. In fact, in all spatial frequencies, contrast sensitivity increases from preoperative levels with best spectacle correction.

Barsam A, Allan BD. Excimer laser refractive surgery versus phakic intraocular lenses for the correction of moderate to high myopia. *Cochrane Database Syst Rev.* 2012;1:CD007679. Epub 2012 Jan 18.

Boxer Wachler BS, Scruggs RT, Yuen LH, Jalali S. Comparison of the Visian ICL and Verisyse phakic intraocular lenses for myopia from 6.00 to 20.00 diopters. *J Refract Surg.* 2009;25(9): 765–770.

Dick HB, Budo C, Malecaze F, et al. Foldable Artiflex phakic intraocular lens for the correction of myopia: two-year follow-up results of a prospective European multicenter study. *Ophthalmology.* 2009;116(4):671–677.

Dougherty PJ, Rivera RP, Schneider D, Lane SS, Brown D, Vukich J. Improving accuracy of phakic intraocular lens sizing using high-frequency ultrasound biomicroscopy. *J Cataract Refract Surg.* 2010;37(1):13–18.

Hassaballa MA, Macky TA. Phakic intraocular lenses outcomes and complications: Artisan vs. Visian ICL. *Eye (Lond).* 2011;25(10):1365–1370.

Kohnen T, Kook D, Morral M, Güell JL. Phakic intraocular lenses: part 2: results and complications. *J Cataract Refract Surg.* 2010;36(12):2168–2194.

Parkhurst GD, Psolka M, Kezirian GM. Phakic intraocular lens implantation in United States military warfighters: a retrospective analysis of early clinical outcomes of the Visian ICL. *J Refract Surg.* 2011;27(7):473–481.

Pérez-Cambrodí RJ, Piñero DP, Ferrer-Blasco T, Cerviño A, Brautaset R. The posterior chamber phakic refractive lens (PRL): a review. *Eye (Lond).* 2013;27:14–21

Summary of safety and effectiveness data. Artisan phakic lens. PMA No. P030028. US Food and Drug Administration website. Available at https://goo.gl/nTYyG2. Accessed November 6, 2016.

Summary of safety and effectiveness data. STAAR Visian ICL (Implantable Collamer Lens). PMA No. P030016. US Food and Drug Administration website. Available at https://goo.gl/jTlZQs. Accessed November 6, 2016.

Complications

Phakic intraocular lens surgery shares the same possible risks and complications as other forms of IOL surgery. However, the most relevant potential complications include raised IOP, persistent anterior chamber inflammation, traumatic PIOL dislocation, cataract formation, and endothelial cell loss. Some of these complications do not manifest for years, thus necessitating long-term follow-up.

Iris-fixated phakic intraocular lens

At 1-year follow-up in an FDA clinical trial of 662 patients who had an iris-fixated PIOL implanted for myopia, 1 patient had a hyphema, 5 had IOL dislocations, and 3 had iritis. Night-vision concerns about glare, starbursts, and halos were reported in 13.5%, 11.8%, and 18.2%, respectively, in patients who did not have these symptoms preoperatively. However, improvement in symptoms occurred 12.9%, 9.7%, and 9.8%, in patients after PIOL implantation. In general, nighttime symptoms were worse in patients with larger pupil diameters.

Stulting and colleagues reported a 3-year follow-up study on 232 eyes of the 662 eyes enrolled in the FDA study. A total of 5 lenses dislocated and required reattachment, and an additional 20 lenses required surgery for insufficient lens fixation. No eyes required IOP-lowering medications after the first month. The mean decrease in endothelial cell density from baseline to 3 years was 4.8%. Six eyes required retinal detachment repair (rate, 0.3% per year), and 3 eyes underwent cataract surgery.

Pop M, Payette Y. Initial results of endothelial cell counts after Artisan lens for phakic eyes: an evaluation of the United States Food and Drug Administration Ophtec Study. *Ophthalmology.* 2004;111(2):309–311.

Stulting RD, John ME, Maloney RK, Assil KK, Arrowsmith PN, Thompson VM; U.S. Verisyse Study Group. Three-year results of Artisan/Verisyse phakic intraocular lens implantation. Results of the United States Food and Drug Administration clinical trial. *Ophthalmology.* 2008;115(3):464–472.

Posterior chamber phakic intraocular lens

In addition to the potential risks associated with implantation of other types of PIOLs, implantation of posterior chamber PIOLs increases the risk of cataract formation and pigmentary dispersion. If the posterior chamber PIOL is too large, vaulting increases, and iris chafing with pigmentary dispersion could result. If the PIOL is too small, the vaulting is reduced, decreasing the chance of chafing but increasing the risk of cataract. Incorrect PIOL vault can necessitate exchange of the implanted lens for one with a better fit.

In an FDA clinical trial for 1 posterior chamber PIOL model, the incidence of nighttime visual symptoms was approximately 10%, but a similar percentage showed improvement in these symptoms after surgery. The incidence of visually significant cataract development in the FDA clinical trial as reported by Sanders and colleagues was 0.4% for anterior subcapsular cataracts and 1% for nuclear sclerotic cataracts.

Kamiya and colleagues reported 4-year follow-up results on 56 eyes of 34 patients with implanted posterior chamber PIOLs. No eyes developed pupillary block or a significant increase in IOP. The mean central endothelial cell loss was 3.7%. Symptomatic cataracts requiring surgery developed in 2 eyes, and asymptomatic anterior subcapsular cataracts developed in 6 other eyes. In a study of more than 500 eyes monitored for an average of 4.7 years, Sanders reported that anterior subcapsular opacities developed in 6%–7% of eyes, and visually significant cataracts developed in 1%–2% of eyes.

The incidence of retinal detachment after posterior chamber PIOL insertion is very low. In a series of 418 eyes that underwent a posterior chamber PIOL procedure, rhegmatogenous retinal detachment developed in 3 eyes (0.7%) at a mean of 19.8 months postoperatively, a rate comparable to the expected natural history of detachment in eyes with similar degrees of myopia.

Al-Abdullah AA, Al-Falah MA, Al-Rasheed SA, Khandekar R, Suarez E, Arevalo JF. Retinal complications after anterior versus posterior chamber phakic intraocular lens Implantation in a myopic cohort. *J Refract Surg.* 2015;1;31(12):814–819.

Kamiya K, Shimizu K, Igarashi A, Hikita F, Komatsu M. Four-year follow-up of posterior chamber phakic intraocular lens implantation for moderate to high myopia. *Arch Ophthalmol.* 2009;127(7):845–850.

Kohnen T, Knorz MC, Cochener B, et al. AcrySof phakic angle-supported intraocular lens for the correction of moderate-to-high myopia: one-year results of a multicenter European study. *Ophthalmology.* 2009;116(7):1314–1321.

Sanders DR. Anterior subcapsular opacities and cataracts 5 years after surgery in the Visian Implantable Collamer Lens FDA trial. *J Refract Surg.* 2008;24(6):566–570.

Sanders DR, Vukich JA, Doney K, Gaston M; Implantable Contact Lens in Treatment of Myopia Study Group. U.S. Food and Drug Administration clinical trial of the Implantable Contact Lens for moderate to high myopia. *Ophthalmology.* 2003;110(2):255–266.

Angle-supported phakic intraocular lens

The complications reported most frequently for angle-supported PIOLs are nighttime glare and halos, pupil ovalization, and endothelial cell loss. The risk of pupillary block is low with the use of modern PIOL designs and of iridotomies when needed.

Glare and halos, the most commonly reported symptoms after angle-supported PIOL insertion, occurred in 18.8%–20.0% of patients, but these symptoms appear to decrease by as much as 50% over a postoperative period of 7 years. Endothelial cell loss occurring 1–7 years after angle-supported PIOL insertion ranges from 4.6% to 8.4%. Pupil ovalization can occur because of iris tuck during insertion, or it can occur over time as a result of chronic inflammation and fibrosis around the haptics within the anterior chamber angle. The incidence of pupil ovalization ranges from 5.9% to 27.5% and is directly related to the postoperative interval studied. Ovalization is more likely when the implant is too large. In contrast, endothelial damage and decentration are most often associated with movement of a lens that is too small.

Knorz and colleagues reported on the 6-month to 3-year results of an angle-supported PIOL in 360 eyes with moderate to high myopia. No eyes experienced pupillary block, pupil ovalization, or retinal detachment. The annualized percentage loss in central and peripheral endothelial cell density from 6 months to 3 years was 0.41% and 1.11%, respectively.

Knorz MC, Lane SS, Holland SP. Angle-supported phakic intraocular lens for correction of moderate to high myopia: Three-year interim results in international multicenter studies. *J Cataract Refract Surg.* 2011;37(3):469–480.

Refractive Lens Exchange

Advantages

Refractive lens exchange has the advantage of greatly expanding the range of refractive surgery beyond what can be achieved with other available methods. The procedure retains the normal contour of the cornea, which may enhance the quality of vision, and it may be used to treat presbyopia as well as refractive error with incorporation of multifocal and/or accommodating IOLs.

Disadvantages

Quality of vision may not be as good with current multifocal IOLs (MFIOLs) as with other forms of vision correction. Patient expectations for excellent uncorrected visual acuity may be higher for RLE than for cataract surgery, underscoring the need for thorough preoperative discussion, close attention to detail preoperatively and intraoperatively, and postoperative treatment of residual refractive error.

Patient Selection

Indications

Refractive lens exchange (RLE) is the removal of the crystalline lens with IOL implantation for the primary purpose of correcting refractive error. RLE may be considered for the correction of myopia, hyperopia, astigmatism, and presbyopia when alternative refractive procedures are not adequate to address the patient's refractive error. RLE is typically used for refractive correction of presbyopic patients and in patients with lens opacity expected to progress quickly. RLE is generally not considered medically necessary and is usually not covered by the patient's insurance. All FDA-approved IOLs are approved specifically for implantation at the time of cataract surgery, and implantation for RLE is considered an off-label use in the United States.

Informed consent

Refractive lens exchange carries risks and complications identical to those for routine cataract extraction with IOL implantation. Potential candidates must be capable of understanding the short-term and long-term risks of the procedure. Patients should be informed that unless they are targeted for residual myopia with monofocal, toric, or accommodating IOLs, or have an MFIOL implanted, they will not have functional near vision without correction. A consent form should be given to the patient prior to surgery to allow ample time for review and signature. A sample consent form for RLE for the correction of hyperopia and myopia is available from the Ophthalmic Mutual Insurance Company (OMIC) at www.omic.com.

Myopia

Refractive lens exchange can be considered in patients with myopia of any level, although it is most commonly used in presbyopic patients with higher myopia, for whom corneal refractive procedures or PIOL implantation are not indicated. Myopia, however, is a significant risk factor for retinal detachment in the absence of lens surgery, and this risk rises with increased axial length. High myopia, defined as an axial length of 26 mm, or greater, is an independent risk factor for subsequent retinal detachment after lens extraction. Thus, a thorough retinal examination, including peripheral retinal evaluation, is indicated in these eyes prior to consideration of RLE.

American Academy of Ophthalmology Retina/Vitreous Panel. Preferred Practice Pattern Guidelines. *Posterior Vitreous Detachment, Retinal Breaks, and Lattice Degeneration.* San Francisco: American Academy of Ophthalmology; 2014. Available at www.aao.org/ppp.

Daien V, Le Pape A, Heve D, Carriere I, Villain M. Incidence, Risk Factors, and Impact of Age on Retinal Detachment after Cataract Surgery in France: A National Population Study. *Ophthalmology.* 2015;122(11):2179–2185.

Haug SJ, Bhisitkul RB. Risk factors for retinal detachment following cataract surgery. *Curr Opin Ophthalmol.* 2012;23(1):7–11.

Hyperopia

If the amount of hyperopia is beyond the range of alternative refractive procedures, RLE might be the only available surgical option. As with correction for myopia, the patient must be informed about the risks of intraocular surgery. A patient with a shallow anterior chamber from a thickened crystalline lens or small anterior segment would not be a candidate for a PIOL and could benefit from the reduced risk of angle-closure glaucoma after RLE. In a highly hyperopic eye with an axial length less than 18 mm, nanophthalmos should be considered. Eyes with these characteristics have a higher risk of uveal effusion syndrome and postoperative choroidal detachment. (See BCSC Section 11, *Lens and Cataract,* for discussion of cataract surgery for a patient with high hyperopia and nanophthalmos.) Patients with hyperopia have a lower risk of retinal detachment than do patients with myopia.

Nanavaty MA, Daya SM. Refractive lens exchange versus phakic intraocular lenses. *Curr Opin Ophthalmol.* 2012;23(1):54–61.

Astigmatism

With the advent of toric IOLs that cover an expanded range, patients with significant astigmatism are also candidates for RLE. In the United States, there are currently no FDA-approved toric MFIOLs, although a toric accommodating IOL has been approved. Thus,

US patients planning to undergo implantation of a nonaccommodating toric IOL must understand the lack of uncorrected near acuity if targeted for distance; patients considering MFIOL implantation should understand that these IOLs will not sufficiently reduce astigmatism. Also, patients need to understand that an additional surgical procedure, usually LASIK, limbal relaxing incisions, or photorefractive keratectomy, may be necessary to maximize spectacle independence. Laser vision correction candidacy should be determined prior to lens-based surgery if it is being considered.

Presbyopia

Discussion of correction of presbyopia, in addition to correction of myopia, hyperopia, and/or astigmatism, should be a component of the preoperative discussion in applicable patients. RLE is occasionally used primarily for the purpose of correcting presbyopia, with the implantation of multifocal or accommodating IOLs or the creation of monovision with lens implants. A patient selecting distance-focused toric or spherical IOLs in both eyes should be informed that reading glasses will be required for functional near vision.

Surgical Planning and Technique

Although RLE is similar to cataract surgery, there are some additional considerations for planning and performing the procedure, as the primary surgical goal is refractive rather than restoration of vision lost due to cataract. In contrast to keratorefractive procedures, which are usually performed bilaterally in the same surgical session, RLE is usually performed as sequential surgery on separate days to minimize the potential for bilateral endophthalmitis. However, practices continue to evolve, and some surgeons are performing bilateral RLE in the same surgical session.

Preoperative corneal topography is essential to detect irregular astigmatism and to identify patients with corneal ectatic disorders, such as keratoconus and pellucid marginal degeneration. Patients with these conditions may still have RLE performed; however, they must understand the limits of vision correction obtainable and that the quality of vision may still suffer postoperatively from their irregular astigmatism. These patients must further understand that they are not good candidates for postoperative treatment with LASIK or photorefractive keratectomy to refine the refractive correction.

Surgeons must identify the degree of corneal versus lenticular astigmatism present, as only the corneal astigmatism will remain postoperatively. The patient should be informed if substantial astigmatism is expected to remain after surgery, and a plan should be devised to correct it in order to optimize the visual outcome. Small amounts of corneal astigmatism (<1.00 D) may be reduced if the incision is placed in the steep meridian.

Limbal relaxing incisions and arcuate keratotomies with either blade or femtosecond laser may be used to correct residual corneal astigmatism of less than 2.00 D (see Chapter 3). Supplemental surface ablation or LASIK could also be considered (see the following discussion on bioptics). Although glasses or contact lenses are an alternative for managing residual astigmatism, refractive surgery patients frequently reject this option.

Some surgeons obtain preoperative retinal OCT to identify potential macular pathology. Careful attention should be paid to the peripheral retinal examination, especially in patients with higher myopia. If relevant pathology is discovered, appropriate treatment or referral to a retina specialist is warranted. In patients with high axial myopia, retrobulbar injections should be performed with caution because of the risk of perforating the globe. Peribulbar, sub-Tenon, topical, and intracameral anesthesia are alternative options.

Most surgeons believe that an IOL should be implanted after RLE in a patient with high myopia rather than leaving the patient with aphakia, even when little or no optical power correction is required. Plano power IOLs are available if indicated. The IOL acts as a barrier to anterior prolapse of the vitreous, maintaining the integrity of the aqueous–vitreous barrier, in the event that Nd:YAG laser posterior capsulotomy is required. Some IOL models also reduce the rate of posterior capsule opacification.

Intraocular Lens Power Calculations in Refractive Lens Exchange

High patient expectations for excellent uncorrected visual acuity (UCVA; also called *uncorrected distance visual acuity, UDVA*) after RLE make accurate IOL power determination crucial. However, IOL power formulas are less accurate at higher levels of myopia and hyperopia. In addition, in high myopia, a posterior staphyloma can make the axial length measurements less reliable. Careful fundus examination and B-scan ultrasound imaging can identify the position and extent of staphylomas. The subject of IOL power determination is covered in greater detail in BCSC Section 3, *Clinical Optics,* and Section 11, *Lens and Cataract.*

In the case of a patient with high hyperopia, biometry may suggest an IOL power beyond what is commercially available. The upper limit of commercially available IOL power is now +40.00 D. A special-order IOL of a higher power may be available or may be designed, but acquiring or designing such a lens usually requires the approval of the institutional review board at the hospital or surgical center, which delays the surgery. Another option is to use a "piggyback" IOL system, in which 2 posterior chamber IOLs are inserted. One IOL is placed in the capsular bag, and the other is placed in the ciliary sulcus. When piggyback IOLs are used, the combined power may need to be increased +1.50 to +2.00 D to compensate for the posterior shift of the posterior IOL. One serious complication of piggyback IOLs is the potential for developing an interlenticular opaque membrane. These membranes cannot be mechanically removed or cleared with the Nd:YAG laser; the IOLs must be removed. Interlenticular membranes have occurred most commonly between 2 acrylic IOLs, especially when both IOLs are placed in the capsular bag. When piggyback lenses are used, they should be of different materials, ideally with one IOL placed in the bag and the other in the sulcus. Piggyback IOLs may also shallow the anterior chamber and increase the risk of iris chafing, especially in smaller eyes.

Hill WE, Byrne SF. Complex axial length measurements and unusual IOL power calculations. *Focal Points: Clinical Modules for Ophthalmologists.* San Francisco: American Academy of Ophthalmology; 2004, module 9.

Shammas HJ. IOL power calculation in patients with prior corneal refractive surgery. *Focal Points: Clinical Modules for Ophthalmologists.* San Francisco: American Academy of Ophthalmology; 2013, module 6.

Complications

The intraoperative and postoperative complications for RLE are identical to those of cataract surgery. See BCSC Section 11, *Lens and Cataract,* Chapter 8, for a comprehensive discussion of this topic.

Monofocal Intraocular Lenses

For some patients, the best IOL choice for implantation at the time of RLE is a monofocal IOL. There are a variety of IOL choices and styles available, and all are utilized in routine cataract surgery as well (see BCSC Section 11, *Lens and Cataract,* for more detail). Patients without significant corneal astigmatism who desire best distance vision only, or individuals who have tolerated monovision well in the past and want it re-created after cataract surgery, are generally the best candidates for monofocal IOL implantation.

Toric Intraocular Lenses

Residual astigmatism after cataract surgery impacts visual function and patient satisfaction. Large population analyses indicate that more than 50% of patients have 0.75 D or more corneal astigmatism at presentation for cataract surgery, and 15%–29% have 1.50 D or more corneal astigmatism. Thus, toric IOLs can address a major need for vision correction after crystalline lens removal. Current toric IOLs in the United States generally come in powers that can correct from 1.00 to 4.00 D of astigmatism at the spectacle plane, and wider power ranges are available outside the United States; however, this range is continually evolving.

Patient Selection

A toric IOL is appropriate for patients with regular corneal astigmatism, currently up to 4.00 D at the corneal plane (United States). Patients with astigmatism exceeding the upper correction limits require additional measures to obtain full correction. In addition to understanding the risks associated with intraocular surgery, patients must be capable of understanding the limitations of a toric IOL. Not all patients with toric IOL implantation achieve spectacle independence for distance vision. Further, patients should be informed that toric IOL implantation will not eliminate the need for reading glasses (unless monovision is planned). The patient also needs to be informed that the IOL may rotate in the capsular bag shortly after surgery and that an additional procedure may be required to reposition it. A silicone toric IOL may be less appropriate for patients who may carry a significant potential of requiring silicone oil for retinal detachment repair in the future; thus, nonsilicone IOLs are more appropriate choices for these patients.

Planning and Surgical Technique

The amount, axis, and regularity of the astigmatism should be measured accurately. First, corneal topography should be examined to determine the regularity and axis of astigmatism and to identify eyes with irregular astigmatism or ectatic disease. Keratometry should be used to confirm the corneal power axis and provide the primary data for corneal astigmatic power. The axis of astigmatism from the refraction should not be the sole source for axis or power determination, but should be considered in context with topographic and keratometric measurements.

Significant disagreement between measurements should prompt re-examination of the clinical data and may also suggest the effect of lenticular astigmatism or posterior corneal astigmatism. Posterior corneal astigmatism may vary widely from patient to patient, but may add 0.3–0.5 D of net against-the-rule astigmatic power in 80% of patients. While technology to accurately measure the posterior corneal astigmatism is evolving, surgeons may use regression formulas, such as the Baylor nomogram, or theoretical formulas, such as the Barrett toric IOL formula (available at www.ascrs.org/barrett-toric-calculator) to help compensate for the tendency of anterior corneal measurements to overestimate the with-the-rule corneal power and underestimate the against-the-rule corneal power. Intraoperative aberrometry may be useful in these cases.

The manufacturers of toric IOLs have online software available to aid in surgical planning. After the surgeon enters data such as keratometry measurements, axes, IOL spherical power generated by A-scan, average surgeon-induced astigmatism, and axis of astigmatism, these programs will generate the recommended power and model lens as well as orientation of the lens.

There are many ways that surgeons mark the cornea prior to surgery. The surgeon should establish and mark the vertical and/or horizontal meridians with the patient in an upright position to avoid potential misalignment resulting from torsional globe rotation, which sometimes occurs in the supine position. Intraoperative alignment systems are available. Cataract surgery with a wound that induces a predictable amount of astigmatism is necessary to achieve the intended benefit of a toric lens. All online toric IOL software requires input of the expected surgically induced astigmatism for lens power calculations.

After the IOL is injected into the capsular bag, the viscoelastic behind the IOL is aspirated and the IOL is rotated into position on the steep meridian. Some surgeons prefer to leave the toric IOL purposely underrotated by 10°–20° and then rotate it into position after all viscoelastic substance has been removed; others position the IOL in its planned orientation and then hold it in place with a variety of techniques while removing the viscoelastic material. If the IOL rotates beyond its appropriate position, it will need to be fully rotated around again, as the 1-piece IOLs tend not to rotate well against their haptics. This maneuver should be performed using irrigation or viscoelastic material to prevent capsule rupture during rotation.

Koch DD, Jenkins R, Weikert MP, Yeu E, Wang L, Correcting astigmatism with toric intraocular lenses: effect of posterior corneal astigmatism. *J Cataract Refract Surg.* 2013; 39(12):1803–1809.

Outcomes

In clinical trials of a 1-piece acrylic toric IOL, data provided by the FDA indicated uncorrected acuity of greater than 20/40 in 93.8% of 198 patients implanted with the IOL (all sizes combined). With the plate-haptic IOL, postoperative astigmatism was less than 0.50 D in 48% of patients and less than 1.00 D in 75%–81% of patients; results were 61.6% and 87.7%, respectively, for the 1-piece acrylic toric IOL.

For those patients with corneal astigmatism greater than that correctable by toric IOLs, surgeons may opt to simultaneously or sequentially correct residual astigmatism with incisional or laser procedures.

Lane SS, Ernest P, Miller KM, Hileman KS, Harris B, Waycaster CR. Comparison of clinical and patient-reported outcomes with bilateral AcrySof toric or spherical control intraocular lenses. *J Refract Surg.* 2009;25(10):899–901.

Complications Specific to Toric Intraocular Lenses

The primary complication of toric IOLs is the possibility of IOL rotation resulting in a misalignment of the astigmatic correction. Full correction is not achieved unless the IOL is properly aligned in the axis of astigmatism. Astigmatism calculations have shown that every 10° off-axis rotation of the lens reduces the correction by approximately one-third. Thus, at 30° the lens is functionally astigmatically neutral, and IOL misalignment greater than 30° can increase the cylindrical refractive error. In the FDA clinical trials for a plate-haptic toric IOL, 76% of lenses were within 10° of preoperative alignment, and 95% were within 30°. In the FDA clinical trials for the 1-piece acrylic toric IOL, the degree of post-operative rotation in 242 implanted eyes was 5° or less in 81.1% and 10° or less in 97.1%. None of the eyes exhibited postoperative rotation greater than 15°.

Typically, a misaligned IOL is recognized within days of the surgery; it should be repositioned before permanent fibrosis occurs within the capsular bag. However, waiting 1 week for some capsule contraction to occur may ultimately help stabilize this IOL. An online calculator is available to help determine the exact amount of IOL rotation necessary to optimize visual outcome (www.astigmatismfix.com).

Visser N, Ruíz-Mesa R, Pastor F, Bauer NJ, Nuijts RM, Montés-Micó R. Cataract surgery with toric intraocular lens implantation in patients with high corneal astigmatism. *J Cataract Refract Surg.* 2011;37(8):1403–1410.

Light-Adjustable Intraocular Lenses

The light-adjustable IOL is a 3-piece silicone-optic posterior chamber IOL that can be ir-radiated with ultraviolet light through a slit-lamp delivery system 1–2 weeks after implantation to induce a change in the shape, and thus the power, of the IOL (Fig 8-5). This lens is not currently FDA approved but is available for use outside the United States. Specific irradiation patterns can be applied to the lens to induce myopic, hyperopic, and astigmatic shifts. In initial work, results indicate that up to 5.00 D of spherical and up to 2.00 D of astigmatic change can be induced. Once final irradiation is performed, the effect is "locked in" and no further adjustments can be made.

Prior to postoperative irradiation, the lens must be protected from sunlight exposure. Further, it seems possible that an error in the irradiation treatment related to centration

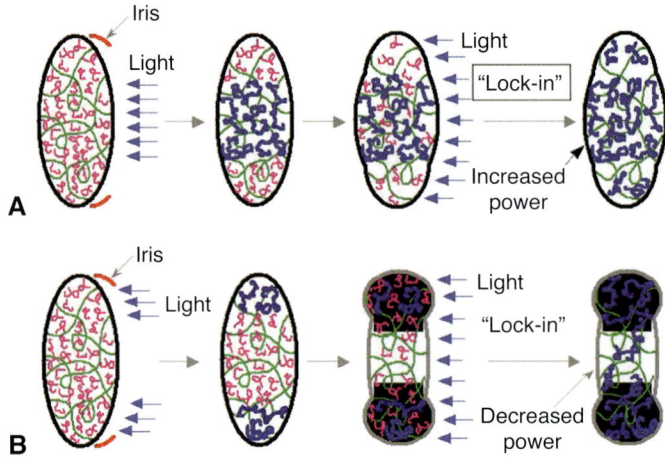

Figure 8-5 Schematic representation of the light-adjustable IOL. **A,** When the IOL is treated with UV light in the center, polymerization occurs and macromers move to the center, increasing the IOL power. **B,** When the IOL is treated with light in the periphery, macromers move to the periphery, decreasing the IOL power. *(Courtesy of Calhoun Vision.)*

or improper data entry could cause irreversible changes in the IOL's visual properties and require IOL exchange surgery. Despite the refractive alterations available initially, after irradiation, the lens is functionally a monofocal IOL with all the limitations that come from that implantation strategy. See also Chapter 9.

Accommodating Intraocular Lenses

Accommodating lenses are another alternative for implantation during refractive lens exchange. Currently, only 1 accommodating IOL and a similar accommodating toric IOL are FDA approved, although others are being investigated. Development is also currently under way for dual-optic IOLs and deformable IOLs. Additional investigational IOLs are discussed in Chapter 9.

Although the accommodating lens was designed to improve distance, intermediate, and near acuity through movement of its hinged haptics during the accommodative process, studies have found limited IOL movement and limited improvement in near acuity for most patients targeted for best distance acuity. Thus, many surgeons are utilizing a "mini-monovision" strategy when implanting the accommodating IOL, leaving the nondominant eye targeted for slight myopia (−0.50 to −0.75 D).

Gooi P, Ahmed IK. Review of presbyopic IOLs: multifocal and accommodating IOLs. *Int Ophthalmol Clin.* 2012;52(2):41–50.

Hoffman RS, Fine IH, Packer M. Accommodating IOLs: current technology, limitations, and future designs. *Current Insight.* San Francisco: American Academy of Ophthalmology. Available at www.aao.org/current-insight/accommodating-iols-current-technology -limitations-. Accessed November 6, 2016.

Multifocal Intraocular Lenses

Multifocal intraocular lenses have the ability to provide appropriate patients with functional vision at near, intermediate, and far distances in each eye. This ability is due to lens multifocality that causes light rays to be split such that different focal points are created where objects will be clearest. However, all have potential trade-offs in vision quality and adverse effects, especially at night, and careful patient selection and counseling are necessary to achieve optimal outcomes. These types of lenses and their outcomes are discussed further in Chapter 9.

Patient Selection

Patients who are likely to be successful candidates for an MFIOL implant after lens surgery tend to be adaptable, less visually demanding, and place a high value on reduced spectacle dependence at all distances. In addition, they should have good potential vision without significant pathology anywhere along the visual axis. Specific preoperative evaluation of macular function and anatomy may be warranted to exclude patients with macular degeneration, epiretinal membrane, or other conditions leading to suboptimal retinal function. Careful attention should be paid to evaluation of the corneal endothelium, as patients with Fuchs dystrophy may not be ideal candidates for MFIOLs. Significant anterior basement membrane dystrophy or tear film abnormality from dry eye syndrome or blepharitis may also adversely affect postoperative performance of these lenses. Patients with more than 0.75 D residual astigmatism after MFIOL implantation frequently have suboptimal vision quality. If this result is expected, strategies to reduce postoperative astigmatism should be evaluated and discussed before IOL implantation. Evidence has shown that patients generally have better visual outcomes if MFIOLs are implanted bilaterally.

> Cionni RJ, Osher RH, Snyder ME, Nordlund ML. Visual outcome comparison of unilateral versus bilateral implantation of apodized diffractive multifocal intraocular lenses after cataract extraction: prospective 6-month study. *J Cataract Refract Surg.* 2009;35(6): 1033–1039.

Surgical Technique

The surgical technique for MFIOL insertion is the same as that used in standard small-incision cataract surgery with a foldable acrylic IOL. MFIOLs are much more sensitive than are monofocal IOLs to minor optic decentration. If the posterior capsule is not intact, IOL decentration is more likely to occur, and adequate fixation for an MFIOL should be determined before implantation.

Outcomes

Patients are most likely to achieve independence from glasses after bilateral implantation of MFIOLs. Recent meta-analyses found bilateral MFIOL implantation associated with significant improvement in both distance and near visual acuity with each type of implant studied.

As patients age, the pupillary diameter may decrease. If the pupillary diameter decreases to less than 2.0 mm, unaided reading ability may diminish. Gentle dilation with topical mydriatic drugs or laser photomydriasis may restore near acuity. Photomydriasis may be performed with an argon or dye photocoagulator, by placing green laser burns circumferentially outside the iris sphincter, or with a Nd:YAG photodisruptor, by creating approximately 4 partial sphincterotomies.

Agresta B, Knorz MC, Kohnen T, Donatti C, Jackson D. Distance and near visual acuity improvement after implantation of multifocal intraocular lenses in cataract patients with presbyopia: a systematic review. *J Refract Surg.* 2012;28:426–435.

Adverse Effects, Complications, and Patient Dissatisfaction With Multifocal Intraocular Lenses

Patient concerns after MFIOL implantation can generally be divided into 2 categories: blurred vision and photic phenomena (glare, halos). Patients may experience both groups of symptoms. These symptoms can occur even after uneventful surgery with a well-centered MFIOL.

Patients with MFIOLs are more likely to have significant glare, halos, and ghosting than are patients with monofocal, toric, or accommodating IOLs. These issues stem from a variety of different etiologies, including residual refractive error, ocular surface disease, or intrinsic IOL problems. The reports of halos intrinsically related to the IOL tend to subside over several months, perhaps from the patient's neural adaptation, but they may be persistent. Because of a reduction in contrast sensitivity, the subjective quality of vision after MFIOL insertion may not be as good as after monofocal IOL implantation. The trade-off of decreased quality of vision in return for reduced dependence on glasses must be discussed fully with the patient preoperatively. With MFIOLs, intermediate vision may be less clear than distance or near acuity.

Some patients never adapt to MFIOLs and require IOL exchange to recover vision. All patients should be counseled as to this possibility before surgery. Patients with MFIOLs appear to be more sensitive to posterior capsule opacification (PCO) than are individuals with monofocal IOLs. These patients benefit from Nd:YAG capsulotomy; however, tolerance of the MFIOL must be determined before undergoing the Nd:YAG capsulotomy, as an open posterior capsule significantly complicates IOL exchange. Intrinsic IOL symptoms usually appear very early if not immediately in the postoperative course and do not generally worsen over time. In contrast, symptoms from PCO are not present initially but gradually worsen over the first few weeks to months after the surgical procedure.

Braga-Mele R, Chang D, Dewey S, et al; ASCRS Cataract Clinical Committee. Multifocal intraocular lenses: relative indications and contraindications for implantation. *J Cataract Refract Surg.* 2014;40(2):313–322.

Packer M, Chu YR, Waltz KL, et al. Evaluation of the aspheric Tecnis multifocal intraocular lens: one-year results from the first cohort of the Food and Drug Administration clinical trial. *Am J Ophthalmol.* 2010;149(4):577–584.

Rosenfeld SI, O'Brien TP. The dissatisfied presbyopia-correcting IOL patient. *Focal Points: Clinical Modules for Ophthalmologists.* San Francisco: American Academy of Ophthalmology; 2011, module 8.

Bioptics

The term *bioptics* was suggested by Zaldivar in the late 1990s. It is used to describe the combination of 2 refractive procedures—1 intraocular and 1 corneal—to treat patients with refractive errors that are suboptimally treated with a single procedure. Examples include extreme myopia, high myopia or hyperopia with significant astigmatism, and MFIOL implantation in patients with significant astigmatism. In these cases, the intraocular procedure is performed first, with keratorefractive surgery performed after both anatomical and refractive stability are achieved, usually 1–3 months after the initial surgery.

Bioptics with LASIK or surface ablation are reasonable alternatives, depending on patient parameters. As new treatment options are developed, the possibilities for other combinations of refractive surgery will increase.

The ability to successfully combine refractive procedures further expands the limits of refractive surgery. The predictability, stability, and safety of LASIK increase when smaller refractive errors are treated. In addition, there is usually sufficient corneal tissue to maximize the treatment zone diameter without exceeding the limits of ablation depth. The LASIK procedure provides the feature of adjustability in the overall refractive operation. These benefits must be balanced against the combined risks of performing 2 surgical procedures rather than 1.

Alfonso JF, Fernández-Vega L, Montés-Micó R, Valcárcel B. Femtosecond laser for residual refractive error correction after refractive lens exchange with multifocal intraocular lens implantation. *Am J Ophthalmol.* 2008;146(2):244–250.

CHAPTER 9

Accommodative and Nonaccommodative Treatment of Presbyopia

▶ *This chapter includes a related video, which can be accessed by scanning the QR code provided in the text or going to www.aao.org/bcscvideo_section13.*

Introduction

Presbyopia, the normal progressive loss of accommodation, affects all individuals beginning in middle age, regardless of any underlying refractive error. This relentless loss of near vision and dependency on glasses for near work may be particularly distressing for individuals with emmetropic vision who have previously enjoyed excellent uncorrected vision at all distances.

Interest in developing a surgical correction for presbyopia has resulted in several treatment options. Some of these techniques rely on scleral modification, some use implantation of presbyopia-correcting intraocular lenses (IOLs), and others depend on the creation of a multifocal cornea by use of lasers or corneal stromal modifications. More recently, the development of corneal inlays has introduced a new option for patients.

Theories of Accommodation

The *Helmholtz hypothesis* or *capsular theory* of accommodation states that during distance vision the ciliary muscle is relaxed and the zonular fibers that cross the circumlental space between the ciliary body and the lens equator are in a state of "resting" tension. With accommodative effort, an anterior movement of the ciliary muscle annular ring and a release of tension on the zonules occur, increasing the accommodative power of the lens. An anterior movement of the ciliary muscle annular ring also takes place during accommodation. The reduced zonular tension allows the elastic capsule of the lens to contract, causing a decrease in equatorial lens diameter and an increase in the curvature of the anterior and posterior lens surfaces. This "rounding up" of the lens yields a corresponding increase in its dioptric power, as is necessary for near vision (Fig 9-1).

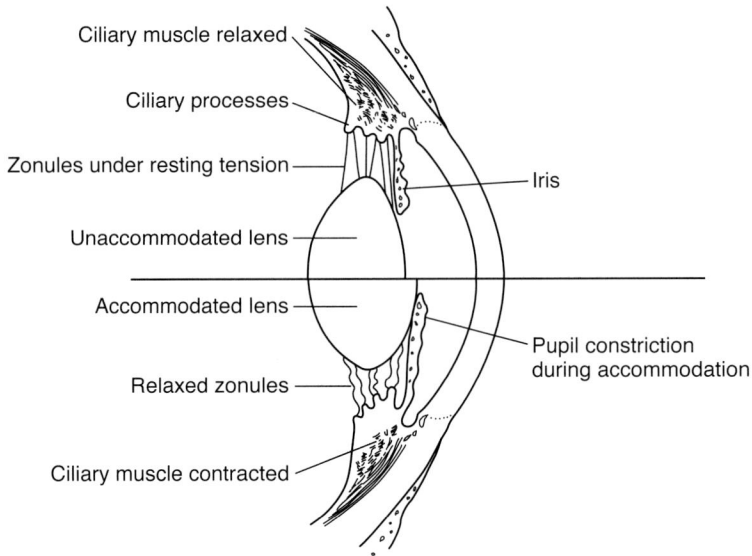

Ciliary muscle relaxed

Ciliary processes

Zonules under resting tension

Iris

Unaccommodated lens

Accommodated lens

Pupil constriction
during accommodation

Relaxed zonules

Ciliary muscle contracted

Figure 9-1 Schematic representation of the Helmholtz theory of accommodation, in which contraction of the ciliary muscle during accommodation *(bottom)* leads to relaxation of the zonular fibers. The reduced zonular tension allows the elastic capsule of the lens to contract, causing an increase in the curvature of the anterior and posterior lens. *(Illustration by Jeanne Koelling.)*

When the accommodative effort ceases, the ciliary muscle relaxes and the zonular tension on the lens equator increases to its resting state. This increased tension on the lens equator causes a flattening of the lens, a decrease in the curvature of the anterior and posterior lens surfaces, and a decrease in the dioptric power of the unaccommodated eye.

In the Helmholtz theory, the equatorial edge of the lens moves away from the sclera during accommodation and toward the sclera when accommodation ends. In this theory, all zonular fibers are relaxed during accommodation and under tension when the accommodative effort ends. According to Helmholtz, presbyopia results from the loss of lens elasticity with age. When the zonules of an older lens are relaxed, the lens does not change its shape to the same degree as a younger lens does; therefore, presbyopia is an aging process that can be reversed only by changing the elasticity of the lens or its capsule.

Diametrically opposed to the Helmholtz hypothesis is the *Schachar theory* of accommodation. Schachar suggested that during accommodation ciliary muscle contraction leads to a selective increase in equatorial zonular tension—rather than to the uniform decrease (anterior, equatorial, and posterior) proposed by the Helmholtz theory—with a subsequent pulling of the equatorial lens outward toward the sclera (Fig 9-2). Schachar postulated that accommodation occurs through the direct effect of zonular tension (as opposed to the passive effect proposed by Helmholtz), causing an increase in lens curvature. In this theory, the loss of accommodation with age is a result of the continued growth of the lens, leading to an increase in lens diameter and a decrease in the lens–ciliary body distance, which in turn cause a loss of zonular tension. Anything that increases resting zonular tension (eg, scleral expansion) should restore accommodation.

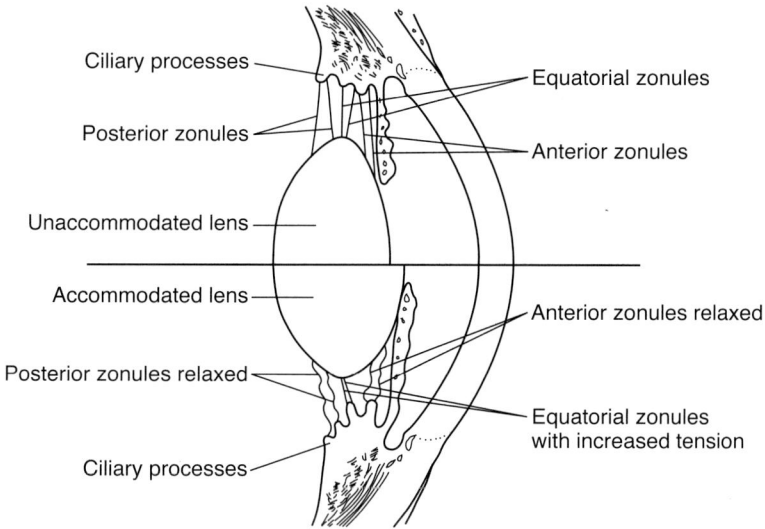

Figure 9-2 Schematic depiction of the Schachar theory of accommodation, which proposes that only the equatorial zonules are under tension during accommodation and that the anterior and posterior zonular fibers serve solely as passive support structures for the lens. *(Illustration by Jeanne Koelling.)*

Schachar proposed that the mechanism for functional lens shape change is equatorial stretching by the zonules, which would decrease the peripheral lens volume and increase the central volume, thereby causing central steepening of the anterior central lens capsule (Fig 9-3). During accommodation and ciliary muscle contraction, tension on the equatorial zonular fibers increases, whereas tension on the anterior and posterior zonules decreases. These actions would allow the lens to maintain a stable position at all times, even as it undergoes changes in shape. Schachar theorized that the anterior and posterior zonules serve as passive support structures for the lens but that the equatorial zonules are what actively determine the optical power of the lens.

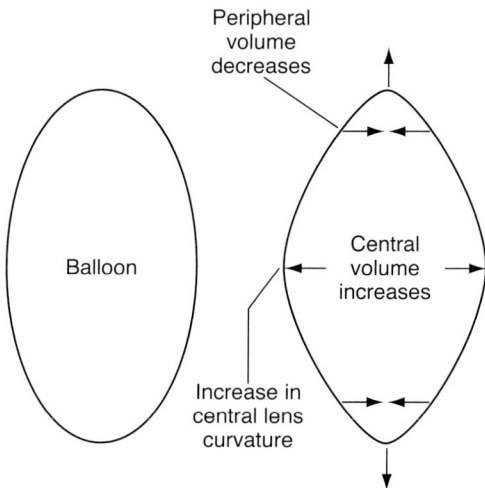

Figure 9-3 The Schachar theory of accommodation proposes that an increase in equatorial zonular tension causes a decrease in peripheral lens volume and, thus, an increase in central lens volume and central lens curvature. *(Illustration by Jeanne Koelling.)*

Evidence from recent studies on human and nonhuman primates contests Schachar's theories of accommodation and presbyopia. Investigations in human tissues and with scanning electron microscopy reveal no zonular insertions (equatorial or otherwise) at the iris root or anterior ciliary muscle. Various imaging techniques have consistently demonstrated that the diameter of the crystalline lens decreases with accommodation so that the equator moves away from the ciliary body. In vitro laser scanning imaging shows that the crystalline lens does not change focal length when increasing and decreasing radial stretching forces are applied. This evidence thus contradicts Schachar's proposal that the lens remains pliable with age and that presbyopia is due solely to lens growth and crowding that prevents optimum ciliary muscle action.

Using model-based reasoning, Goldberg proposed another theory of accommodation with the help of a computer-animated 3-dimensional (3-D) model of the eye and the accommodative system. Goldberg's *theory of reciprocal zonular action* describes 3 components of the zonules and posits that a synchronized movement among the ciliary body, zonules, and anterior hyaloid complex leads to a shift in the posterior lenticular curvature and refractive power (Video 9-1).

VIDEO 9-1 Theory of reciprocal zonular action.
Courtesy of Daniel B. Goldberg, MD.
Access all Section 13 videos at www.aao.org/bcscvideo_section13.

Glasser A, Kaufman PL. The mechanism of accommodation in primates. *Ophthalmology.* 1999; 106(5):863–872.

Goldberg DB. Computer-animated model of accommodation and theory of reciprocal zonular action. *Clin Ophthalmol.* 2011;5:1559–1566.

Schachar RA. Cause and treatment of presbyopia with a method for increasing the amplitude of accommodation. *Ann Ophthalmol.* 1992;24(12):445–447, 452.

Strenk SA, Strenk LM, Koretz JF. The mechanism of presbyopia. *Prog Retin Eye Res.* 2005; 24(3):379–393.

Accommodative Treatment of Presbyopia

Scleral Surgery

Several scleral surgical procedures have been evaluated for use in the reduction of presbyopia. They share the objective of attempting to increase zonular tension by weakening or altering the sclera over the ciliary body to allow for its passive expansion. Thornton first proposed weakening the sclera by creating 8 or more scleral incisions over the ciliary body (anterior ciliary sclerotomy, ACS). Results were mixed, and any positive effect appeared short-lived. A prospective study of ACS using a 4-incision technique was discontinued because of significant adverse events, including anterior segment ischemia. In 2001, the American Academy of Ophthalmology stated that ACS was ineffective and a potentially dangerous treatment for presbyopia. Another method involving the placement of scleral expansion bands is under study (Fig 9-4). The LaserACE procedure (Ace Vision Group Inc., Silver Lake, OH) employs a laser to increase the plasticity of the sclera over the ciliary body in order to increase the efficiency of accommodation. This technique is under investigation.

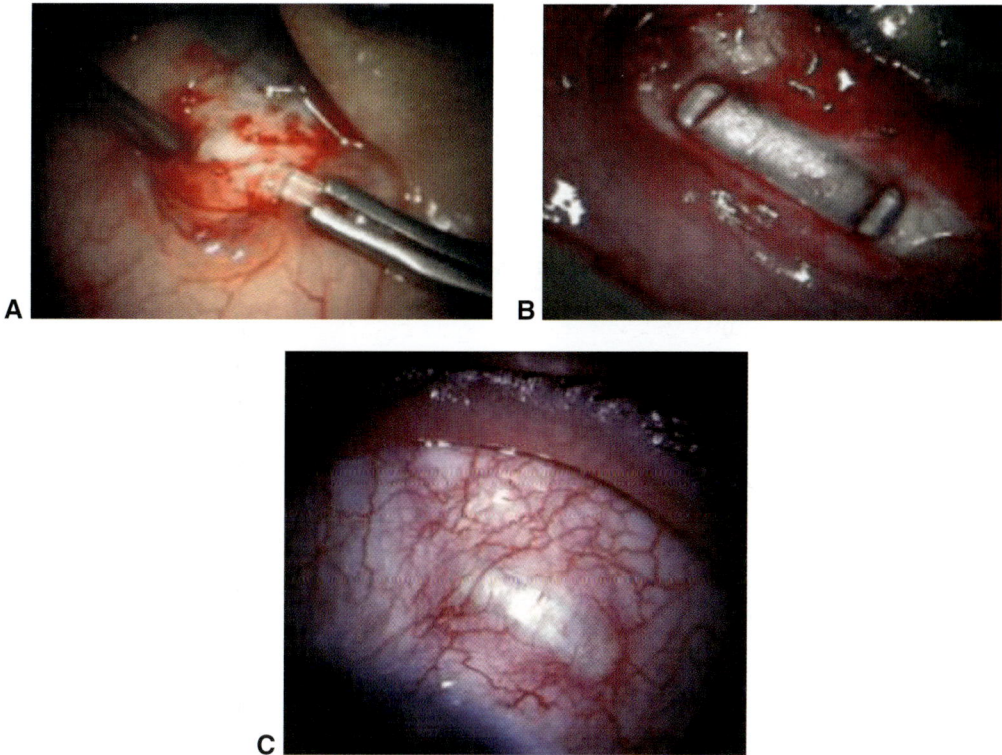

Figure 9-4 **A,** The scleral expansion band is inserted in a scleral tunnel over the ciliary body parallel to the limbus. **B,** The appearance of the band after placement, prior to conjunctival closure. **C,** The appearance of the well-healed band. *(Courtesy of Refocus Group.)*

Hamilton DR, Davidorf JM, Maloney RK. Anterior ciliary sclerotomy for treatment of pres-byopia: a prospective controlled study. *Ophthalmology.* 2002;109(11):1970–1977.

Kleinmann G, Kim HJ, Yee RW. Scleral expansion procedure for the correction of presbyopia. *Int Ophthalmol Clin.* 2006;46(3):1–12.

Accommodating Intraocular Lenses

Accommodating IOLs attempt to restore a significant amount of true accommodation to patients with surgically induced pseudophakia. Accommodating IOLs were designed fol-lowing the observation that some patients who received silicone-plate IOLs reported bet-ter near vision than that expected from their refractive result. Investigations revealed that, during ciliary muscle contraction, forward displacement of the IOL led to an increase in the IOL's effective power and thus an improvement in near vision. However, some studies have questioned the amplitude of true accommodation that can be expected solely on the basis of anterior displacement of the IOL optic. Other factors, such as pupil size, with-the-rule astigmatism, and mild myopia, may also contribute to unaided near visual acuity and increased depth of focus.

Some IOLs that use this accommodative approach are modified silicone plate–haptic lenses (Fig 9-5). These lenses may allow anterior movement of the lens during accom-modation. Another possibility is that ciliary body contraction causes a steepening of the

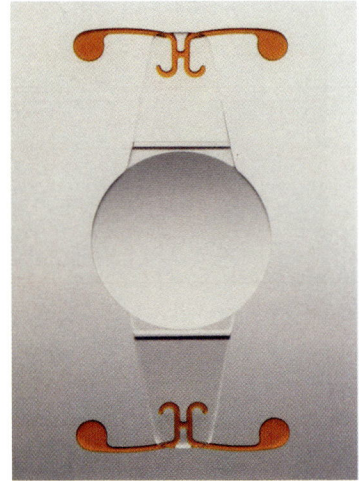

Figure 9-5 Example of an intraocular lens with a flexible hinge in the haptic at the proximal end and a polyamide footplate at the distal end. The footplate functions to maximize contact with the capsule and ciliary body, and the hinge transfers the horizontal force into an anteroposterior movement of the optic. *(Courtesy of Eyeonics, acquired by Bausch + Lomb.)*

anterior optic surface, allowing for better near vision. Although the exact cause of the movement is unclear, it appears to be a combination of posterior chamber pressure on the back surface of the IOL and ciliary body pressure on the IOL that vaults the optic forward. The anterior displacement is postulated to result in an effective increase in optical power and near vision.

Findl O, Kiss B, Petternel V, et al. Intraocular lens movement caused by ciliary muscle contraction. *J Cataract Refract Surg.* 2003;29(4):669–676.

Langenbucher A, Huber S, Nguyen NX, Seitz B, Gusek-Schneider GC, Küchle M. Measurement of accommodation after implantation of an accommodating posterior chamber intraocular lens. *J Cataract Refract Surg.* 2003;29(4):677–685.

Nonaccommodative Treatment of Presbyopia

Monovision

In the United States, monovision is the technique used most frequently for the nonspectacle correction of presbyopia. In this approach, the refractive power of 1 eye is adjusted to improve near vision. Monovision may be achieved with contact lenses, laser in situ keratomileusis (LASIK), surface ablation (photorefractive keratectomy [PRK]), conductive keratoplasty (CK), or even lens surgery. Historically, the term *monovision* typically referred to the use of a distance contact lens in 1 eye and a near contact lens in the other. A power difference between the eyes of 1.25–2.50 diopters (D) was targeted on the basis of near visual acuity demands. Many refractive surgeons target mild myopia (−0.50 to −1.50 D) for the near-vision eye in the presbyopic and prepresbyopic population. The term *modified monovision,* or *mini-monovision,* is more appropriate for this lower level of myopia for the near-vision eye. Mini-monovision is associated with only a mild decrease in distance vision, retention of good stereopsis, and a significant increase in the intermediate zone of functional vision. The intermediate zone is where many visual functions used in daily life occur (eg, looking at a computer screen, store shelves, or a car dashboard). For many patients, this compromise is an attractive alternative to constantly reaching for reading glasses. Selected patients who want better near vision may prefer greater monovision correction (–1.50 to –2.50 D) despite the accompanying decrease in distance vision and stereopsis. The clinician should counsel the patient that leaving 1 eye undercorrected may lead to glare and halos when driving at night. This can be corrected by giving patients driving glasses.

Patient selection

Appropriate patient selection and education are fundamental to the overall success of monovision treatment. Although monovision can be demonstrated with trial lenses in the examination room, a contact lens trial period at home is often more useful. Patients whose vision is neither presbyopic nor approaching presbyopia are typically not good candidates for monovision, as they are usually seeking optimal bilateral distance visual acuity. However, patients in their mid- to late 30s should be counseled about impending presbyopia and the option of monovision.

The best candidates for monovision are patients with myopia who are older than 40 years and who, because of their current refractive error, retain some useful uncorrected near vision. These patients have always experienced adequate near vision simply by removing their glasses and therefore understand the importance of near vision. Patients who do not have useful uncorrected near vision (ie, patients with myopia worse than –4.50 D, high astigmatism, or hyperopia; or contact lens wearers) may be more accepting of the need for reading glasses after refractive surgery. For most patients, refractive surgeons routinely aim for mild myopia (–0.50 to –0.75 D, occasionally up to –1.50 D) in the nondominant eye. It is prudent to give the patient a trial with contact lenses to ascertain patient acceptance and the exact degree of near vision desired. Patients should understand that loss of accommodation is progressive and that, as a result, monovision may not be permanent and corrective glasses may eventually be required.

Reinstein DZ, Carp GI, Archer TJ, Gobbe M. LASIK for presbyopia correction in emmetropic patients using aspheric ablation profiles and a micro-monovision protocol with the Carl Zeiss Meditec MEL 80 and VisuMax. *J Refract Surg*. 2012;28(8):531–541.

Rocha KM, Vabre L, Chateau N, Krueger RR. Expanding depth of focus by modifying higher-order aberrations induced by an adaptive optics visual simulator. *J Cataract Refract Surg*. 2009;35(11):1885–1892.

Conductive Keratoplasty

As discussed in Chapter 7, CK is a nonablative, collagen-shrinking procedure approved for the correction of low levels of hyperopia (+0.75 to +3.25 D). This procedure has been approved by the US Food and Drug Administration (FDA) for the treatment of presbyopia in individuals with hyperopic or emmetropic vision.

Multifocal Intraocular Lens Implants

The number of IOL options for patients undergoing cataract surgery has increased in recent years. Patients may select a traditional monofocal IOL with a refractive target of emmetropia, mild myopia, or monovision, or they may opt for a multifocal or accommodating IOL for greater range of focus.

Several multifocal IOLs (MFIOLs) are FDA approved in the United States. Since the first IOL was introduced, lens design has evolved to include *zonal refractive* and *apodized diffractive IOLs*. The zonal refractive lens design uses refractive power changes from the center of the lens to the periphery to provide distance and near correction. In contrast, diffractive lens designs employ a series of concentric rings to form a diffraction grating (see BCSC Section 3, *Clinical Optics*) to create 2 separate focal points for distance and near vision (Fig 9-6). Some diffractive lenses are apodized, meaning that the diffractive step heights are gradually tapered to yield a more even distribution of light, theoretically allowing for a smoother transition among images from distance to intermediate and near targets. An example of a zonal refractive lens is the ReZoom lens (Johnson & Johnson Vision, Santa Ana, CA), no longer available in the United States. Various styles are available in Europe. Examples of this type of lens include the M-*flex* T (Rayner, Hove, United Kingdom) and the LENTIS Mplus (Oculentis GmbH, Berlin, Germany) (Fig 9-7). IOLs with extended depth of focus (EDOF) and trifocal optics are also available in Europe; examples are the TECNIS Symfony (Johnson & Johnson Vision), FineVision (PhysIOL, Liège, Belgium), and the AT LISA tri (Carl Zeiss Meditec AG, Jena, Germany).

Maisel WH. TECNIS Symfony extended range of vision intraocular lens - P980040/S065.
US Food and Drug Administration website. Available at https://goo.gl/7pzDz0. Accessed
November 6, 2016.

Patient selection

The clinician should have a comprehensive discussion with each patient regarding the benefits and visual outcomes of MFIOLs to ensure that the patient has realistic expectations. The preoperative examination is equally crucial as it is critical to rule out any macular or

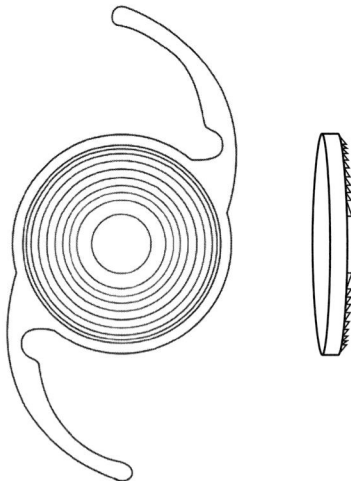

Figure 9-6 Example of a diffractive multifocal intraocular lens. *Left,* schematic of the frontal view. *Right,* schematic of the side view. *(Left image courtesy of Abbott Medical Optics Inc.)*

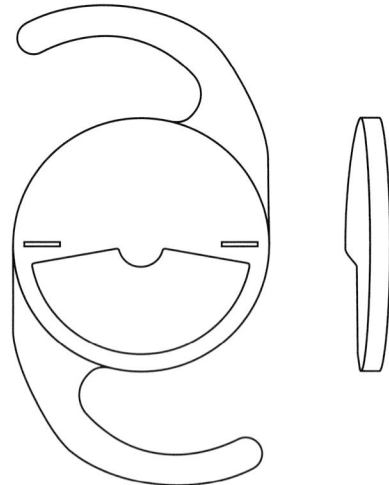

Figure 9-7 Example of a zonal refractive multifocal intraocular lens. *Left,* a schematic frontal view. *Right,* a schematic lateral view of the rotationally asymmetric, multifocal sector lens, which is made from a combination of 2 spherical surfaces of differing radii. *(Illustration by Mark Miller from information courtesy of Oculentis GmbH.)*

other ocular diseases preoperatively, as MFIOLs are contraindicated in eyes with preexisting poor vision potential. In addition, any ocular abnormality that could increase systemic ocular aberrations (eg, corneal scarring, irregular astigmatism, dry eye) may significantly decrease image quality with these lenses. The clinician should carefully consider the possibility of patient dissatisfaction with the quality of vision after MFIOL implantation.

Complications

Patients with suboptimal results or who are dissatisfied with the quality of vision should undergo a comprehensive evaluation from the ocular surface to the macula. The clinician should exclude possible causes of vision disturbance, such as dry eye, residual refractive error, decentered lens or pupil, irregular astigmatism, vitreous opacities, cystoid macular edema, or epiretinal membrane. Postoperative capsular opacification is of greater concern with MFIOLs because minimal changes in the capsule can cause early deterioration in vision. To achieve optimal vision, Nd:YAG laser capsulotomy may be required earlier or more frequently in patients with MFIOLs than in patients with monofocal IOLs. However, if IOL exchange is being contemplated, Nd:YAG laser capsulotomy should be deferred. Other possible causes of vision disturbance should be excluded before an IOL exchange is considered. MFIOLs may cause glare and halos around lights at night, although newer MFIOLs incorporate technology that substantially reduces (but does not generally eliminate) these optical phenomena. Symptoms may be reduced through the use of nighttime driving glasses or instillation of topical brimonidine drops to reduce mesopic pupil size. In addition, most of these symptoms will decrease over time through neuroadaptation.

Custom or Multifocal Ablations

An excimer laser may be used to create a multifocal cornea. Prompted by the observation that, following excimer ablation, the uncorrected near vision of many patients improved more than expected (Fig 9-8), ophthalmologists began to investigate the potential for improving near vision without significantly compromising distance vision. To this end, the following ablation patterns have been employed:

- a small, central steep zone ablation, in which the central portion of the cornea is used for near vision and the midperiphery is used for distance vision
- an inferior near-zone ablation
- an inferiorly decentered hyperopic ablation
- a central distance ablation with an intermediate/near midperipheral ablation

Some of these patterns generate simultaneous near and distance images, whereas others rely on pupillary constriction (accommodative convergence) to concentrate light rays through the steeper central ablation.

Although the excimer laser offers some potential advantages, the results of multifocal corneal ablations are still under investigation.

Alarcón A, Anera RG, del Barco LJ, Jiménez JR. Designing multifocal corneal models to correct presbyopia by laser ablation. *J Biomed Opt.* 2012;17(1):018001. doi:10.1117/1. JBO.17.1.018001.

Pallikaris IG, Panagopoulou SI. PresbyLASIK approach for the correction of presbyopia. *Curr Opin Ophthalmol.* 2015;26(4):265–272.

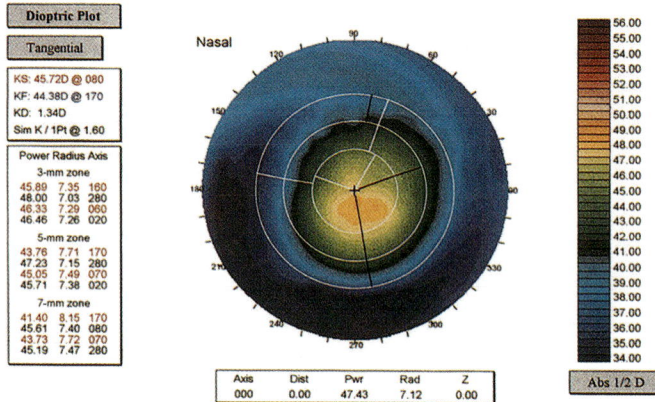

Figure 9-8 Multifocal ablation. Corneal topographic map showing a multifocal pattern after hyperopic laser in situ keratomileusis in a 62-year-old patient with preoperative hyperopia of +4.00 diopters (D). Postoperatively, the uncorrected distance visual acuity at distance is 20/25^{-2} and at near is Jaeger score J1. Manifest refraction of −0.25 + 0.75 D × 20 yields visual acuity of 20/20. Corneal topography demonstrates central hyperopic ablation *(green)* with relative steepening in the lower portion of the pupillary axis *(orange)*, which provides the near add for reading vision. *(Courtesy of Jayne S. Weiss, MD.)*

Corneal Intrastromal Femtosecond Laser Treatment

Femtosecond lasers may also be used to treat presbyopia. This minimally invasive approach is available in several countries outside the United States (but is not currently FDA approved) and does not involve incisions or flap creation. In this procedure, known as IntraCor, the femtosecond laser makes concentric rings within the stroma, starting in the center with a ring diameter of 1.8 mm, and proceeding with subsequent rings toward the periphery. The formation of these rings produces a localized biomechanical change that reshapes the cornea to create multifocality. The procedure is typically performed only in the nondominant eye. Studies have demonstrated that this procedure can benefit patients with hyperopic presbyopia (+0.50 D to +1.25 D), as the treatment causes an increase in the corneal true net power as well as a potential gain of 4–5 lines of near vision. It is important to counsel patients that uncorrected near vision is not significantly improved at 1 month postoperatively but that it is improved by 6 months in most cases.

Holzer MP, Knorz MC, Tomalla M, Neuhann TM, Auffarth GU. Intrastromal femtosecond laser presbyopia correction: 1-year results of a multicenter study. *J Refract Surg.* 2012;28(3):182–188.

Menassa N, Fitting A, Auffarth GU, Holzer MP. Visual outcomes and corneal changes after intrastromal femtosecond laser correction of presbyopia. *J Cataract Refract Surg.* 2012;38(5):765–773.

Ruiz LA, Cepeda LM, Fuentes VC. Intrastromal correction of presbyopia using a femtosecond laser system. *J Refract Surg.* 2009;25(10):847–854.

Thomas BC, Fitting A, Khoramnia R, Rabsiber TM, Auffarth GU, Holzer MP. Long-term outcomes of intrastromal femtosecond laser presbyopia correction: 3-year results. *Br J Ophthalmol.* 2016 Feb 22. doi:10.1136/bjophthalmol-2015-307672. Epub ahead of print.

Corneal Inlays

Corneal inlays improve near vision by several different mechanisms: changing corneal curvature, increasing depth of field via a small central aperture, or changing the refractive index of the cornea (see Fig 4-1B). The KAMRA corneal inlay (AcuFocus Inc, Irvine, CA) has been used successfully and is commercially availability in 49 countries. It was FDA approved in 2015 and is the first inlay to be available in the United States. It is 5 μm thick with a 3.8-mm outer diameter and a 1.6-mm central aperture. It "corrects" presbyopia via a pinhole effect, providing near vision in the nondominant eye in which it is implanted. Another inlay is the Flexivue Microlens (Presbia, Dublin, Ireland), a small, hydrophilic acrylic clear inlay with an index of refraction different from that of the cornea. A small hole in the center allows for distance vision and nutritional circulation. The Raindrop Near Vision Inlay (Revision Optics, Lake Forest, CA) is a hydrogel inlay 2 mm in diameter and 32 μm thick centrally. As a hydrogel, it allows nutrients and oxygen to pass through and, when placed centrally, causes central corneal steepening, resulting in variable power from center of the cornea to the periphery.

All currently available inlays are implanted only in the nondominant eye, which should have a stable refractive spherical equivalent of −1.00 to 0.00 D at the time of surgery. This value either can be the baseline refractive error or can be achieved with laser refractive surgery, such as LASIK, performed at least 1 month prior to implantation of the inlay. The inlay is typically placed in a corneal pocket created by a femtosecond laser, allowing for better centration, lower risk of corneal striae, and minimal impact on the peripheral corneal nerve innervation. The inlay must be centered on the visual axis, as even a slightly decentered placement can significantly affect the visual outcome.

Neuroadaptation to these inlays may take months. Because the procedure is performed only in the nondominant eye, some adverse visual effects (night halos) may be less perceptible in binocular viewing conditions. One of the benefits of corneal inlays is that they can be removed with few to no long-term sequelae. See Chapter 4 for more details.

Bouzoukis DI, Kymionis GD, Limnopoulou AN, Kounis GA, Pallikaris IG. Femtosecond laser–assisted corneal pocket creation using a mask for inlay implantation. *J Refract Surg.* 2011;27(11):818–820.

Garza EB, Gomez S, Chayet A, Dishler J. One-year safety and efficacy results of a hydrogel inlay to improve near vision in patients with emmetropic presbyopia. *J Refract Surg.* 2013; 29(3):166–172.

Limnopoulou AN, Bouzoukis DI, Kymionis GD, et al. Visual outcomes and safety of a refractive corneal inlay for presbyopia using femtosecond laser. *J Refract Surg.* 2013;29(1):12–18.

Lindstrom RL, Macrae SM, Pepose JS, Hoopes PC Sr. Corneal inlays for presbyopia correction. *Curr Opin Ophthalmol.* 2013;24(4):281–287.

Tomita M, Kanamori T, Waring GO IV, et al. Simultaneous corneal inlay implantation and laser in situ keratomileusis for presbyopia in patients with hyperopia, myopia, or emmetropia: six-month results. *J Cataract Refract Surg.* 2012;38(3):495–506.

US Food and Drug Administration. KAMRA Inlay - P120023. Approval April 17, 2015. Available at https://goo.gl/xzJHzY. Accessed November 6, 2016.

Waring GO IV. Correction of presbyopia with a small aperture corneal inlay. *J Refract Surg.* 2011;27(11):842–845.

Other Intraocular Lens Innovations on the Horizon

In addition to single-plate accommodating IOLs, which are thought to work via lens effectivity secondary to a change in the position of the optic in the eye, lenses with dual-optic elements connected by a system of springlike struts have been developed and are under clinical investigation (Fig 9-9). During accommodation, the lens system confined within the capsular bag undergoes a change in the separation of the 2 optics, resulting in increased effective lens power. The lens can be implanted into the eye through a 3.5-mm incision.

Another type of lens is made from a thermoplastic acrylic gel that can be customized to any size, shape, or power specified by the physician. The hydrophobic acrylic material is chemically bonded to wax, which melts inside the eye at body temperature and allows the predetermined shape and power of the material to emerge. Theoretically, compression of this pliable lens by the capsular bag allows adjustment of its effective power in a manner analogous to the way the crystalline lens adjusts. Examples of deformable IOLs in preliminary stages of development are the FlexOptic IOL (Abbott Medical Optics), FluidVision IOL (PowerVision, Belmont, CA), and NuLens accommodating IOL (NuLens Ltd, Herzliya Pituach, Israel). The NuLens changes its power rather than its position in the eye. It incorporates a small chamber of silicone gel and a posterior piston with an aperture.

In addition, flexible polymers are being designed for injection into a nearly intact capsular bag following extraction of the crystalline lens through a tiny, laterally placed capsulorrhexis.

The Light Adjustable Lens (LAL) (Calhoun Vision, Pasadena, CA) is made from a macromer silicone matrix with smaller, embedded photosensitive molecules that allow for postoperative customization of the power via tunable ultraviolet light treatment (see Chapter 8 for more details).

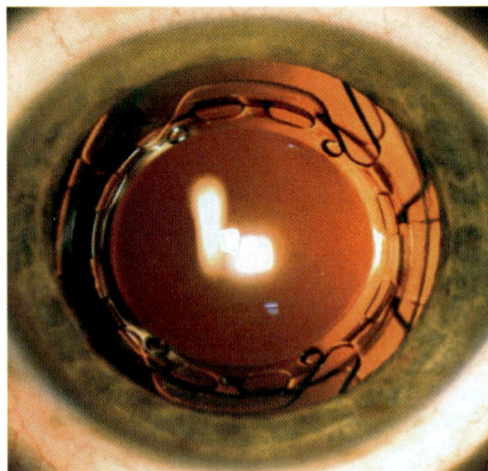

Figure 9-9 Clinical photograph of an implanted dual-optic accommodating intraocular lens, which has a high-plus anterior optic connected by spring haptics to a posterior optic with variable negative power. The 3-dimensional design mimics the natural lens, and its response to the contraction and relaxation of the ciliary muscle increases paraxial power and provides accommodation. *(Courtesy of Ivan Ossma, MD.)*

CHAPTER 10

Refractive Surgery in Ocular and Systemic Disease

Introduction

Over the past 3 decades, the field of refractive surgery has evolved into a subspecialty with finely tuned, computer- and laser-assisted procedures that play an important role in the surgical armamentarium of today's ophthalmologists. As the spectrum of indications for refractive surgery has grown, so has the prevalence of patients with concomitant known ocular or systemic diseases who wish to undergo these procedures.

During this period, many patients excluded from the original United States Food and Drug Administration (US FDA) clinical trials have been successfully treated with refractive surgery, and some formerly absolute contraindications have been changed to relative contraindications. With increased experience, laser in situ keratomileusis (LASIK) and photorefractive keratectomy (PRK) have been performed safely and effectively in patients with ocular or systemic diseases. Nevertheless, the use of these procedures on patients whose conditions would have excluded them from participation in the original FDA protocols is considered off-label. Performing off-label surgery is neither illegal nor medically incorrect if, in the surgeon's judgment, the benefit of a surgical procedure outweighs the potential risk to a patient. However, it is the surgeon's ethical, legal, and medical responsibility to explain the concept of off-label surgery to the patient, to determine whether the procedure meets the standard of care in the community, and emphasize to the patient the unknown risk associated as a result of using an off-label non–FDA-approved protocol.

In higher-risk patients, unilateral surgery may offer the advantage of providing assurance that one eye is doing well before surgery is performed on the second eye. In addition, when deciding whether a patient with connective tissue disease or immunosuppression is an appropriate candidate for refractive surgery, the surgeon may find that consultation with the patient's primary physician or rheumatologist provides important information about the patient's systemic health.

The process of consent should be altered, not only to inform the patient, but also to document the patient's understanding of the additional risks and limitations of postoperative results associated with any coexisting ocular or systemic diseases. The refractive surgeon may choose to supplement the standard written consent with additional points to highlight specific concerns. The ophthalmologist should assiduously avoid the high-risk refractive surgery patient who volunteers to sign any preoperative consent because

"I know these complications won't happen to me." Such patients have not heard or understood the informed consent discussion.

American Academy of Ophthalmology Refractive Management/Intervention Panel. Preferred Practice Pattern Guidelines. *Refractive Errors & Refractive Surgery.* San Francisco: American Academy of Ophthalmology; 2013. Available at www.aao.org/ppp.

Bowers KS, Woreta F. Update on contraindications for laser-assisted in situ keratomileusis and photorefractive keratectomy. *Curr Opin Ophthalmol.* 2014;25(4):251–257.

Ocular Conditions

Ocular Surface Disease

Dry eye after LASIK is the most common and anticipated complication of refractive surgery, although symptoms are typically self-limited. During creation of the flap, corneal nerves are severed, which may result in corneal anesthesia lasting 3–6 months and may less frequently persist for years. As a result, many patients develop keratopathy, decreased tear production, and related symptoms as a result of the neurotrophic state of their cornea. Patients who had dry eyes prior to surgery, or whose eyes were marginally compensated before surgery, may experience more severe symptoms postoperatively. These individuals demonstrate tear-film and ocular surface disruption and often report fluctuating vision between blinks throughout the day. In a review of 109 patients who had undergone LASIK surgery, Levinson and colleagues found that dry eye symptoms and blepharitis were the most common diagnoses among patients dissatisfied with the procedure, even for patients with relatively good postoperative vision outcomes. Fortunately, in the great majority of these patients, symptoms resolve 3–6 months after surgery but those whose symptoms persist are among the least satisfied in this series.

Ophthalmologists may take several steps to reduce the incidence and severity of dry eye symptoms after refractive surgery. One of the most important is to screen patients carefully for dry eye and tear-film abnormalities and to treat them aggressively before surgery. Many patients seeking refractive surgery are actually dry eye patients who are intolerant of contact lens wear because of their preexisting dry eye disease. Any history of contact lens intolerance should suggest the possibility of underlying dry eye.

Any refractive surgery candidate with signs or symptoms of dry eye should be thoroughly evaluated. Patient history should include questions about collagen vascular diseases and conjunctival cicatrizing disorders; these conditions are relative contraindications to refractive procedures and should be addressed prior to any surgical consideration (see Chapter 2).

External examination should include evaluation of eyelid anatomy and function for conditions such as incomplete blink, lagophthalmos, entropion, ectropion, and eyelid notching. On slit-lamp examination, the ophthalmologist should note anterior and posterior blepharitis, tear-film quantity and quality, and the presence of conjunctivochalasis, subconjunctival fibrosis, or symblepharon. Screening questionnaires to highlight or elicit dry eye–related symptoms could help start the discussion and lead to further workup. Ancillary testing for dry eyes (eg, Schirmer testing, tear breakup time, fluorescein corneal staining, lissamine green or rose bengal conjunctival staining) should be performed on all patients considering refractive surgery. Corneal topography should be reviewed for evidence of irregularity or patchy, poor image quality often seen in the presence of an unstable tear film. A screening evaluation in patients considering refractive surgery may also include other testing. An immunoassay for matrix metalloproteinase 9 levels, as an inflammatory biomarker in the tear film, and tear osmolarity measurement, as an indicator of tear deficiency, could be helpful in screening for ocular surface disease. Imaging the quality of the tear lipid layer and the health of the meibomian gland structure and function are other tools for screening at-risk patients. Once the at-risk patient is identified, aggressive preoperative treatment often leads to better outcomes, fewer complications, and patients more satisfied with the results of surgery.

Treatment of ocular surface disease with aqueous deficiency may include topical tear replacement, punctal occlusion, and use of topical anti-inflammatory drugs, such as corticosteroids or cyclosporine (see BCSC Section 8, *External Disease and Cornea*). Topical cyclosporine improves dry eye and refractive outcomes in patients with dry eye who are undergoing LASIK and surface ablation. Patients with ocular surface disease and blepharitis or meibomitis should be instructed in the use of hygienic eyelid scrubs and dietary supplements, such as flaxseed or omega-3 fish oils, to improve the tear film. Meibomian gland expression, oral or topical medications (eg, doxycycline or azithromycin), and a short course of topical corticosteroids may help improve the quality of the tear film and optimize the ocular surface prior to surgery. A delay in surgery may be necessary to allow time for treatment response. In addition, patients must be cautioned that their dry eye condition may worsen postoperatively. Such an occurrence may result in additional discomfort or decreased vision and may be permanent.

American Academy of Ophthalmology Cornea/External Disease Panel. Preferred Practice Pattern Guidelines. *Blepharitis.* San Francisco: American Academy of Ophthalmology; 2013. Available at www.aao.org/ppp.

American Academy of Ophthalmology Cornea/External Disease Panel. Preferred Practice Pattern Guidelines. *Dry Eye Syndrome.* San Francisco: American Academy of Ophthalmology; 2013. Available at www.aao.org/ppp.

Bower KS, Sia RK, Ryan DS, Mines MJ, Dartt DA. Chronic dry eye in photorefractive keratectomy and laser in situ keratomileusis: Manifestations, incidence, and predictive factors. *J Cataract Refract Surg.* 2015;41(12):2624–2634.

Levinson BA, Rapuano CJ, Cohen EJ, Hammersmith KM, Ayres BD, Laibson PR. Referrals to the Wills Eye Institute Cornea Service after laser in situ keratomileusis: reasons for patient dissatisfaction. *J Cataract Refract Surg.* 2008;34(1)32–39.

Salib GM, McDonald MB, Smolek M. Safety and efficacy of cyclosporine 0.05% drops versus unpreserved artificial tears in dry-eye patients having laser in situ keratomileusis. *J Cataract Refract Surg.* 2006;32(5):772–778.

Herpes Simplex Virus Infection

Many surgeons avoid laser vision correction in patients with a history of herpes simplex virus (HSV) keratitis because of the risk of recurrent disease induced by the surgery. Trauma from the lamellar dissection or exposure to the excimer laser may reactivate the virus and cause recurrent HSV keratitis. However, some authors have concluded that the recurrence reflects simply the natural course of the disease rather than reactivation due to excimer laser ablation.

The role of excimer laser ablation in inciting recurrence of HSV keratitis has been investigated in the laboratory. Rabbits infected with HSV type 1 demonstrated viral reactivation after exposure of the corneal stroma to 193-nm ultraviolet radiation during PRK and LASIK. Pretreatment with systemic valacyclovir before the laser treatment decreased the rate of recurrence in the rabbit model. In another study, a rabbit latency model demonstrated that systemic valacyclovir reduced ocular shedding of HSV after LASIK.

Reactivation of HSV keratitis has been reported in humans after radial keratotomy (RK), phototherapeutic keratectomy (PTK), PRK, and LASIK. Fagerholm and colleagues reported a 25% incidence of postoperative HSV keratitis 17 months after PTK for surface irregularities from prior HSV infections, compared with an 18% recurrence rate in an equivalent time period prior to PTK. The authors concluded that the procedure does not seem to significantly increase the incidence of recurrences.

A retrospective review of 13,200 PRK-treated eyes with no history of corneal HSV revealed a 0.14% incidence of HSV keratitis. Of these cases, 16.5% occurred within 10 days of the procedure; the authors postulated that this finding may indicate a direct effect of the excimer ultraviolet laser. In 78% of cases, HSV keratitis occurred within 15 weeks, which could be related to the corticosteroid therapy.

Reactivation of herpes zoster ophthalmicus was also reported in 1 case after LASIK, in association with vesiculo-ulcerative lesions on the tip of the nose. The few cases in which herpes zoster ophthalmicus was reactivated responded to topical and oral antiviral treatment with excellent recovery of vision. There are anecdotal reports of flap interface inflammation resembling diffuse lamellar keratitis after LASIK in patients with herpes simplex or herpes zoster keratitis. In these cases, topical corticosteroids may also be required.

Due to the potential for vision loss from recurrence of HSV keratitis, some refractive surgeons consider prior herpetic keratitis a contraindication to refractive surgery. Others may consider performing PRK, PTK, or LASIK in patients with a history of HSV keratitis who have not had any recent recurrences and who have good corneal sensation, minimal or no corneal vascularization or scarring, and normal best-corrected visual acuity (BCVA; also called *corrected distance visual acuity, CDVA*). Preoperative and postoperative prophylaxis with systemic antiviral drugs should be strongly considered in these patients. Results of the Herpetic Eye Disease Study (HEDS) showed only a 50% reduction in the risk of recurrence with a prophylactic dose of oral acyclovir over the course of 1 year in patients with latent HSV even with no inciting factors, such as treatment with an excimer laser. Patients with pronounced corneal hypoesthesia or anesthesia, vascularization, thinning and scarring, or recent herpetic attacks should not be considered candidates for refractive surgery. Any patient with a history of herpes simplex or herpes zoster keratitis must be counseled about the continued risk of recurrence and its concomitant potential for vision loss after excimer laser vision correction.

Asbell PA. Valacyclovir for the prevention of recurrent herpes simplex virus eye disease after excimer laser photokeratectomy. *Trans Am Ophthalmol Soc.* 2000;98:285–303.

de Rojas Silva V, Rodriguez-Conde R, Cobo-Soriano R, Beltrán J, Llovet F, Baviera J. Laser in situ keratomileusis in patients with a history of ocular herpes. *J Cataract Refract Surg.* 2007;33(11):1855–1859.

Fagerholm P, Ohman L, Orndahl M. Phototherapeutic keratectomy in herpes simplex keratitis. Clinical results in 20 patients. *Acta Ophthalmol (Copenh).* 1994;72(4):457–460.

Jain V, Pineda R. Reactivated herpetic keratitis following laser in situ keratomileusis. *J Cataract Refract Surg.* 2009;35(5):946–948.

Levy J, Lapid-Gortzak R, Klemperer I, Lifshitz T. Herpes simplex virus keratitis after laser in situ keratomileusis. *J Refract Surg.* 2005;21(4):400–402.

Keratoconus

Keratoconus is generally considered a contraindication to LASIK and surface ablation. Weakening of the cornea, as a result of the loss of structural integrity involved in creating the LASIK flap, and removal of tissue significantly increase the risk of exacerbation of ectasia. Although advanced stages of keratoconus can be diagnosed by slit-lamp examination, more sensitive analyses using corneal topography and corneal pachymetry can reveal findings early in the disease process. No specific agreed-upon test or measurement is diagnostic of a corneal ectatic disorder, but corneal topography and corneal pachymetry should be part of the evaluation. Subtle corneal thinning, curvature, or elevation changes can be overlooked on slit-lamp evaluation.

In cases of forme fruste keratoconus where the fellow eye is seemingly normal, studies have suggested several risk factors for progression to keratoconus in the fellow eye and post-LASIK ectasia in either eye. These include interocular asymmetry of inferior corneal steepening or asymmetric bow-tie topographic patterns with skewed steep radial axes above and below the horizontal meridian (Fig 10-1). Keratoconus suspect patients

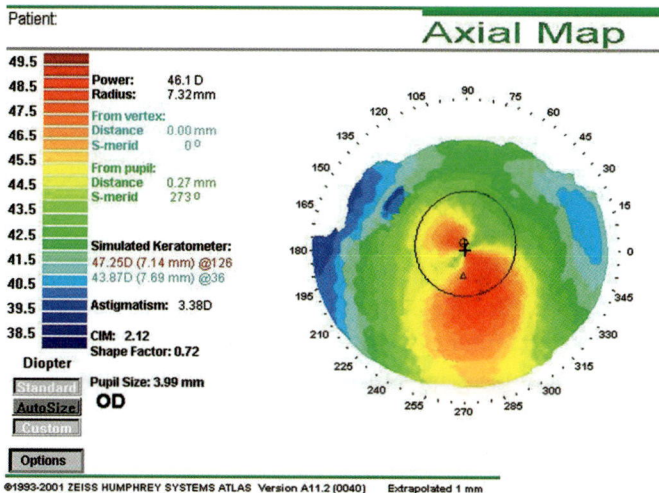

Figure 10-1 Corneal topographic map indicating keratoconus with asymmetric irregular steepening. *(Courtesy of Eric D. Donnenfeld, MD.)*

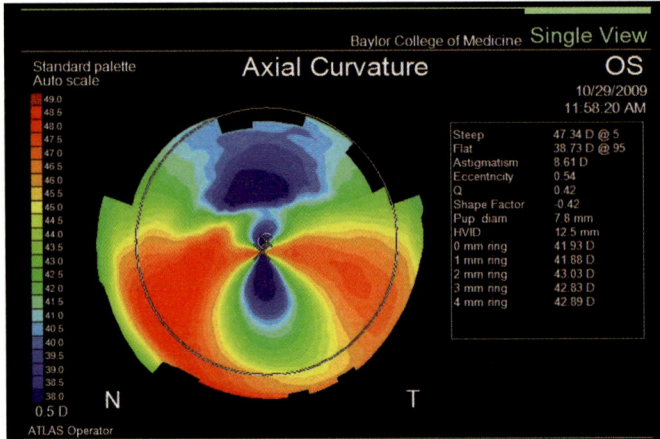

Figure 10-2 Topography of pellucid marginal degeneration showing the "crab-claw" appearance. N = nasal; T = temporal. *(Courtesy of M. Bowes Hamill, MD.)*

have the aforementioned features in either or both eyes. LASIK using current technology should not be considered in such patients. Patients with an inferior "crab-claw" pattern accompanied by central flattening are at risk of developing pellucid marginal degeneration or a "low-sagging cone" variety of keratoconus, even in the absence of clinical signs (Fig 10-2). This pattern may be designated "pellucid suspect," and LASIK should be avoided in eyes that exhibit it.

Global pachymetry measurements may help rule out forme fruste keratoconus. Posterior curvature evaluation with newer corneal imaging technology may also prove significant (Fig 10-3). Often, the refractive surgeon is the first physician to detect and inform a patient of the existence of corneal ectasia. The patient may have excellent vision with glasses or contact lenses and may be seeking the convenience of a more permanent correction through LASIK. It is important that the ophthalmologist clearly convey that, although the presence of forme fruste keratoconus does not necessarily indicate the presence of a progressive disease, refractive surgery should not be performed because of the potential for unpredictable results and vision loss. The patient should also be informed of the importance of follow-up for any signs of progression, as corneal crosslinking (CCL) may be an option for stabilization of their corneal condition.

Intrastromal corneal ring segments are FDA approved for keratoconus (see Chapter 4). CCL with riboflavin administration and ultraviolet-A exposure shows promising early results and may prove effective in preventing and treating corneal ectasia (see Chapter 7 and BCSC Section 8, *External Disease and Cornea*). Although some early case reports have suggested that combining CCL treatments with PRK may offer some benefit to keratoconus patients, the clinical experience remains preliminary.

Alessio G, L'Abbate M, Sborgia C, La Tegola MG. Photorefractive keratectomy followed by cross-linking versus cross-linking alone for management of progressive keratoconus: two-year follow-up. *Am J Ophthalmol.* 2013;155(1):54–65.

Ambrósio R Jr, Alonso RS, Luz A, Coca Velarde LG. Corneal-thickness spatial profile and corneal-volume distribution: tomographic indices to detect keratoconus. *J Cataract Refract Surg.* 2006;32(11):1851–1859.

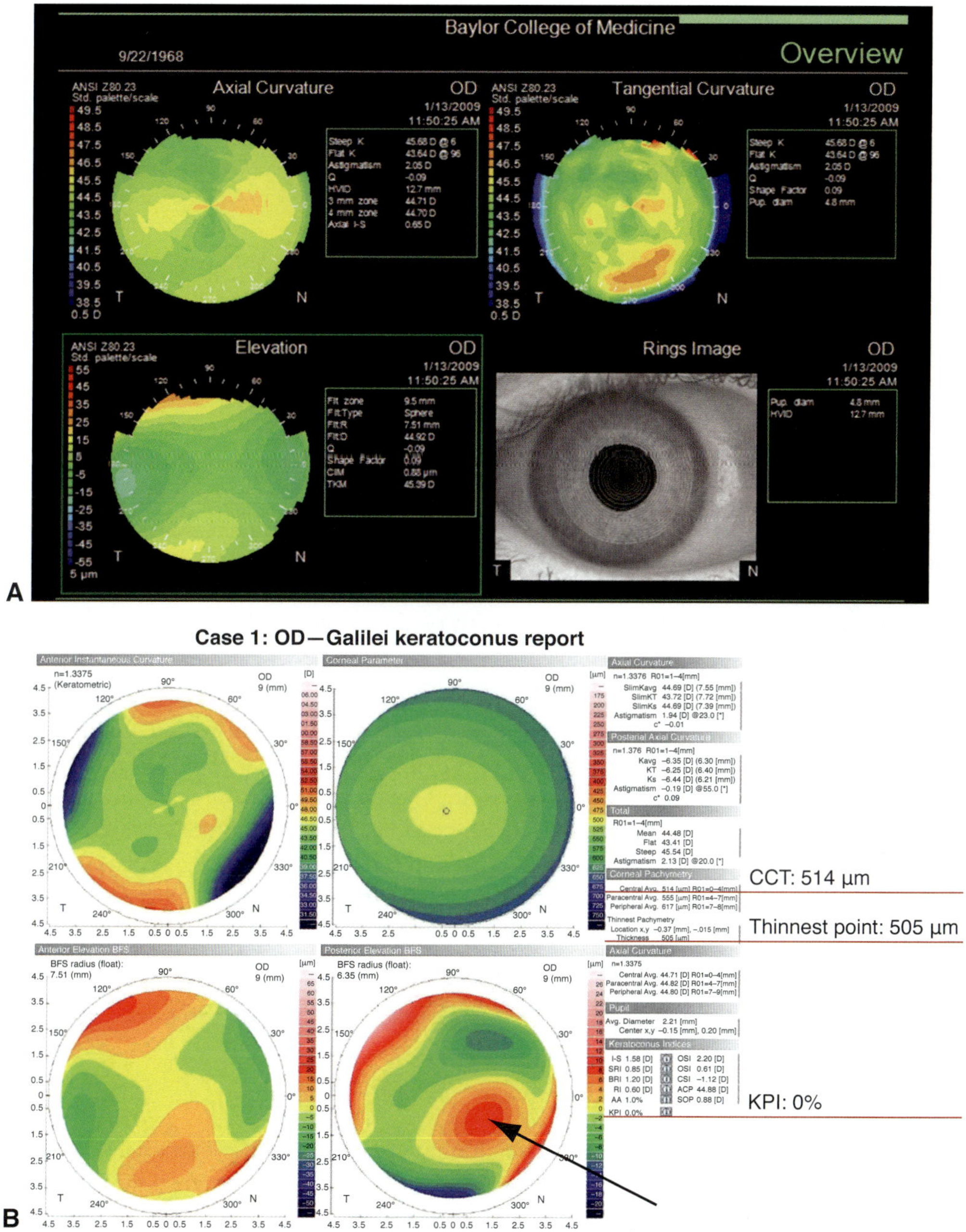

Figure 10-3 A 40-year-old man wishes to correct his myopia and high astigmatism. He does not wear contact lenses. His manifest refraction is −4.00 +3.00 × 4 OD and −3.75 +3.00 × 168 OS; corrected distance visual acuity is 20/20 OU. Both eyes appear normal on slit-lamp examination. **A,** Although the topographic examination appears normal on first glance, there is subtle inferior steepening that requires close inspection to appreciate. **B,** A clearly abnormal hot spot *(arrow)* is apparent on the Galilei dual Scheimpflug analyzer posterior elevation map, which may be concerning for keratoconus suspect. Technologies that evaluate regional corneal thickness and posterior corneal elevation in addition to anterior curvature may improve the identification of patients with early keratoconus. CCT = central corneal thickness; KPI = keratoconus prediction index. *(Courtesy of Douglas D. Koch, MD.)*

Belin MW, Asota IM, Ambrósio R, Khachikian SS. What's in a name: keratoconus, pellucid marginal degeneration, and related thinning disorders. *Am J Ophthalmol.* 2011;152(2): 157–162.

Binder PS, Lindstrom RL, Stulting RD, et al. Keratoconus and corneal ectasia after LASIK. *J Cataract Refract Surg.* 2005;31(11):2035–2038.

Kılıç A, Colin J. Advances in the surgical treatment of keratoconus. *Focal Points: Clinical Modules for Ophthalmologists.* San Francisco: American Academy of Ophthalmology; 2012: module 2.

Randleman JB, Russell B, Ward MA, Thompson KP, Stulting RD. Risk factors and prognosis for corneal ectasia after LASIK. *Ophthalmology.* 2003;110(2):267–275.

Saad A, Gatinel D. Topographic and tomographic properties of forme fruste keratoconus corneas. *Invest Ophthalmol Vis Sci.* 2010;51(11):5546–5555.

Other Corneal Dystrophies

Basement membrane dystrophy (also called *map-dot-fingerprint dystrophy*) is a common corneal dystrophy that can be an incidental finding in many asymptomatic patients. In determining the safety of refractive surgery in these eyes, one must ensure that the irregularity in the epithelium is not impacting the refractive error being treated, nor is it causing visually significant irregularity in the central corneal surface. If the eye is deemed stable to proceed with laser refractive surgery, surface ablation may be the preferred approach. In addition, surface treatment may help reduce irregular astigmatism and recurrent erosions, which are frequent in these patients.

The experience and published reports of refractive surgery in patients with Fuchs endothelial dystrophy are limited. Among the small number of patients with mild guttae and family history of Fuchs dystrophy who, following LASIK, were evaluated and reported on, the majority developed progressive corneal edema, loss of endothelial cells, and loss of BCVA. The progressive nature of this disease and the fluctuations in the corneal refractive power due to the fluctuating edema make these eyes difficult to stabilize for accurate measurements and postoperative management.

Moshirfar M, Feiz V, Feilmeier MR, Kang PC. Laser in situ keratomileusis in patients with corneal guttata and family history of Fuchs' endothelial dystrophy. *J Cataract Refract Surg.* 2005;31(12):2281–2286.

Post–Penetrating Keratoplasty

Refractive unpredictability after penetrating keratoplasty (PKP) is extremely common owing to the inherent imprecision of the operation. Most series document a mean postoperative astigmatism of 4.00–5.00 D. In many cases, these refractive errors are not amenable to spectacle correction, and 10%–30% of patients require rigid gas-permeable contact lens correction to achieve good vision after PKP. However, contact lens fitting may not be successful in this patient population due to abnormal corneal curvature or the patient's inability to tolerate or manipulate a contact lens.

Surgical alternatives for the correction of post-PKP astigmatism include astigmatic keratotomy, compression sutures, and wedge resections. In a series of 201 corneal transplants for keratoconus, 18% of patients required refractive surgery to correct the astigmatism.

Although these procedures can significantly decrease corneal cylinder and are highly effective, they have minimal effect on spherical equivalent. In addition, they can be unpredictable and may destabilize the graft–host wound.

Phakic eyes with significant corneal astigmatism after suture removal could undergo crystalline lens replacement with a toric intraocular lens if the astigmatism is regular centrally and has stabilized. Patients with significant anisometropia after PKP surgery may be candidates for intraocular lens (IOL) exchange or piggyback IOL implantation (see Chapter 8). These alternatives require another intraocular procedure, which increases the risk of endothelial decompensation, glaucoma, and cystoid macular edema and may incite graft rejection.

Given the successful use of the excimer laser in treating myopia and astigmatism, PRK has been studied and used to treat post-PKP refractive errors. PRK has the disadvantages associated with epithelial removal in a corneal transplant and may result in corneal haze when high refractive errors are treated. With the use of prophylactic topical mitomycin C, PRK has become a more acceptable treatment option for refractive errors after PKP. Although the refractive results are often good, PRK in patients who had past PKP is generally less predictable and less effective than it is for naturally occurring astigmatism and myopia.

LASIK after PKP is subject to the same patient-selection constraints as conventional LASIK. Without extenuating circumstances, patients with monocular vision or patients with limited vision potential in the fellow eye usually are poor candidates. In addition, patients with a wound-healing disorder, significant dry eye syndrome, or a collagen-vascular disease should be offered other options. Finally, patients should have realistic expectations for their rehabilitation after post-PKP LASIK. The goal of LASIK following PKP is to return the patient to spectacle-corrected binocularity or to enable the patient to wear contact lenses successfully, as the accuracy of the procedure is less predictable than that of conventional LASIK. Also, note that there are no FDA-approved procedures at this time to treat irregular astigmatism. Preoperative evaluation of the post-PKP patient who is considering refractive surgery should include the original indications for the PKP. It has been the experience of many surgeons that patients with low endothelial cell counts may be at increased risk of flap dislocation after LASIK because of impairment of the endothelial cell pump function.

Optimal timing of refractive surgery after PKP is controversial. All sutures should be removed, and the refraction should be stable. To avoid wound dehiscence, many surgeons wait at least 1 year after PKP, and an additional 4 months after all sutures are removed, before performing the refractive surgery. An interval of at least 18–24 months after PKP provides sufficient wound healing in most cases. No matter how much time has elapsed since the PKP surgery, the entirety of the graft–host wound should be carefully inspected to identify areas of variability in coaptation of the graft–host junction. Complications that can occur with a LASIK procedure include a small but significant risk of keratoplasty wound dehiscence during application of the vacuum ring used to create the LASIK flap, or during PRK or astigmatic keratotomy procedures.

Refraction and corneal topography should be stable, as documented by 2 consecutive readings on separate visits at least 1 month apart. Areas of stromal thinning should be confirmed to avoid exacerbation or, in extreme cases, perforation during LASIK flap creation. Refractive surgery should be avoided if the corneal graft shows evidence of inflammation, diffuse vascularization, ectasia, inadequate healing of the graft–host interface, refractive instability, or if there are signs of rejection or endothelial decompensation.

Because eye alignment under the laser is crucial for accurate treatment of astigmatism, some surgeons mark the vertical or horizontal axis of the cornea at the slit lamp before placing the patient under the laser. If the corneal curvature is very steep, cutting a thicker flap during the microkeratome pass may decrease the risk of buttonhole formation. PRK should also be considered in steep corneas to avoid flap complications.

Another potential problem specific to post-PKP LASIK is that the creation of a lamellar flap may itself cause a change in the amount and axis of the astigmatism. Therefore, some surgeons perform LASIK in 2 stages. In the first stage, the flap is cut and laid back down. Several weeks later, after the curvature and refraction have stabilized, the second stage is performed, where the flap is lifted and laser ablation is applied. Some reports describe minimal refractive changes after flap creation, and some surgeons prefer to perform LASIK in 1 stage to avoid increasing the potential for the complications associated with performing 2 separate procedures, including infection, graft rejection, and epithelial ingrowth. Flap retraction and necrosis have been reported in patients undergoing LASIK after keratoplasty.

The mean percentage reduction of astigmatism after LASIK following PKP ranges from 54.0% to 87.9%. Although most series report improvement in uncorrected visual acuity (UCVA; also called *uncorrected distance visual acuity, UDVA*), up to 42.9% of patients require enhancement because of cylindrical undercorrection. In addition, up to 35% of patients in some series have lost 1 line of BCVA. Corneal graft rejection has been described after PRK; thus, higher and more prolonged dosing with topical corticosteroids should be prescribed for post-PKP refractive surgery patients to decrease this risk.

Alió JL, Javaloy J, Osman AA, Galvis B, Tello A, Haroun HE. Laser in situ keratomileusis to correct post-keratoplasty astigmatism: 1-step vs 2-step procedure. *J Cataract Refract Surg.* 2004;30(11):2303–2310.

Fares U, Sarhan AR, Dua HS. Management of post-keratoplasty astigmatism. *J Cataract Refract Surg.* 2012;38(11):2029–2039.

Hardten DR, Chittcharus A, Lindstrom RL. Long term analysis for the correction of refractive errors after penetrating keratoplasty. *Cornea.* 2004;23(5):479–489.

Huang PY, Huang PT, Astle WF, et al. Laser-assisted subepithelial keratectomy and photorefractive keratectomy for post-penetrating keratoplasty myopia and astigmatism in adults. *J Cataract Refract Surg.* 2011;37(2):335–340.

Kollias AN, Schaumberger MM, Kreutzer TC, Ulbig MW, Lackerbauer CA. Two-step LASIK after penetrating keratoplasty. *Clin Ophthalmol.* 2009;3:581–586.

Sharma N, Sinha R, Vajpayee RB. Corneal lamellar flap retraction after LASIK following penetrating keratoplasty. *Cornea.* 2006;25(4):496.

Ocular Hypertension and Glaucoma

An estimated 9%–28% of patients with myopia have primary open-angle glaucoma (POAG). Consequently, it is likely that some patients with glaucoma will request refractive surgery.

Of particular concern in patients with ocular hypertension or POAG is the effect of the acute rise in intraocular pressure (IOP) to more than 65 mm Hg when suction is applied while the stromal flap is cut for LASIK or the epithelial flap for epipolis LASIK (epi-LASIK). There have been reports of new visual field defects arising immediately after LASIK that are attributed to mechanical compression or ischemia of the optic nerve head from the temporary increase in IOP.

Evaluation of a patient with ocular hypertension or POAG includes a complete history and ocular examination with peripheral visual field testing and corneal pachymetry. A history of poor IOP control, nonadherence to treatment, maximal medical therapy, or prior surgical interventions may suggest progressive disease, which may contraindicate refractive surgery. The surgeon should also note the status of the angle, the presence and amount of optic nerve cupping, and the degree of visual field loss, especially if split fixation is present.

Several reports have confirmed that central corneal thickness affects the Goldmann applanation tonometry (GAT) and the Tono-Pen (Reichert Technologies, Depew, NY) measurement of IOP (see the section Glaucoma After Refractive Surgery in Chapter 11). The principle of applanation tonometry assumes a corneal thickness of 520 μm. Studies have demonstrated that thinner-than-normal corneas give falsely low IOP readings, whereas thicker corneas give falsely high readings. For example, IOP is underestimated by approximately 5.2 mm Hg in a cornea with a central thickness of 450 μm. Although all reports agree that central corneal thickness affects GAT IOP measurement, there is no consensus on a specific formula to compensate for this effect in clinical practice.

In the treatment of myopia, LASIK and surface ablation procedures remove tissue to reduce the steepness of the cornea; this sculpting process creates a thinner central cornea, which leads to artifactually low IOP measurements postoperatively. Such inaccurately low central applanation tonometry measurements hinder the diagnosis of corticosteroid-induced glaucoma after keratorefractive procedures, resulting in optic nerve cupping, visual field loss, and decreased visual acuity (Fig 10-4).

Because of the difficulty that PRK and LASIK cause in the accurate measurement of IOP, these refractive procedures should not be considered for a patient whose IOP is poorly controlled. Furthermore, patients should be advised of the effect of refractive surgery on their IOP measurements and urged to inform future ophthalmologists about their surgery. Patients should be referred to a glaucoma specialist when indicated.

Patients with ocular hypertension can often safely undergo refractive surgery. Such patients must be counseled preoperatively that refractive surgery treats only the refractive error and not the natural history of the ocular hypertension, which can sometimes progress to glaucoma, accompanied by optic nerve cupping and visual field loss. The ophthalmologist should pay particular attention to the risk factors for progression to glaucoma, including older age, reduced corneal thickness, increased cup–disc ratio, family history of glaucoma, and elevated IOP. Each patient needs to understand that after excimer laser ablation, it is more difficult to accurately assess IOP.

The decision about whether to perform refractive surgery in a patient with glaucoma is controversial. There are no long-term studies on refractive surgery in this population. LASIK is contraindicated in any patient with marked optic nerve cupping, visual field loss, or visual acuity loss. The refractive surgeon may ask the patient to sign an ancillary

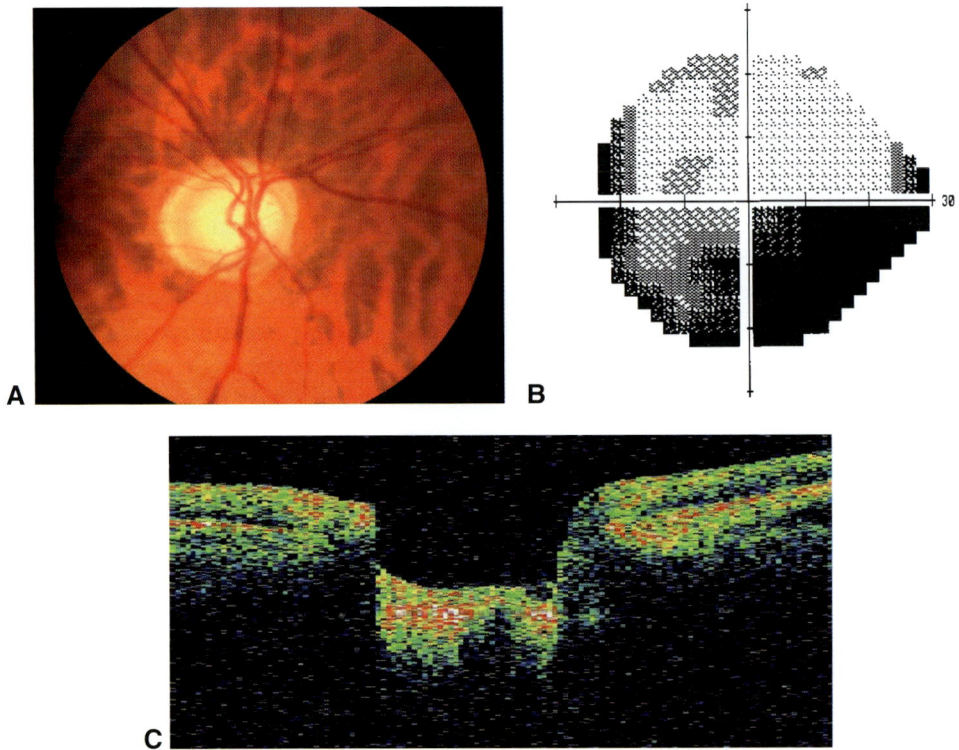

Figure 10-4 Glaucomatous optic nerve atrophy in a patient with "normal" intraocular pressure (IOP) after laser in situ keratomileusis (LASIK). **A,** Fundus photograph demonstrating increased cup–disc ratio in a patient who received a diagnosis of glaucoma 1 year after LASIK. The patient had decreased vision, with corrected distance visual acuity of 20/40 and IOP of 21 mm Hg. **B,** Humphrey 24-2 visual field with extensive inferior arcuate visual field loss corresponding to thinning of the superior optic nerve rim. **C,** Optical coherence tomography image demonstrates marked optic nerve cupping. *(Parts A and B courtesy of Jayne S. Weiss, MD; part C courtesy of Steven I. Rosenfeld, MD.)*

consent form that documents the patient's understanding that POAG may cause progressive vision loss independent of any refractive surgery and that IOP elevation during a LASIK or epi-LASIK procedure, or following LASIK or surface ablation (often due to a corticosteroid response), can cause glaucoma progression.

The surgeon should be aware that placement of a suction ring may not be possible if there is a functioning filtering bleb or a tube shunt. In rare cases in which both filtering surgery and LASIK are being planned, it is preferable to perform LASIK before the filter is placed. Suction time should be minimized to decrease the chance of optic nerve damage from the transient increase in IOP. Alternatively, PRK or laser subepithelial keratomileusis (LASEK) may be preferable because each avoids the IOP rise associated with LASIK flap creation. The surgeon must exercise caution when using postoperative corticosteroids because of their potential for elevating IOP. The patient should be informed as to when to resume postoperative topical medications for glaucoma. Finally, to avoid trauma to the flap, IOP should generally not be checked for at least 72 hours.

Bashford KP, Shafranov G, Tauber S, Shields MB. Considerations of glaucoma in patients undergoing corneal refractive surgery. *Surv Ophthalmol.* 2005;50(3):245–251.

Brandt JD, Beiser JA, Kass MA, Gordon MO. Central corneal thickness in the Ocular Hypertension Treatment Study (OHTS). *Ophthalmology.* 2001;108(10):1779–1788.

Brandt JD, Gordon MO, Gao F, Beiser JA, Miller JP, Kass MA; Ocular Hypertension Treatment Study Group. Adjusting intraocular pressure for central corneal thickness does not improve prediction models for primary open-angle glaucoma. *Ophthalmology.* 2012;119(3): 437–442.

Bushley DM, Parmley VC, Paglen P. Visual field defect associated with laser in situ keratomileusis. *Am J Ophthalmol.* 2000;129(5):668–671.

Chang DH, Stulting RD. Change in intraocular pressure measurements after LASIK. *Ophthalmology.* 2005;112(6):1009–1016.

Choplin NT, Schallhorn SC, Sinai M, Tanzer D, Tidwell JL, Zhou Q. Retinal nerve fiber layer measurements do not change after LASIK for high myopia as measured by scanning laser polarimetry with custom compensation. *Ophthalmology.* 2005;112(1):92–97.

Hamilton DR, Manche EE, Rich LF, Maloney RK. Steroid-induced glaucoma after laser in situ keratomileusis associated with interface fluid. *Ophthalmology.* 2002;109(4):659–665.

Lewis RA. Refractive surgery and the glaucoma patient. Customized corneas under pressure. *Ophthalmology.* 2000;107(9):1621–1622.

Morales J, Good D. Permanent glaucomatous visual loss after photorefractive keratectomy. *J Cataract Refract Surg.* 1998;24(5):715–718.

Pepose JS, Feigenbaum SK, Qazi MA, Sanderson JP, Roberts CJ. Changes in corneal biomechanics and intraocular pressure following LASIK using static, dynamic, and noncontact tonometry. *Am J Ophthalmol.* 2007;143(1):39–47.

Schallhorn JM, Schallhorn, SC, Ou Y. Factors that influence intraocular pressure changes after myopic and hyperopic LASIK and photorefractive keratectomy: a large population study. *Ophthalmology.* 2014;122(3):471–479.

Shaikh NM, Shaikh S, Singh K, Manche E. Progression to end-stage glaucoma after laser in situ keratomileusis. *J Cataract Refract Surg.* 2002;28(2):356–359.

Sharma N, Sony P, Gupta A, Vajpayee RB. Effect of laser in situ keratomileusis and laser-assisted subepithelial keratectomy on retinal nerve fiber layer thickness. *J Cataract Refract Surg.* 2006;32(3):446–450.

Yang CC, Wang IJ, Chang YC, Lin LL, Chen TH. A predictive model for postoperative intraocular pressure among patients undergoing laser in situ keratomileusis (LASIK). *Am J Ophthalmol.* 2006;141(3):530–536.

Retinal Disease

High myopia

Patients with high myopia are at increased risk of retinal tears and detachment. A thorough, dilated retinal examination (including scleral depression, if indicated) should be performed on all patients with high myopia, and a referral to a retina specialist should be considered for patients with predisposing retinal pathology. One study of 4800 consecutive patients in a private refractive surgery practice found that 52 (1.1%) had posterior segment pathology that required intervention. Another study of 29,916 myopic and hyperopic eyes undergoing LASIK demonstrated that 1.5% of patients required preoperative treatment of retinal pathology.

Brady J, O'Keefe M, Kilmartin D. Importance of fundoscopy in refractive surgery. *J Cataract Refract Surg.* 2007;33(9):1602–1607.

Retinal detachment

Patients with high myopia should be counseled that refractive surgery corrects only the refractive aspect of the myopia and not the natural history of the highly myopic eye with its known complications. Such patients remain at risk of retinal tears and detachment throughout their lives, despite refractive surgery.

Although no causal link has been established between retinal detachment and excimer laser refractive surgery, the potential adverse effects should be considered. The rapid increase and then decrease in IOP could theoretically stretch the vitreous base, and the acoustic shock waves from the laser could play a role in the development of a posterior vitreous detachment. Although the actual risk to eyes with high myopia or preexisting retinal pathology has not been determined through well-controlled, long-term studies, current data suggest that radial keratotomy, surface ablation, and LASIK do not appear to increase the incidence of retinal detachment. The occurrence of retinal detachment after LASIK ranges from 0.034% to 0.250%. In a series of 1554 eyes that underwent LASIK for myopia with a mean refractive error of –13.52 ± 3.38 D, retinal detachments developed in 4 eyes (0.25%) at 11.25 ± 8.53 months after the procedure. Three of the eyes had retinal flap tears, and 1 eye had an atrophic hole. There was no statistically significant difference in BCVA before and after conventional retinal reattachment surgery. A myopic shift did result from the scleral buckle, however.

In a study of 38,823 eyes with a mean myopia of –6.00 D, the frequency of rhegmatogenous retinal detachments at a mean of 16.3 months after LASIK was 0.8%. The eyes that developed retinal detachments had a mean preoperative myopia of –8.75 D. In a retrospective review, Blumenkranz reported that the frequency of retinal detachment after excimer laser treatment was similar to the frequency in the general population, averaging 0.034% over 2 years. It would be important for the LASIK surgeon to let the operating retinal surgeon know that LASIK has previously been performed on the patient, because of the potential for flap dehiscence during retinal detachment surgery, especially during corneal epithelial scraping.

Highly myopic eyes undergoing phakic IOL procedures are at risk of retinal detachment from the underlying high myopia, as well as from the intraocular surgery. A retinal detachment rate of 4.8% was reported in a study of phakic IOLs used to correct high myopia.

Arevalo JF. Posterior segment complications after laser-assisted in situ keratomileusis. *Curr Opin Ophthalmol.* 2008;19(3):177–184.

Arevalo JF, Ramirez E, Suarez E, Cortez R, Ramirez G, Yepez JB. Retinal detachment in myopic eyes after laser in situ keratomileusis. *J Refract Surg.* 2002;18(6):708–714.

Blumenkranz MS. LASIK and retinal detachment: should we be concerned? [editorial]. *Retina.* 2000;5:578–581.

Qin B, Huang L, Zeng J, Hu J. Retinal detachment after laser in situ keratomileusis in myopic eyes. *Am J Ophthalmol.* 2007;144(6):921–923.

Sakurai E, Okuda M, Nozaki M, Ogura Y. Late-onset laser in situ keratomileusis (LASIK) flap dehiscence during retinal detachment surgery. *Am J Ophthalmol.* 2002;134(2):265–266.

Previous retinal detachment surgery

Patients who have had prior scleral buckle surgery or vitrectomy may seek refractive surgery because of resultant myopia. Prior retinal detachment surgery can result in a myopic shift because of axial elongation of the eye from indentation of the scleral buckle. Refractive surgery can be considered in selected cases that have symptomatic anisometropia with good BCVA. The surgeon should determine whether the scleral buckle or conjunctival scarring will interfere with placement of the suction ring in preparation for creation of the LASIK flap. If it will, PRK may be considered instead of LASIK. Preoperative pathology, including preexisting macular pathology, will continue to limit UCVA and BCVA after refractive surgery. There are no published long-term series of the results of excimer laser vision correction in patients with prior retinal detachment surgery. Both the patient and the surgeon should realize that the final visual results may not be as predictable as after other refractive surgeries. Patients should also be aware that if the scleral buckle needs to be removed, the refractive error could change dramatically. Unexpected corneal steepening has been reported in patients undergoing LASIK with previously placed scleral buckles.

> Barequet IS, Levy J, Klemperer I, et al. Laser in situ keratomileusis for correction of myopia in eyes after retinal detachment surgery. *J Refract Surg.* 2005;21(2):191–193.

Amblyopia and Strabismus in Adults and Children

Amblyopia and anisometropic amblyopia

Amblyopia is defined as a decrease in visual acuity without evidence of organic eye disease, typically resulting from unequal visual stimulation during the period of visual development. The prevalence of amblyopia is 2%–4% of the US population; up to half of these cases represent anisometropic amblyopia. Patients with anisometropia greater than 3.00 D between the 2 eyes are likely to develop amblyopia that may be more resistant to traditional amblyopia therapy, such as glasses, contact lenses, patching, or atropine penalization therapy, partly because of the significant amount of induced aniseikonia.

Evaluation of a patient with amblyopia should include a thorough medical history to identify any known cause of amblyopia, a history of ocular disease or surgery, assessment of ocular alignment and motility, and a comprehensive anterior segment and retinal examination. Patients should be referred to a strabismus specialist when indicated. Preoperative counseling of a patient with amblyopia must emphasize that, even after refractive surgery, the vision in the amblyopic eye will not be as good as that in the nonamblyopic eye. The patient should also understand that BCVA will be the same, or nearly so, with or without refractive surgery.

Typically, refractive surgery is performed in this group of patients to treat high anisometropia or astigmatism in 1 eye or high refractive error in both eyes. Laser vision correction and phakic IOL implantation have been successfully performed in the more myopic, amblyopic eye in adult patients with anisometropic amblyopia. Some studies suggest that postoperative BCVA may even improve modestly compared with preoperative levels in a subset of adults who undergo refractive surgery. In a study examining phakic IOL implantation in patients with greater than 3.00 D of anisometropia, an average of 3 lines of vision were gained; 91% of eyes gained more than 1 line, and no eyes lost BCVA. This improvement in vision was attributed to an increase in magnification and a decrease in optical aberrations, rather than an actual improvement in the amblyopia.

Performing refractive surgery in the normal eye of the adult patient with amblyopia, however, is controversial. The decision to do so depends on many factors, including the level of BCVA in the amblyopic eye and the normal eye as well as the ocular alignment. To increase safety, unilateral surgery in the amblyopic eye followed by surgery in the non-amblyopic eye can be considered. However, ocular alignment deviation has been reported after unilateral LASIK for high myopia because of focus disparity causing esodeviation and impairment of fusion. In some cases, a preoperative contact lens trial may help in assessing this potential risk.

Consider a patient with anisometropic amblyopia whose vision is corrected to 20/40 with –7.00 D in the right eye and to 20/20 with –1.00 D in the left eye. This patient may be an excellent candidate for refractive surgery in the amblyopic right eye because he or she probably cannot tolerate glasses to correct the anisometropic amblyopia and may not tolerate contact lenses. Even if the post-LASIK UCVA were worse than 20/40 in the amblyopic eye, it would be better than the pre-LASIK UCVA of counting fingers.

If the postoperative UCVA in the amblyopic right eye improved to 20/40, the patient could be considered for laser vision correction in the left eye for –1.00 D. However, if the patient had presbyopia, some surgeons would discourage further intervention and discuss potential advantages of the low myopia. In a younger patient with accommodation, some surgeons would inform the patient of the potential risks associated with treating the better eye but would perform the excimer laser vision correction.

If BCVA in the amblyopic eye were 20/200 or worse, the patient would be considered legally blind if he or she were to lose significant vision after laser refractive surgery in the normal eye. In such cases, refractive surgery in the amblyopic eye may or may not offer much benefit, and refractive surgery in the nonamblyopic eye should be regarded as contraindicated in most cases. In the extenuating circumstances for which such surgery might be considered, the physician and patient should have an extensive discussion about the potential risks. Generally, if the patient would not be happy with the vision in the amblyopic eye alone in the event that something adverse happened to the better eye, then refractive surgery should not be performed on the better eye.

Persistent diplopia has been reported after bilateral LASIK in a patient with anisometropic amblyopia and a history of intermittent diplopia in childhood. Preoperatively, this type of patient can adjust to the disparity of the retinal image sizes with spectacle correction. Refractive surgery, however, can result in a dissimilar retinal image size that the patient cannot fuse, resulting in diplopia. This type of diplopia cannot be treated by prisms or muscle surgery.

Alió JL, Ortiz D, Abdelrahman A, de Luca A. Optical analysis of visual improvement after correction of anisometropic amblyopia with a phakic intraocular lens in adult patients. *Ophthalmology*. 2007;114(4):643–647.

Kim SK, Lee JB, Han SH, Kim EK. Ocular deviation after unilateral laser in situ keratomileusis. *Yonsei Med J*. 2000;41(3):404–406.

Sakatani K, Jabbur NS, O'Brien TP. Improvement in best corrected visual acuity in amblyopic adult eyes after laser in situ keratomileusis. *J Cataract Refract Surg.* 2004; 30(12):2517–2521.

Refractive surgery in children

In children, refractive surgery is controversial because their eyes and refractive status continue to change. Additional studies on the growing eye and the long-term effect of excimer laser treatment and phakic IOLs on the corneal endothelium and lens are needed to better assess the outcome of refractive surgery in children. Consequently, these procedures are typically regarded as investigational.

However, the literature is replete with reports of the successful performance of PRK, LASEK, LASIK, and phakic IOL implantation in children, mostly 8 years and older, when conventional therapies have failed. Most of these children underwent treatment for anisometropic amblyopia in the more myopic eye. In these studies, refractive error was decreased and visual acuity was maintained or improved in moderately amblyopic eyes. Refractive surgery did not improve BCVA or stereopsis in older children with densely amblyopic eyes. The limited effect on visual acuity was generally attributed to the fact that the children were beyond amblyogenic age. In 1 study, general anesthesia was used during performance of PRK in 40 children, aged 1–6 years, who were unable to wear glasses or contact lenses for high myopia or anisometropic amblyopia from myopia. Patients were treated for existing amblyopia, and mean BCVA improved from 20/70 to 20/40. The study found that posttreatment corneal haze developed in 60% of eyes. Most patients demonstrated "increasing corneal clarity" within 1 year, although 2 of 27 patients required PTK for the corneal haze. Regression of effect was attributed to a vigorous healing response and the axial myopic shift associated with growth.

Several studies have reported successful implantation of phakic IOLs in children with high anisometropia and amblyopia. This technique eliminates the previously mentioned corneal-wound-healing problems associated with keratorefractive procedures and may be considered when the refractive error is high and other traditional methods of amblyopia therapy have failed. Depending on the type of phakic IOL, however, other potentially serious complications may ensue, including progressive corneal endothelial cell loss, cataract formation, pupillary block glaucoma, and persistent inflammation, as well as the usual risks associated with intraocular surgery. Thus, phakic IOLs should be considered investigational in children. Larger clinical trials are necessary to adequately evaluate the safety and efficacy of this technique in this age group. Furthermore, these patients should be monitored for endothelial evaluation through the years.

Astle WF, Huang PT, Ells AL, Cox RG, Deschenes MC, Vibert HM. Photorefractive keratectomy in children. *J Cataract Refract Surg.* 2002;28(6):932–941.

Astle WF, Huang PT, Ereifej I, Paszuk A. Laser-assisted subepithelial keratectomy for bilateral hyperopia and hyperopic anisometropic amblyopia in children: one-year outcomes. *J Cataract Refract Surg.* 2010;36(2):260–267.

Daoud YJ, Hutchinson A, Wallace DK, Song J, Kim T. Refractive surgery in children: treatment options, outcomes, and controversies. *Am J Ophthalmol.* 2009;147(4): 573–582.e2.

Lesueur LC, Arne JL. Phakic intraocular lens to correct high myopic amblyopia in children. *J Refract Surg*. 2002;18(5):519–523.

Paysse EA, Coats DK, Hussein MA, Hamill MB, Koch DD. Long-term outcomes of photorefractive keratectomy for anisometropic amblyopia in children. *Ophthalmology*. 2006;113(2): 169–176.

Phillips CB, Prager TC, McClellan G, Mintz-Hittner HA. Laser in situ keratomileusis for treated anisometropic amblyopia in awake, autofixating pediatric and adolescent patients. *J Cataract Refract Surg*. 2004;30(12):2522–2528.

Tychsen L, Packwood E, Berdy G. Correction of large amblyopiogenic refractive errors in children using the excimer laser. *J AAPOS*. 2005;9(3):224–233.

Accommodative esotropia

Uncorrected hyperopia can stimulate an increase in accommodation, leading to accommodative convergence. Esotropia arises from insufficient fusional divergence. Traditional treatment includes correction of hyperopia with glasses or contact lenses and muscle surgery for any residual esotropia (see BCSC Section 6, *Pediatric Ophthalmology and Strabismus*). While glasses or contact lenses are being worn, the esotropia is usually not manifest. As a child ages, the hyperopia typically decreases, with concomitant resolution of the accommodative esotropia. If significant hyperopia persists, glasses or contact lenses continue to be needed to control the esotropia.

Before refractive surgery, it is important to perform an adequate cycloplegic refraction (using cyclopentolate, 1%) on patients younger than 35 years who have intermittent strabismus or phoria. Accurate refraction is necessary to avoid inducing postoperative hyperopia. Otherwise, the postoperative hyperopia may result in a new onset of esotropia with an accommodative element.

Several studies performed outside the US report the use of PRK and LASIK for adults with accommodative esotropia. In one of the studies, orthophoria or microesotropia was achieved after LASIK for hyperopia in accommodative esotropia in a series of 9 patients older than 18 years. A second study demonstrated a reduction in the mean esotropia of 21 prism diopters (Δ) prior to LASIK to 3.7Δ after surgery. However, another study of LASIK in accommodative esotropia in patients aged 10–52 years found that 42% of these patients had no reduction in their esotropia.

Brugnoli de Pagano OM, Pagano GL. Laser in situ keratomileusis for the treatment of refractive accommodative esotropia. *Ophthalmology*. 2012;119(1):159–163.

Hoyos JE, Cigales M, Hoyos-Chacón J, Ferrer J, Maldonado-Bas A. Hyperopic laser in situ keratomileusis for refractive accommodative esotropia. *J Cataract Refract Surg*. 2002;28(9): 1522–1529.

Systemic Conditions

Human Immunodeficiency Virus Infection

Little has been written about refractive surgery in patients with known human immunodeficiency virus (HIV) infection, and individual opinions vary. Note that the FDA recommends that patients with an immunodeficiency disease not undergo LASIK, regardless of the excimer platform, because the risk outweighs the benefit.

In a survey of members of the International Society of Refractive Surgery, 51% of respondents considered HIV-seropositive patients who did not have definite acquired immune deficiency syndrome (AIDS) to be acceptable refractive surgery candidates. Only 13% thought that patients with definite AIDS were candidates for refractive surgery, whereas 44% believed that the presence of AIDS was an absolute contraindication to refractive surgery. Some surgeons advise such patients against undergoing refractive surgery because of concerns about postoperative complications, including the increased risk of infection associated with immunosuppression. However, only 1 case of keratitis (a bilateral infection with *Staphylococcus aureus*) following LASIK in an HIV-seropositive patient has been reported.

An additional concern is the potential for aerosolizing live virus during laser ablation, which could pose a risk to laser-suite personnel. Because refractive surgeons may operate on patients who do not know they are infected with viruses such as HIV or one of the hepatitis viruses, universal precautions must be followed with all patients.

In 1 study, excimer laser ablation of a cornea infected with pseudorabies virus, a porcine-enveloped herpesvirus similar to HIV and HSV, did not appear capable of causing infection by transmission through the air. The authors concluded that excimer laser ablation of the cornea in a patient infected with HIV is unlikely to pose a health hazard to the surgeon or assistants. Another study demonstrated that, after excimer laser ablation of infected corneal stroma, polymerase chain reaction did not detect viable varicella virus (200 nm in diameter) but did detect viable polio particles (70 nm in diameter).

Inhaled particles greater than or equal to 5 μm in diameter are deposited in the bronchial, tracheal, nasopharyngeal, and nasal walls, and particles less than 2 μm in diameter are deposited in the bronchioles and alveoli. Even if viral particles are not viable, the excimer laser plume produces particles with a mean diameter of 0.22 μm. Although the health effects of inhaled particles from the plume have not yet been determined, there have been anecdotal reports of respiratory ailments such as chronic bronchitis in high-volume excimer laser refractive surgeons. Canister filter masks can exclude particles down to a diameter of 0.1 μm and may be more protective than conventional surgical masks. In addition, evacuation of the laser plume potentially decreases the amount of breathable debris.

If a surgeon is considering performing excimer laser ablation in an HIV-infected patient who is not immunocompromised and has normal results on eye examination, extra precautions are warranted. The surgeon should counsel the patient about the visual risks of HIV infection and the lack of long-term follow-up results for refractive surgery in this population. The surgeon may also consider consulting with the physicians managing the patient's underlying disease, including specialists in infectious diseases. The surgeon may choose to treat 1 eye at a time on separate days and schedule the patient as the last patient of the day. In addition, the surgeon may consider implementing additional precautions for the operating room staff, such as wearing filter masks during the procedure and evacuating the laser plume.

Aref AA, Scott IU, Zerfoss EL, Kunselman AR. Refractive surgical practices in persons with human immunodeficiency virus positivity or acquired immune deficiency syndrome. *J Cataract Refract Surg.* 2010;36(1):153–160.

Hagen KB, Kettering JD, Aprecio RM, Beltran F, Maloney RK. Lack of virus transmission by the excimer laser plume. *Am J Ophthalmol.* 1997;124(2):206–211.

Diabetes Mellitus

In 2014, the Centers for Disease Control and Prevention reported a prevalence of 12.3% for diabetes mellitus in US adults aged 20 years and older—about 28.9 million people. A patient with diabetes mellitus who is considering refractive surgery should have a thorough preoperative history and examination, and the surgeon should pay special attention to the presence of active diabetic ocular disease. The blood sugar of a diabetic patient must be well controlled at the time of examination to ensure an accurate refraction. A history of laser treatment for proliferative diabetic retinopathy or cystoid macular edema indicates visually significant diabetic complications that typically contraindicate refractive surgery. Ocular examination should include inspection of the corneal epithelium to check the health of the ocular surface, identification of cataract if present, and detailed retinal examination. Preoperative corneal sensation should be assessed because corneal anesthesia can impede epithelial healing.

A retrospective review 6 months after LASIK in 30 eyes of patients with diabetes mellitus revealed a complication rate of 47%, compared with a complication rate of 6.9% in the control group. The most common problems in this study were related to epithelial healing and included epithelial loosening and defects. A loss of 2 or more lines of BCVA was reported in less than 1% of both the diabetes mellitus and control groups. However, 6 of the 30 eyes in the diabetes mellitus group required a mean of 4.3 months to heal because of persistent epithelial defects. The authors concluded that the high complication rate in these patients was explained by unmasking subclinical diabetic keratopathy.

Another retrospective review of 24 patients with diabetes mellitus who underwent LASIK demonstrated that 63% achieved UCVA of 20/25 or better. Three of the 24 eyes had an epithelial defect after surgery, and epithelial ingrowth developed in 2 of these eyes. No eye lost BCVA. In contrast, Cobo-Soriano and colleagues evaluated 44 diabetic patients (both insulin-dependent and non–insulin-dependent) who underwent LASIK in a retrospective, observational, case-controlled study and reported no significant difference in perioperative and postoperative complications, including epithelial defects, epithelial ingrowth, and flap complications between diabetic patients and control subjects.

In light of these contradictory reports, refractive surgeons should exercise caution in the selection of patients with diabetes mellitus for refractive surgery. Intraoperative technique should be adjusted to ensure maximal epithelial health. To reduce corneal toxicity, the surgeon should use the minimal amount of topical anesthetic (preferably in the form of nonpreserved drops) immediately before performing the procedure. Patients with diabetes mellitus should be counseled preoperatively about the increased risk of postoperative complications and the possibility of a prolonged healing time after LASIK. They should also be informed that the procedure treats only the refractive error and not the natural history of the diabetes mellitus, which can lead to future diabetic ocular complications and associated vision loss.

Centers for Disease Control and Prevention. *National Diabetes Statistics Report: Estimates of Diabetes and Its Burden in the United States, 2014.* Atlanta, GA: U.S. Department of Health and Human Services; 2014.

Cobo-Soriano R, Beltrán J, Baviera J. LASIK outcomes in patients with underlying systemic contraindications: a preliminary study. *Ophthalmology.* 2006;113(7):1118.e1–e8.

Fraunfelder FW, Rich LF. Laser-assisted in situ keratomileusis complications in diabetes mellitus. *Cornea.* 2002;21(3):246–248.

Halkiadakis I, Belfair N, Gimbel HV. Laser in situ keratomileusis in patients with diabetes. *J Cataract Refract Surg.* 2005;31(10):1895–1898.

Jabbur NS, Chicani CF, Kuo IC, O'Brien TP. Risk factors in interface epithelialization after laser in situ keratomileusis. *J Refract Surg.* 2004;20(4):343–348.

Connective Tissue and Autoimmune Diseases

Most surgeons consider active, uncontrolled connective tissue diseases, such as rheumatoid arthritis, systemic lupus erythematosus, and polyarteritis nodosa, to be contraindications to refractive surgery. Reports in the literature have discussed corneal melting and perforation following cataract extraction in patients with these conditions, as well as corneal scarring after PRK in a patient with systemic lupus erythematosus.

However, 2 retrospective series suggest that refractive surgery may be considered in patients with well-controlled connective tissue or autoimmune disease. One retrospective study of 49 eyes in 26 patients with inactive or stable autoimmune disease who underwent LASIK revealed no postoperative corneal melting or persistent epithelial defects. Another retrospective study of 62 eyes of patients with autoimmune or connective tissue disorders who had undergone LASIK revealed that these eyes had a somewhat worse refractive outcome than eyes of control subjects but did not sustain any severe complications such as corneal melting, laceration, or interface alterations.

Because the risk from an underlying disease cannot be quantified, increased caution should be exercised if refractive surgery is considered in patients with well-controlled autoimmune or connective tissue disease. It should be emphasized that the problems associated with autoimmune diseases may not present for many years, especially with significant ocular surface disease and dry eye. Consultation with the treating physician, unilateral surgery, and ancillary informed consent should be considered.

Alió JL, Artola A, Belda JI, et al. LASIK in patients with rheumatic diseases: a pilot study. *Ophthalmology.* 2005;112(11):1948–1954.

Cobo-Soriano R, Beltrán J, Baviera J. LASIK outcomes in patients with underlying systemic contraindications: a preliminary study. *Ophthalmology.* 2006;113(7):1118.e1–e8.

Simpson RG, Moshirfar M, Edmonds JN, Christiansen SM, Behunin N. Laser in situ keratomileusis in patients with collagen vascular disease: a review of the literature. *Clin Ophthalmol.* 2012;6:1827–1837.

Smith RJ, Maloney RK. Laser in situ keratomileusis in patients with autoimmune diseases. *J Cataract Refract Surg.* 2006;32(8):1292–1295.

CHAPTER 11

Considerations After Refractive Surgery

The number of patients who have had refractive surgery continues to grow, and ophthalmologists are increasingly confronted with the management of post–refractive surgery patients with other ocular conditions, such as cataract, glaucoma, retinal detachment, corneal opacities, and irregular astigmatism. Calculation of the intraocular lens (IOL) power presents a particular challenge in this population.

Intraocular Lens Calculations After Refractive Surgery

Although numerous formulas have been developed to calculate IOL power prior to cataract surgery for eyes that have undergone refractive surgery, these cases are still prone to refractive surprises. Currently, there is no infallible way to calculate IOL power for a patient who has undergone refractive surgery. Although the measurement of axial length should remain accurate after refractive surgery, determining the keratometric power of the post–refractive surgery cornea is problematic. The difficulty arises from several factors. Small, effective central optical zones after refractive surgery (especially after radial keratotomy [RK]) can lead to inaccurate measurements because keratometers and Placido disk–based corneal topography units measure the corneal curvature several millimeters away from the center of the cornea and possibly outside the modified treated zone. In addition, the relationship between the anterior and posterior corneal curvatures may be considerably altered after refractive surgery (especially after laser ablative procedures), leading to inaccurate results. Generally, if standard keratometry readings are used to calculate IOL power for a previously myopic, post–refractive surgery eye, the postoperative refractive error will be hyperopic, because the keratometry readings are erroneously steeper than the true central corneal power.

A variety of methods have been developed to better estimate the central corneal power after refractive surgery. None is perfectly accurate, and different methods can lead to disparate values. As many methods as possible should be used to calculate corneal power, and these estimates should be compared with each other, with standard keratometric readings, and with corneal topographic central power and simulated K readings.

Newer corneal topography and tomography systems not based on the Placido disk imaging claim to directly measure the central corneal curvature; such technology may make direct calculation of IOL power after refractive surgery more accurate. In addition, intraoperative wavefront aberrometer systems use Talbot-Moiré–based interferometry to obtain real-time aphakic IOL calculations—an approach that has been shown to increase accuracy and improve refractive outcomes in cataract surgery.

Prior to cataract surgery, patients need to be informed that IOL power calculations are less accurate when performed after refractive surgery and that, despite maximum preoperative effort by the surgeon, additional surgery, such as surface ablation, laser in situ keratomileusis (LASIK), IOL exchange, or implantation of a piggyback IOL, may be required to attain a better refractive result if the patient is unwilling to consider corrective glasses or contact lenses to correct the refractive outcome. Cataract surgery done after RK frequently induces short-term corneal swelling with flattening and hyperopic shift. For this reason, in the event of a refractive "surprise," an IOL exchange should not be performed in post-RK eyes until the cornea and refraction stabilize, which may take several weeks to months. Corneal curvature does not tend to change as much following cataract surgery performed after photorefractive keratectomy (PRK) or LASIK; thus, it may be possible to plan and perform an IOL exchange or refractive surgical procedures earlier in these patients.

Eyes With Known Pre– and Post–Refractive Surgery Data

One method for calculating IOL power following refractive surgery is the *clinical history method,* in which pre–refractive surgery refraction and keratometry values, if available, combined with the current refraction and keratometry readings, are used to approximate the true post–refractive keratometry values for the central cornea. Unfortunately, even with these measurements, this approach has not been proven to be accurate. Despite this, pre–refractive surgery information should be kept by both the patient and the surgeon. To assist in retaining these data, the American Academy of Ophthalmology has developed the K-Card with its partner, the International Society of Refractive Surgery. The card is available in PDF form on the Academy website (www.aao.org/patient-safety-statement/kcard).

The key concept is to understand what changes occur on the corneal surface with refractive surgery. To use the historical method, the ophthalmologist should have the pre–refractive surgery refraction and keratometry readings, and the change in spherical equivalent can be calculated at the spectacle plane or, better yet, at the corneal plane. The post–refractive surgery refraction must be stable and obtained several months after the refractive surgery but before the onset of induced myopia from the developing nuclear sclerotic cataract. For example:

Preoperative average keratometry: 44.00 D
Preoperative spherical equivalent refraction (vertex distance 12 mm): –8.00 D
Preoperative refraction at the corneal plane: $-8.00 \text{ D}/(1 - [0.012 \times -8.00 \text{ D}]) = -7.30 \text{ D}$
Postoperative spherical equivalent refraction (vertex distance 12 mm): –1.00 D
Postoperative refraction at the corneal plane: $-1.00 \text{ D}/(1 - [0.012 \times -1.00 \text{ D}]) = -0.98 \text{ D}$
Change in manifest refraction at the corneal plane: $-7.30 \text{ D} - (-0.98 \text{ D}) = -6.32 \text{ D}$
Postoperative estimated keratometry: $44.00 - 6.32 \text{ D} = 37.68 \text{ D}$

Eyes With No Preoperative Information

When no preoperative information is available, the *hard contact lens method* can be used to calculate corneal power. This method is not very useful in clinical practice. The best-corrected visual acuity (BCVA; also called *corrected distance visual acuity, CDVA*) needs to be at least 20/80 for this approach to work. First, a baseline manifest refraction is performed and then a plano hard contact lens of known base curve (power) is placed on the eye, and another manifest refraction is performed. If the manifest refraction does not change, then the cornea has the same power as the contact lens. If the refraction is more myopic, the contact lens is steeper (more powerful) than the cornea by the amount of change in the refraction; the reverse holds true if the refraction is more hyperopic. For example:

> Current spherical equivalent manifest refraction: –1.00 D
> A hard contact lens of known base curve (8.7 mm) and power (37.00 D) is placed
> Overrefraction: +2.00 D
> Change in refraction: +2.00 D – (–1.00 D) = +3.00 D
> Calculation of corneal power: 37.00 D + 3.00 D = 40.00 D

The ASCRS Online Post-Refractive Intraocular Lens Power Calculator

A particularly useful resource for calculating IOL power in a post–refractive surgery patient has been developed by Warren Hill, MD; Li Wang, MD, PhD; and Douglas D. Koch, MD. It is available on the website of the American Society of Cataract and Refractive Surgery (ASCRS) (www.ascrs.org) and directly at http://iolcalc.ascrs.org.

To use this IOL calculator, the surgeon selects the appropriate prior refractive surgical procedure and enters the patient data, if known (Fig 11-1). The IOL powers, calculated by a variety of formulas, are displayed at the bottom of the form, and the surgeon can compare the results to select the best IOL power for the individual situation. This spreadsheet is updated with new formulas and information as they become available and, at this time, probably represents the best option for calculation of IOL powers in post–refractive surgery patients. For more detailed IOL power calculation information, see BCSC Section 3, *Clinical Optics*.

Awwad ST, Manasseh C, Bowman RW, et al. Intraocular lens power calculation after myopic laser in situ keratomileusis: estimating the corneal refractive power. *J Cataract Refract Surg.* 2008;34(7):1070–1076.

Chen M. An evaluation of the accuracy of the ORange (Gen II) by comparing it to the IOL-Master in the prediction of postoperative refraction. *Clin Ophthalmol.* 2012;6:397–401.

Chokshi AR, Latkany RA, Speaker MG, Yu G. Intraocular lens calculations after hyperopic refractive surgery. *Ophthalmology.* 2007;114(11):2044–2049.

Fram NR, Masket S, Wang L. Comparison of intraoperative aberrometry, OCT-based IOL formula, Haigis-L, and Masket formulae for IOL power calculations after laser vision correction. *Ophthalmology.* 2015;122(6):1096–101.

Hill WE, Byrne SF. Complex axial length measurements and unusual IOL power calculations. *Focal Points: Clinical Modules for Ophthalmologists.* San Francisco: American Academy of Ophthalmology; 2004, module 9.

Masket S, Masket SE. Simple regression formula for intraocular lens power adjustment in eyes requiring cataract surgery after excimer laser photoablation. *J Cataract Refract Surg.* 2006; 32(3):430–434.

IOL Calculator for Eyes with Prior Myopic LASIK/PRK
(Your data will not be saved. Please print a copy for your record.)

Please enter all data available and press "Calculate"

Doctor Name [ ]   Patient Name [ ]   Patient ID [ ]

Eye [ ]   IOL Model [ ]   Target Ref (D) [ ]

Pre-LASIK/PRK Data:

Refraction*   Sph(D) [ ]   Cyl(D)* [ ]   Vertex (If empty, 12.5 mm is used) [ ]

Keratometry   K1(D) [ ]   K2(D) [ ]

Post-LASIK/PRK Data:

Refraction*§   Sph(D) [ ]   Cyl(D)* [ ]   Vertex(If empty, 12.5 mm will be used) [ ]

Topography   EyeSys EffRP [ ]   Tomey ACCP / Nidek#ACP/APP [ ]   Galilei TCP [ ]   ○ TCP2 / ○ TCP1

Atlas Zone value   Atlas 9000 4mm zone [ ]   Pentacam TNP_Apex_4.0 mm Zone [ ]

Atlas Ring Values   0mm [ ]   1mm [ ]   2mm [ ]   3mm [ ]

OCT (RTVue or Avanti XR)   Net Corneal Power [ ]   Posterior Corneal Power [ ]   Central Corneal Thickness [ ]

Optical/Ultrasound Biometric Data:

Ks   K1(D) [ ]   K2(D) [ ]   Device Keratometric Index (n) ● 1.3375 ○ 1.332 ○ Other [ ]

    AL(mm) [ ]   ACD(mm) [ ]   Lens Thick (mm) [ ]   WTW (mm) [ ]

Lens Constants**   A-const(SRK/T) [ ]   SF(Holladay1) [ ]

    Haigis a0 (If empty, converted value is used) [ ]   Haigis a1 (If empty, 0.4 is used) [ ]   Haigis a2 (If empty, 0.1 is used) [ ]

*If entering "Sph(D)", you must enter a value for "Cyl(D)", even if it is zero.
§Most recent stable refraction prior to development of a cataract.
Magellan ACP or OPD-Scan III APP 3-mm manual value (personal communication Stephen D. Klyce, PhD).
**Enter any constants available; others will be calculated from those entered. If ultrasonic AL is entered, be sure to use your ultrasound lens constants. It is preferable to use optimized a0, a1, and a2 Haigis constants.

[Calculate]   [Reset Form]

IOL calculation formulas used: Double-K Holladay 1[1], Shammas-PL[2], Haigis-L[3], OCT-based[4], & Barrett True K[5]

Using ΔMR		Using no prior data	
[1]Adjusted EffRP	--	[2]Wang-Koch-Maloney	--
[2]Adjusted Atlas 9000 (4mm zone)	--	[2]Shammas	--
[1]Adjusted Atlas Ring Values	--	[3]Haigis-L	--
Masket Formula	--	[1]Galilei	--
Modified-Masket	--	[2]Potvin-Hill Pentacam	--
[1]Adjusted ACCP/ACP/APP	--	[4]OCT	--
[5]Barrett True K	--	[5]Barrett True K No History	--

Average IOL Power (All Available Formulas): --

Min: --

Max: --

Figure 11-1 The data screen of the post-keratorefractive IOL power calculator of the ASCRS. The surgeon enters the patient's pre–refractive surgery data (if known) and the current data into the data form. After the "calculate" button at the bottom of the form is clicked, the IOL power calculated by a variety of formulas is displayed. (Note: In this illustration, accessed January 19, 2017, the "calculate" button was activated with no patient data entered so as to show the final appearance of the screen; the form itself is updated periodically and available at http://iolcalc.ascrs.org.) *(Used with permission from the American Society of Cataract and Refractive Surgery.)*

Shammas HJ. Intraocular lens power calculation in patients with prior refractive surgery. *Focal Points: Clinical Modules for Ophthalmologists.* San Francisco: American Academy of Ophthalmology; 2013, module 6.

Wang L, Hill WE, Koch DD. Evaluation of intraocular lens power prediction methods using the American Society of Cataract and Refractive Surgeons Post-Keratorefractive Intraocular Lens Power Calculator. *J Cataract Refract Surg.* 2010;36(9):1466–1473.

Retinal Detachment Repair After LASIK

Even if the eyes of patients with high myopia become emmetropic as a result of refractive surgery, these patients need to be informed that their eyes remain at increased risk of retinal detachment. For this reason, symptoms such as floaters or photopsias warrant a thorough retinal evaluation with scleral depression to ensure that there are no peripheral retinal tears or holes. In addition, if vitreoretinal surgery or laser is deemed necessary, the vitreoretinal surgeon should ask about prior refractive surgery. Eyes undergoing retinal detachment repair after LASIK are prone to flap problems, including flap dehiscence, microstriae, and macrostriae. The surgeon may find it helpful to mark the edge of the flap prior to surgery to aid in flap replacement in case the flap is dislodged. The risk of flap problems increases dramatically if the epithelium is debrided during the retinal detachment repair. If flap dehiscence occurs, the flap should be carefully repositioned and the interface irrigated. A bandage contact lens may be placed at the end of the procedure.

Postoperatively, the patient should be observed closely for signs of flap problems such as epithelial ingrowth and diffuse lamellar keratitis, especially if an epithelial defect was present on the flap. After retinal detachment repair, the intraocular pressure (IOP) needs to be monitored, especially when an intraocular gas bubble is used, keeping in mind that IOP measurements may read falsely low after refractive surgery because of corneal thinning. In addition, elevated IOP can cause a diffuse lamellar keratitis–like picture or even a fluid cleft between the flap and the stroma, resulting in a misleading, extremely low IOP measurement (see Chapter 6). These problems are discussed in greater detail later in the chapter in the section Glaucoma After Refractive Surgery.

Qin B, Huang L, Zeng J, Hu J. Retinal detachment after laser in situ keratomileusis in myopic eyes. *Am J Ophthalmol.* 2007;144(6):921–923.

Wirbelauer C, Pham DT. Imaging interface fluid after laser in situ keratomileusis with corneal optical coherence tomography. *J Cataract Refract Surg.* 2005;31(4):853–856.

Corneal Transplantation After Refractive Surgery

Corneal transplantation is occasionally required after refractive surgery. Reasons for needing a corneal graft after refractive surgery include significant corneal scarring, irregular astigmatism, corneal ectasia, and corneal edema. Issues unrelated to refractive surgery, such as trauma, infectious keratitis, or corneal edema after cataract surgery, can also necessitate corneal transplant surgery. Each type of refractive surgical procedure is unique in the reasons a graft may be required and in ways to avoid problems with the corneal transplant. Corneal transplantation techniques and indications are discussed in greater detail in BCSC Section 8, *External Disease and Cornea.*

After RK, a graft may be required because of trauma resulting in incisional rupture, central scarring not responsive to phototherapeutic keratectomy, irregular astigmatism, contact lens intolerance, or progressive hyperopia. The RK incisions can gape or dehisce during penetrating keratoplasty trephination, preventing creation of an even, uniform, and deep trephination. One method for avoiding RK wound gape or dehiscence during keratoplasty is to mark the cornea with the trephine and then reinforce the RK incisions with interrupted sutures outside the trephine mark prior to trephination. If the RK incisions open during the corneal transplant surgery, then X, mattress, or lasso sutures may be required to close these stellate wounds.

Corneal transplantation may also be required after excimer laser surface ablation. However, because of the 6- to 8-mm ablation zones typically used, the corneal periphery is generally not thinned, and transplantation in this situation is usually straightforward.

After LASIK, corneal transplantation may be required to treat central scarring (eg, after infection or with a buttonhole) or corneal ectasia. A significant challenge in this scenario is that most LASIK flaps are larger than a typical trephine size (8 mm). Trephination through the flap increases the risk that the flap peripheral to the corneal transplant wound may separate. This complication may be avoidable through careful trephination and use of a gentle suture technique that incorporates the LASIK flap under the corneal transplant suture. Femtosecond laser trephination theoretically may decrease the risk of flap separation during trephination.

A few cases have been reported of inadvertent use of donor tissue that had undergone prior LASIK. The risk of this untoward event will increase as the donor pool includes more individuals who have undergone LASIK or surface ablation. Eye banks need to develop better methods to screen out such donor corneas. If a post-LASIK eye is inadvertently used for corneal transplantation, the patient should be informed. A regraft may be required to address significant anisometropia or irregular astigmatism.

Corneal transplantation is occasionally required in a patient with intrastromal corneal ring segments. The polymethyl methacrylate ring segments are typically placed near the edge of a standard corneal transplant, so the ring segments may be removed prior to grafting, or—because the ring segments lie within the central 7 mm of the cornea—they may also be left in place and removed in toto with the host tissue or removed at the time of trephination.

Though rare, corneal transplantation after laser thermokeratoplasty or conductive keratoplasty may be required. Trephination should be straightforward in such cases, and the thermal scars should generally be incorporated into the corneal button. Even if the scars are not incorporated and remain peripheral to the new cornea, they should not significantly affect wound architecture, graft healing, or corneal curvature.

Contact Lens Use After Refractive Surgery

Indications

Contact lenses can be used before and after refractive surgery. For example, a patient with presbyopia can use a temporary trial with soft contact lenses to experience monovision before undergoing surgery, thus reducing the risk of postoperative dissatisfaction. Contact lenses can also be used preoperatively in a patient with a motility abnormality (eg, eso-tropia or exotropia) to simulate expected vision after refractive surgery and to ensure that diplopia does not become manifest.

In the perioperative period, hydrophilic soft contact lenses can help promote epithelial healing or prevent flap-related complications. Rigid gas-permeable (RGP) contact lenses are more effective than are soft lenses to correct reduced vision due to residual irregular astigmatism, and they can be a useful adjunct after RK and LASIK. Night-vision problems caused by a persistent, uncorrected refractive error or irregular astigmatism may also be reduced by using contact lenses. However, if the symptoms are related to higher-order aberrations, they may persist despite contact lens use.

General Principles

Contact lenses for refractive purposes should not be fitted until surgical wounds and serial refractions are stable. The most practical approach to fitting an RGP lens after refractive surgery is to do a trial fitting with overrefraction.

The clinician needs to discuss with the patient in understandable terms the challenges of contact lens fitting after refractive surgery and align the patient's expectations with reality. A patient who successfully wore contact lenses before refractive surgery is more likely to be a successful contact lens wearer postoperatively than is one who never wore contact lenses.

Contact Lenses After Radial Keratotomy

Centration is a challenge in fitting contact lenses after RK because the corneal apex is displaced to the midperiphery (Fig 11-2). Frequently used fitting techniques involve referring to the preoperative keratometry readings and basing the initial lens trial on the average keratometry values. Contact lens stability is achieved by adjusting the lens diameter. In general, larger-diameter lenses take advantage of the eyelid to achieve stability. However, they also increase the effective steepness of the lens due to increased sagittal depth. If the preoperative keratometry reading is not available, the ophthalmologist can use a paracentral or midperipheral curve, as measured with postoperative corneal topography, as a starting point.

When a successful fit cannot be obtained with a standard RGP lens, a reverse-geometry lens can be used. The secondary curves can be designed to be as steep as necessary to achieve a stable fit. The larger the optical zone, the flatter the fit.

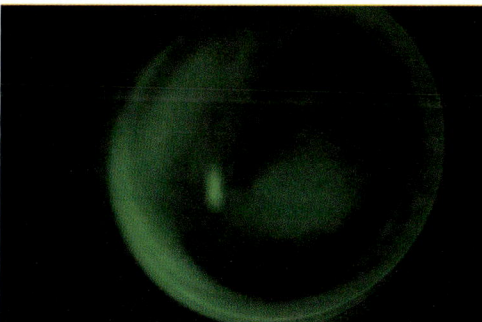

Figure 11-2 Fluorescein staining pattern in a contact lens patient who had undergone RK and LASIK shows pooling centrally and touch in the midperiphery. This pattern is the result of central corneal flattening and steepening in the midperiphery. *(Courtesy of Robert S. Feder, MD.)*

Hydrophilic soft lenses can also be used after RK. Toric soft lenses can be helpful when regular astigmatism is present. Soft lenses are less helpful in eyes with irregular astigmatism because they are less able to mask an irregular surface. Lens designs such as hybrid contacts, which consist of an RGP center surrounded by a soft contact lens skirt, and scleral RGP lenses, which vault the cornea and contact the perilimbal conjunctiva/sclera, may be helpful for patients with significant irregular astigmatism who are intolerant of conventional RGP lenses.

Whenever contact lenses are prescribed for post-RK eyes, as in the preceding scenarios, the ophthalmologist should continue to monitor the cornea to check for neovascularization of the wounds. Should neovascularization occur, contact lens wear should cease. Once the vessels have regressed, refitting can commence.

Contact Lenses After Surface Ablation

Immediately after surface ablation, a soft contact lens is placed on the cornea as a bandage to help promote epithelialization and reduce discomfort. The lens is worn until the corneal epithelium has healed. Healing time depends on the size of the epithelial defect but in general takes between 4 and 7 days. A tight-fitting lens should be removed if there is evidence of corneal hypoxia (eg, corneal edema, folds in the Descemet membrane, or iritis).

Contact Lenses After LASIK

The indications for contact lens fitting after LASIK are similar to those following other types of refractive surgery. The corneal contour is usually stable by 3 months after LASIK for myopia; however, it may take up to 6 months for the cornea to stabilize after LASIK for hyperopia.

A soft contact lens may be used immediately after LASIK surgery to promote epithelialization and to prevent epithelial ingrowth. It is generally used for several days on an extended-wear basis and then removed by the surgeon. Daily-wear contact lenses for refractive purposes should not be considered until the surgeon believes the risk of flap displacement is low.

Glaucoma After Refractive Surgery

The force required for applanation of a Goldmann tonometer is proportional to the central corneal thickness. As a result, an eye that has a thin central cornea may have an artifactually low IOP as measured by Goldmann applanation tonometry (GAT). Patients with normal-tension glaucoma have significantly thinner corneas than do patients with primary open-angle glaucoma. When a correction factor based on corneal thickness is applied, more than 30% of glaucoma patients demonstrate abnormally high IOP. The correction factor needed may be lower for measurements taken with the Tono-Pen (Reichert Technologies, Depew, NY) and the pneumotonometer.

For IOP measured with GAT, an artifactual IOP reduction occurs following surface ablation and LASIK for myopia, both of which reduce central corneal thickness. Similar inaccuracies in IOP measurement can occur after surface ablation and LASIK for hyperopia. After excimer laser refractive surgery, the mean reduction in IOP measurement is 0.63 mm Hg per diopter of correction, with a wide standard deviation. Postoperatively, some patients may demonstrate no change in IOP measurement, whereas others may exhibit an increase. In general, the reduction of measured IOP is greater after LASIK than after surface ablation. Surface ablation patients with a preoperative refractive error of less than 5.00 D may have a negligible decrease in IOP measurements.

Topical corticosteroids that are used after refractive surgery pose a serious risk of corticosteroid-induced IOP elevation, particularly because an accurate IOP measurement is difficult to obtain. By 3 months postoperatively, up to 15% of surface ablation patients may have IOP above 22 mm Hg. If the elevated IOP is not recognized early enough, optic nerve damage and visual field loss can occur.

If topical corticosteroids are used postoperatively for an extended time, periodic, careful disc evaluation is essential. Optic nerve and nerve fiber layer imaging may facilitate the evaluation. Periodic visual field assessment may be more effective than IOP measurement for identifying at-risk patients before severe visual field loss occurs (see Chapter 10, Fig 10-4).

Refractive surgery patients who develop glaucoma are initially treated with IOP-lowering medications, and their IOP is carefully measured. If medication or laser treatment does not adequately reduce the IOP, glaucoma surgery may be recommended. Patients who have had refractive surgery should be warned prior to glaucoma surgery of the potential for transient vision loss from inflammation, hypotony, or change in refractive error. The glaucoma surgeon should be made aware of the patient's previous LASIK in order to avoid trauma to the corneal flap. For additional information on glaucoma management, see BCSC Section 10, *Glaucoma*.

Belin MW, Hannush SB, Yau CW, Schultze RL. Elevated intraocular pressure–induced interlamellar stromal keratitis. *Ophthalmology*. 2002;109(10):1929–1933.

Brandt JD, Beiser JA, Kass MA, Gordon MO. Central corneal thickness in the Ocular Hypertension Treatment Study (OHTS). *Ophthalmology*. 2001;108(10):1779–1788.

Chang DH, Stulting RD. Change in intraocular pressure measurements after LASIK: the effect of refractive correction and the lamellar flap. *Ophthalmology*. 2005;112(6):1009–1016.

Hamilton DR, Manche EE, Rich LF, Maloney RK. Steroid-induced glaucoma after laser in situ keratomileusis associated with interface fluid. *Ophthalmology*. 2002;109(4):659–665.

Kaufmann C, Bachmann LM, Thiel MA. Comparison of dynamic contour tonometry with Goldmann applanation tonometry. *Invest Ophthalmol Vis Sci*. 2004;45(9):3118–3121.

Yang CC, Wang IJ, Chang YC, Lin LL, Chen TH. A predictive model for postoperative intraocular pressure among patients undergoing laser in situ keratomileusis (LASIK). *Am J Ophthalmol*. 2006;141(3):530–536.

CHAPTER **12**

Emerging Technologies

▶ *This chapter includes a related video, which can be accessed by scanning the QR code provided in the text or going to www.aao.org/bcscvideo_section13.*

Over the past 20 years, a wide variety of surgical techniques and technologies have evolved to reduce dependence on contact lenses or glasses for use in routine daily activities. As a new frontier, the field of refractive surgery is expected to see continued innovation and progress. To give the reader a glimpse of the possible future, this chapter highlights some refractive surgical procedures that are not currently approved by the US Food and Drug Administation (FDA). These procedures include all-femtosecond laser keratorefractive surgery as well as corneal crosslinking (CCL) for ectatic disorders combined with additional refractive intervention to achieve visual rehabilitation with greater spectacle and contact lens independence.

Refractive Lenticule Extraction

In 1996, investigators first described the use of a picosecond laser to generate an intrastromal lenticule that was removed manually after the flap was lifted. The main drawbacks of this procedure, which was a precursor to modern refractive lenticule extraction (commonly referred to as ReLEx) were the relatively low precision and accuracy of the laser. In 1998, the first studies involving this technology were performed in rabbit eyes and in partially sighted eyes.

Following the debut of the VisuMax femtosecond laser (Carl Zeiss Meditec, Jena, Germany) in 2007, the intrastromal lenticule method was reintroduced in a procedure named femtosecond lenticule extraction (commonly referred to as FLEx) This procedure involved intrastromal dissection of a refractive lenticule as well as creation of a corneal flap and was performed exclusively by femtosecond laser. The refractive results were similar to those observed in laser in situ keratomileusis (LASIK), but the visual recovery time was longer.

More recently, a method called small-incision lenticule extraction (SMILE), has been developed. It is also a form of lenticule extraction but has the advantage of being performed entirely within a pocket, thereby avoiding the need for a flap. Conformité Européenne (CE) marking was achieved in 2009. SMILE received FDA approval in September 2016 after US pivotal studies.

Blum M, Kunert KS, Engelbrecht C, Dawczynski J, Sekundo W. [Femtosecond lenticule extraction (FLEx)—results after 12 months in myopic astigmatism]. *Klin Monbl Augenheilkd.* 2010; 227(12):961–965. German.

Krueger RR, Juhasz T, Gualano A, Marchi V. The picosecond laser for nonmechanical laser in situ keratomileusis. *J Refract Surg.* 1998;14(4):467–469.

Sekundo W, Kunert KS, Blum M. Small incision corneal refractive surgery using the small incision lenticule extraction (SMILE) procedure for the correction of myopia and myopic astigmatism: results of a 6-month prospective study. *Br J Ophthalmol.* 2011;95(3): 335–339.

Shah R, Shah S. Effect of scanning patterns on the results of femtosecond laser lenticule extraction refractive surgery. *J Cataract Refract Surg.* 2011;37(9):1636–1647.

Vestergaard A, Ivarsen A, Asp S, Hjortdal JØ. Femtosecond (FS) laser vision correction procedure for moderate to high myopia: a prospective study of ReLEx® FLEx and comparison with a retrospective study of FS-laser in situ keratomileusis. *Acta Ophthalmol.* 2013;91(4): 355–362.

Indications and Preoperative Evaluation

The SMILE procedure (as of the printing of this book) is approved for use in the reduction or elimination of myopia –1.00 D to –8.00 D, with ≤–0.50 D cylinder and MRSE –8.25 D in the eye to be treated in patients aged 22 years or older with documentation of stable manifest refraction over the past year. Preoperative evaluation is similar to that for patients undergoing photoablative procedures, such as LASIK or photorefractive keratectomy (PRK); as in all refractive procedures involving tissue removal, a primary goal is to exclude patients with corneal ectatic diseases and susceptibility to postoperative ectasia.

Ambrósio R Jr, Ramos I, Lopes B, et al. Ectasia susceptibility before laser vision correction. *J Cataract Refract Surg.* 2015;41(6):1335–1336.

Moshirfar M, McCaughey MV, Reinstein DZ, Shah R, Santiago-Caban L, Fenzl CR. Small-incision lenticule extraction. *J Cataract Refract Surg.* 2015;41(3):652–665.

Surgical Technique

During SMILE, the femtosecond laser creates first the lower interface of the intrastromal lenticule (using an *out-to-in* direction, in order to minimize the length of time that the patient's central vision is blurred), then the upper interface of the lenticule (using an *in-to-out* direction). The surgeon then makes a tunnel incision (usually superotemporal) measuring 2–3 mm, connecting the cap interface to the corneal surface (Video 12-1). The total time to generate the incisions is between 20 and 35 seconds, regardless of the magnitude of the refractive error. A spatula is then inserted through the tunnel incision to separate residual lenticular attachments, first within the anterior lamella and then within the posterior plane. Once both planes have been separated, microforceps are used to extract the intrastromal lenticule.

VIDEO 12-1 Small incision lenticule extraction procedure.
Courtesy of Renato Ambrósio Jr, MD, PhD.
Access all Section 13 videos at www.aao.org/bcscvideo_section13.

Ivarsen A, Asp S, Hjortdal J. Safety and complications of more than 1500 small-incision lenticule extraction procedures. *Ophthalmology.* 2014;121(4):822–828.

Moshirfar M, McCaughey MV, Reinstein DZ, Shah R, Santiago-Caban L, Fenzl CR. Small-incision lenticule extraction. *J Cataract Refract Surg.* 2015;41(3):652–665.

Reinstein DZ, Archer TJ, Gobbe M. Small incision lenticule extraction (SMILE) history, fundamentals of a new refractive surgery technique and clinical outcomes. *Eye Vis (Lond).* 2014 Oct 16;1:3.

Outcomes

Several studies have compared refractive outcomes of SMILE with those of LASIK. Overall, studies have shown that SMILE results are nearly identical to those of femtosecond laser–assisted LASIK. Currently, the disadvantage of SMILE is its slightly slower visual recovery on postoperative day 1. In a study comparing SMILE with femtosecond laser–assisted LASIK, the uncorrected visual acuity (UCVA; also called *uncorrected distance visual acuity, UDVA*) in the LASIK group was at first statistically better than in the SMILE group, but at 6 months, no difference in vision was observed between the 2 groups. Incidentally, spherical aberration was lower in the SMILE group. Another study reported that 84% of eyes in each group achieved a UCVA of 20/20; however, 12% in the SMILE group and 4% in the LASIK group achieved a UCVA of 20/15. Higher-order aberrations, postoperative dry eye difficulty, and glare were significantly more common in the LASIK group.

Ganesh S, Gupta R. Comparison of visual and refractive outcomes following femtosecond laser–assisted LASIK with SMILE in patients with myopia or myopic astigmatism. *J Refract Surg.* 2014;30(9):590–596.

Liu M, Chen Y, Wang D, et al. Clinical outcomes after SMILE and femtosecond laser–assisted LASIK for myopia and myopic astigmatism: a prospective randomized comparative study. *Cornea.* 2016;35(2):210–216.

Complications

Studies have reported a low incidence of complications related to SMILE. Because the procedure can be technically challenging, most of the complications described in the literature occurred early in the learning curve. In a study enrolling 1800 eyes treated with SMILE, perioperative complications included epithelial abrasions (occurring in 6.0% of eyes), difficult lenticule extraction (1.9%), small tears at the incision (1.8%), and cap perforation (0.22%); a major tear occurred in 1 eye (0.06%). However, none of these patients reported late visual symptoms. Postoperative complications included trace haze (8.0%), epithelial dryness on postoperative day 1 (5.0%), interface inflammation secondary to central abrasion (0.3%), and minor interface infiltrates (0.3%). Topographic irregular astigmatism was described in 1.0% of eyes, resulting in reduced 3-month best-corrected visual acuity (BCVA; also called *corrected distance visual acuity, CDVA*), or ghost images. Another complication unique to SMILE is the presence of a lenticule remnant in the interface. Postoperative ectasia has also been reported.

Dong Z, Zhou X. Irregular astigmatism after femtosecond laser refractive lenticule extraction. *J Cataract Refract Surg.* 2013;39(6):952–954.

Ivarsen A, Asp S, Hjortdal J. Safety and complications of more than 1500 small-incision lenticule extraction procedures. *Ophthalmology.* 2014;121(4):822–828.

Re-treatment After SMILE

There are many options for performing re-treatments after SMILE. The choice is often dictated by the primary cap thickness and the availability of the technology. The cap may be converted into a flap and a thin-flap LASIK procedure may be performed. PRK may also be performed to re-treat SMILE patients.

Riau AK, Ang HP, Lwin NC, Chaurasia SS, Tan DT, Mehta JS. Comparison of four different VisuMax circle patterns for flap creation after small incision lenticule extraction. *J Refract Surg*. 2013;29(4):236–244.

Zhao J, Yao P, Chen Z, et al. Enhancement of femtosecond lenticule extraction for visual symptomatic eye after myopia correction. *BMC Ophthalmol*. 2014 May 18;14:68.

Comparison With LASIK

Because SMILE does not involve creation of a flap, the procedure has potential advantages over LASIK. Therefore, flap-related complications are avoided. In addition to reduced aberrations, dry eye difficulty, and glare, SMILE offers the relative preservation of biomechanical stability due to the absence of a flap and the maintenance of anterior stroma lamellae. The procedure may be particularly appropriate for patients who are involved in contact sports or high-risk professions.

Corneal Crosslinking Plus Refractive Procedures

Corneal crosslinking (CCL) has been gaining popularity internationally as a first-line treatment for keratoconus and other ectatic disorders of the cornea (see Chapter 7). However, the primary objective of the procedure is to stabilize a progressive ectatic condition; the patient will likely be relegated to using optical correction (glasses or contact lenses) to optimize visual acuity.

Visual rehabilitation of ectasia must achieve stabilization (using CCL) while reducing corneal irregularity and minimizing the residual refractive error. The term *corneal crosslinking plus* refers to CCL plus additional procedures such as PRK, phototherapeutic keratectomy (PTK), intracorneal ring segment (ICRS) implantation, conductive keratoplasty (CK), and phakic intraocular lens (PIOL) implantation.

Kymionis GD. Corneal collagen cross linking—plus. *Open Ophthalmol J*. 2011 Feb 11;5:10. doi:10.2174/1874364101105010010.

Photorefractive or Phototherapeutic Keratectomy and Corneal Crosslinking

Topography-guided PRK (T-PRK) may be performed either after CCL or simultaneously. One study showed that same-day simultaneous T-PRK and CCL is superior to sequential CCL and T-PRK beyond 6 months. It is believed that CCL followed by T-PRK 6 months later would remove the stiffened crosslinked cornea, thereby reducing the benefits of CCL; thus, simultaneous T-PRK and CXL is preferred. Similarly, another study demonstrated significant improvement in mean spherical equivalent refraction, defocus aberration, UCVA and BCVA, and keratometric parameters in patients undergoing simultaneous T-PRK and CCL.

The primary variables in combined T-PRK and CXL are the maximal ablation depth and the postoperative corneal thickness. Most surgeons choose a maximum ablation depth of 50 μm and a minimal postoperative corneal thickness of 350–400 μm. Although some surgeons advocate the use of mitomycin C 0.02% to prevent haze, others believe that it is not necessary.

In patients with keratoconus, the epithelium is not uniform in thickness; rather, it is thinner directly above the cone. Therefore, manual removal of the epithelium over the central 6–8 mm will "unmask" the corneal stromal irregularity. In contrast, transepithelial PTK has the advantage of removing the thinned epithelium, Bowman layer, and stroma over the cone apex. Thus, the procedure may be able to regularize the anterior corneal surface while allowing the patient's epithelium to act as a masking agent.

Kanellopoulos AJ. Comparison of sequential vs same-day simultaneous collagen cross-linking and topography-guided PRK for treatment of keratoconus. *J Refract Surg.* 2009; 25(9):S812–S818.

Kymionis GD, Kontadakis GA, Kounis GA, et al. Simultaneous topography-guided PRK followed by corneal collagen cross-linking for keratoconus. *J Refract Surg.* 2009;25(9): S807–S811.

Stojanovic A, Zhang J, Chen X, Nitter TA, Chen S, Wang Q. Topography-guided transepithelial surface ablation followed by corneal collagen cross-linking performed in a single combined procedure for the treatment of keratoconus and pellucid marginal degeneration. *J Refract Surg.* 2010;26(2):145–152.

Intracorneal Ring Segment Implantation and Corneal Crosslinking

Although ICRS implantation flattens the cone and regularizes the corneal topography, the procedure might not halt the progression of the ectatic process. Combining ICRS implantation and CCL may achieve both goals, however. Variations in technique relate to the number of segments used, the location of the segments, and the timing of the procedures.

One study reported that inferior-segment Intacs (Addition Technology, Lombard, IL) implantation with CCL resulted in better keratoconus improvement than Intacs implantation alone. Another study demonstrated that ICRS implantation followed by CCL resulted in better outcomes than CCL followed by ICRS.

Chan CC, Sharma M, Wachler BS. Effect of inferior-segment Intacs with and without C3-R on keratoconus. *J Cataract Refract Surg.* 2007;33(1):75–80.

Coskunseven E, Jankov MR 2nd, Hafezi F, Atun S, Arslan E, Kymionis GD. Effect of treatment sequence in combined intrastromal corneal rings and corneal collagen crosslinking for keratoconus. *J Cataract Refract Surg.* 2009;35(12):2084–2091.

Phakic Intraocular Lens Implantation and Corneal Crosslinking

Several reports have demonstrated the benefits of PIOL implantation in conjunction with CCL. In patients with keratoconus, toric posterior chamber PIOLs and foldable iris-claw

PIOLs both have shown improved refractive outcomes with good safety (no loss of BCVA and no significant decrease in endothelial cell count). Neither of these PIOLs has been approved by the US FDA.

Kymionis GD, Grentzelos MA, Portaliou DM, et al. Corneal collagen cross-linking (CXL) combined with refractive procedures for the treatment of corneal ectatic disorders: CXL plus. *J Refract Surg.* 2014;30(8):566–576.

Basic Texts

Refractive Surgery

Azar DT, Gatinel D, Hoang-Xuan T, eds. *Refractive Surgery*. 2nd ed. Philadelphia: Elsevier/ Mosby; 2007.

Boyd BF, Agarwal S, Agarwal A, Agarwal A, eds. *LASIK and Beyond LASIK: Wavefront Analysis and Customized Ablations*. Thorofare, NJ: Slack; 2001.

Feder R. *The LASIK Handbook: A Case-Based Approach*. 2nd ed. Philadelphia: Lippincott Williams & Wilkins; 2013.

Garg A, Rosen E, Lin JT, et al, eds. *Mastering the Techniques of Customized LASIK*. New Delhi: Jaypee Brothers; 2007.

Hardten DR, Lindstrom RL, Davis EA, eds. *Phakic Intraocular Lenses: Principles and Practice*. Thorofare, NJ: Slack; 2003.

Probst LE, ed. *LASIK: Advances, Controversies, and Custom*. Thorofare, NJ: Slack; 2003.

Troutman RC, Buzard KA. *Corneal Astigmatism: Etiology, Prevention, and Management*. St Louis: Mosby; 1992.

Wang MX, ed. *Refractive Lens Exchange: A Surgical Treatment for Presbyopia*. Thorofare, NJ: Slack; 2015.

Related Academy Materials

The American Academy of Ophthalmology is dedicated to providing a wealth of high-quality clinical education resources for ophthalmologists.

Print Publications and Electronic Products

For a complete listing of Academy products related to topics covered in this BCSC Section, visit our online store at https://store.aao.org/clinical-education/topic/refractive-mgmt-intervention.html. Or call Customer Service at 866.561.8558 (toll free, US only) or +1 415.561.8540, Monday through Friday, between 8:00 AM and 5:00 PM (PST).

Online Resources

Visit the Ophthalmic News and Education (ONE®) Network at aao.org/onenetwork to find relevant videos, online courses, journal articles, practice guidelines, self-assessment quizzes, images, and more. The ONE Network is a free Academy-member benefit.

Access free, trusted articles and content with the Academy's collaborative online encyclopedia, EyeWiki, at aao.org/eyewiki.

Requesting Continuing Medical Education Credit

The American Academy of Ophthalmology is accredited by the Accreditation Council for Continuing Medical Education (ACCME) to provide continuing medical education for physicians.

The American Academy of Ophthalmology designates this enduring material for a maximum of 10 *AMA PRA Category 1 Credits™*. Physicians should claim only the credit commensurate with the extent of their participation in the activity.

To claim *AMA PRA Category 1 Credits™* upon completion of this activity, learners must demonstrate appropriate knowledge and participation in the activity by taking the posttest for Section 13 and achieving a score of 80% or higher.

To take the posttest and request CME credit online:

1. Go to www.aao.org/cme-central and log in.
2. Click on "Claim CME Credit and View My CME Transcript" and then "Report AAO Credits."
3. Select the appropriate media type and then the Academy activity. You will be directed to the posttest.
4. Once you have passed the test with a score of 80% or higher, you will be directed to your transcript. *If you are not an Academy member, you will be able to print out a certificate of participation once you have passed the test.*

CME expiration date: June 1, 2020. *AMA PRA Category 1 Credits™* may be claimed only once between June 1, 2017, and the expiration date.

For assistance, contact the Academy's Customer Service department at 866.561.8558 (US only) or + 1 415.561.8540 between 8:00 am and 5:00 pm (PST), Monday through Friday, or send an e-mail to customer_service@aao.org.

Study Questions

Please note that these questions are *not* part of your CME reporting process. They are provided here for your own educational use and identification of any professional practice gaps. The required CME posttest is available online (see "Requesting CME Credit"). Following the questions are a blank answer sheet and answers with discussions. Although a concerted effort has been made to avoid ambiguity and redundancy in these questions, the authors recognize that differences of opinion may occur regarding the "best" answer. The discussions are provided to demonstrate the rationale used to derive the answer. They may also be helpful in confirming that your approach to the problem was correct or, if necessary, in fixing the principle in your memory. The Section 13 faculty thanks the Self-Assessment Committee for reviewing these self-assessment questions.

1. A Placido disk–based corneal topographer uses what technology?
   a. scanning slit beam of light swept across the cornea
   b. laser reflected off the retina and captured by a lenslet array
   c. image of a series of concentric rings reflected off the cornea
   d. ultrasonic image of the corneal surface

2. What finding will affect Placido disk–based topography measurements of the corneal curvature?
   a. dry eye
   b. latent hyperopia
   c. senile furrow degeneration
   d. previous photorefractive keratectomy (PRK)

3. Which variable will affect the depth of laser ablation required to treat a specific degree of myopia?
   a. corneal density
   b. ambient humidity in the laser suite
   c. optical zone diameter
   d. central keratometric power

4. When considering a patient's candidacy for laser in situ keratomileusis (LASIK), what is the minimum residual stromal bed thickness?
   a. 250 μm
   b. 225 μm
   c. 200 μm
   d. 175 μm

5. What condition might prevent a 25-year-old patient from being a good candidate for PRK?
   a. pregnancy
   b. posterior polymorphous corneal dystrophy
   c. high myopia
   d. asthma

6. Cycloplegic refraction is recommended as part of the preoperative evaluation for myopic LASIK to prevent which result?
   a. regression
   b. overcorrection
   c. ectasia
   d. diplopia

7. Prior to refractive surgery, how long should patients be advised to avoid use of rigid contact lenses?
   a. 1 week
   b. 3 weeks
   c. 6 weeks
   d. 12 weeks

8. Changing what characteristic of an arcuate keratotomy procedure may result in an overcorrection?
   a. incision placed at a smaller optical zone
   b. incision placed at a larger optical zone
   c. shorter incision length
   d. shallower incision

9. What complication of radial keratotomy (RK) commonly occurs 10 years after the procedure?
   a. nuclear sclerotic cataract
   b. ocular hypertension
   c. progressive hyperopia
   d. globe perforation

10. Intrastromal corneal ring segments may be implanted to improve vision in what condition?
    a. herpetic keratitis
    b. keratoconus
    c. recurrent corneal erosions
    d. stromal corneal dystrophy

11. Intrastromal corneal ring segments are made from what material?
    a. hydrophilic gel
    b. silicone
    c. polymethyl methacrylate (PMMA)
    d. glass

12. Alloplastic corneal inlays can be used to treat what condition?
    a. myopia
    b. presbyopia
    c. keratoconus
    d. aniridia

13. What is the mechanism of action of presbyopic inlays?
    a. induced multifocality
    b. pinhole effect
    c. increased corneal thickness
    d. reduced corneal refractive power

14. What advantages does the femtosecond laser for lamellar flap creation for LASIK surgery offer compared to microkeratome use?
    a. reduced procedure time
    b. lower total treatment cost
    c. more predictable flap thickness
    d. increased iris registration success

15. What is an important preoperative step prior to the laser ablation in the LASIK procedure?
    a. Apply topical anesthetic at least 5 times 15 minutes prior to surgery.
    b. Cover the eye that is not being treated to block fixation.
    c. Perform a retrobulbar block to prevent pain during the flap creation.
    d. Place asymmetrical marks on the cornea to help with flap alignment.

16. What postoperative pain management after PRK carries the least toxicity?
    a. commercially available topical anesthetics every 2 hours after the procedure
    b. topical nonsteroidal anti-inflammatory drugs (NSAIDs) every 2 hours after the procedure
    c. sparingly used nonpreserved topical NSAIDs
    d. topical mitomycin C twice a day for 36 hours after the procedure

17. What optical effect is observed following wavefront-guided and wavefront-optimized ablations, compared to conventional excimer laser ablations?

    a. improved contrast sensitivity

    b. increased nighttime glare and halos

    c. increased postoperative higher-order aberrations

    d. increased postoperative spherical aberration

18. Regarding corneal haze after PRK, what is the primary natural history or mechanism of action?

    a. The haze usually presents several days after PRK.

    b. The severity of haze is greater in lower corrections.

    c. The haze results from deposits from increased keratocyte activity.

    d. The haze typically does not improve over time.

19. Which individuals may be at a higher risk for an excimer laser overcorrection?

    a. individuals who are younger

    b. individuals who have lower refractive errors

    c. individuals who are older

    d. individuals with minimal stromal bed exposure during the surgery

20. What vitamin is responsible for generation of singlet oxygen in corneal crosslinking?

    a. thiamine (B_1)

    b. niacin (B_3)

    c. riboflavin (B_2)

    d. pantothenic acid (B_{12})

21. What postoperative complication of corneal crosslinking is more likely with inadequate riboflavin saturation in a very thin cornea?

    a. improvement in best-corrected visual acuity

    b. endothelial cell damage with resultant corneal edema

    c. altered index of refraction with change in spectacle correction

    d. corneal steepening

22. Which preoperative testing is required prior to phakic IOL implantation but is unnecessary in patients considering LASIK?

    a. Schirmer test

    b. anterior chamber depth measurements

    c. corneal topography

    d. Worth 4-dot test

23. What preoperative test is most crucial for determining the available strategies for astigmatism correction in evaluating a patient for a refractive lens exchange?
    a. manual keratometry
    b. simulated keratometry from an autorefractor or topographer
    c. corneal topography
    d. Scheimpflug measurement of lenticular astigmatism

24. When offering monovision for a patient who desires near and distance vision with contact lenses, refractive surgery, or cataract surgery, what refractive error differential typically provides the best balance of distance and near vision, with good tolerance?
    a. The nondominant eye is corrected for distance and the dominant eye with a target refraction of −3.25 D.
    b. The dominant eye is corrected for distance and the nondominant eye with a target refraction of −1.25 D to −2.50 D.
    c. The nondominant eye is corrected for distance and the dominant eye with a target refraction of −0.50 D.
    d. The dominant eye is corrected for distance and the nondominant eye with a target refraction of −0.50 D.

25. A 65-year-old woman undergoes cataract surgery with implantation of a multifocal IOL (MFIOL). Two weeks postoperatively, she notes that she is experiencing glare and halos around lights at night. What is the most appropriate next step?
    a. Remove and replace the MFIOL with a monofocal IOL because the multifocal lens is probably causing the halos and glare.
    b. Proceed with Nd:YAG laser capsulotomy.
    c. Evaluate the ocular surface thoroughly to rule out tear dysfunction.
    d. Plan a return to the operating room to reposition the IOL, as decentration may be the cause.

26. Corneal inlays are approved by the Food and Drug Administration to treat what condition?
    a. early to moderate presbyopia
    b. early signs of keratoconus
    c. ectasia after LASIK
    d. progressive hyperopia after RK

27. A 45-year-old patient with myopia desires monovision correction with LASIK. The nondominant eye is chosen for near vision and has a refraction of −5.00 sphere. Assuming no nomogram adjustment is required, what is the most appropriate laser treatment setting?
    a. +3.50 sphere
    b. −6.50 sphere
    c. −3.50 sphere
    d. +6.50 sphere

28. What is the most common complication of dry eyes after LASIK?

    a. diffuse lamellar keratitis

    b. epithelial basement membrane dystrophy

    c. dislocation of the flap

    d. decreased vision

29. What is an absolute contraindication for performing LASIK?

    a. dry eyes

    b. history of herpes simplex keratitis

    c. autoimmune disease

    d. predicted residual corneal bed less than 250 μm

30. What clinical presentations would be an absolute contraindication to performing LASIK surgery?

    a. myopic patient with keratometry readings of 39.00 diopters (D)

    b. hyperopic patient with keratometry readings of 46.00 D

    c. patient with active, uncontrolled connective tissue or autoimmune disease

    d. patient with a predicted residual corneal bed less than 275 μm

31. A patient has a history of strabismus without diplopia. What is a possible result of performing PRK?

    a. reduced accommodative convergence in hyperopic PRK, resulting in lessening of esotropia.

    b. alleviated need for prism correction

    c. significantly improved best-corrected visual acuity in older children with dense amblyopia

    d. persistent diplopia that can be treated with extraocular muscle surgery

32. A 42-year-old man with adult-onset diabetes mellitus reports worsening vision at distance over the past 6 months. The patient has not worn eyeglasses or contact lenses in the past, but asks about the possibility of LASIK surgery to correct his vision. During the past 2 years, the patient states that his glucose levels have ranged between 175 to 350 mg/dL, and the most recent $HgbA_{1c}$ was 8.5. Best-corrected visual acuity is 20/15 in each eye (OD: −2.50 sphere; OS: −2.00 sphere) and the ophthalmologic evaluation is otherwise normal. What is the most appropriate initial treatment?

    a. contact lens fitting

    b. eyeglass correction

    c. improving glucose control and scheduling a repeat refraction

    d. LASIK surgery

33. A 22-year-old man is referred for a LASIK evaluation. He has noted worsening visual acuity over the past 3 years, which has required several eyeglass prescription changes. He states that he had good vision with soft contact lenses as a teenager, but he cannot see well with his current soft contact lens prescription. A manifest refraction reveals 3 diopters of nonorthogonal astigmatism, and manual keratometry shows irregular mires. What test is most appropriate for establishing a diagnosis of forme fruste keratoconus?

    a. corneal pachymetry

    b. corneal topography

    c. cycloplegic refraction

    d. slit-lamp photography

34. A patient presents with nuclear cataracts in both eyes. He has a history of a bilateral 16-incision RK procedure with a 3-mm optical zone. His vision is limited to 20/60 best distance vision in both eyes related to the cataracts, and he undergoes cataract surgery and IOL implantation. At his 2-week postoperative visit, his vision is corrected to 20/25+ with a measured refractive error of +1.50 −0.50 × 120. He is very unhappy with his uncorrected vision, as he had hoped for either an emmetropic or a slight myopic outcome. What is the next best option for this patient?

    a. Perform an IOL exchange, as it appears the choice of IOL power was incorrect, leaving him hyperopic.

    b. Plan surface ablation to correct his hyperopic outcome.

    c. Inform him that this is a typical outcome in RK eyes and that there is nothing more than can be done and glasses are the best option.

    d. Assure him that with time and as the swelling of the cornea resolves, the hyperopia may lessen, requiring follow-up and monitoring.

35. A 28-year-old woman undergoes LASIK for myopic astigmatism with great success, achieving uncorrected distance vision of 20/20 1 week after LASIK. She returns 3 years later, reporting blurring of her distance vision. She is noted to have uncorrected distance vision of 20/50 in her right eye and 20/60 in the left, with a refractive error of −1.25 +0.75 × 89 in the right eye and −1.00 +1.25 × 100 in the left eye. What is the next best option for this patient?

    a. Proceed with flap lift and touchup to treat the regression of her initial LASIK treatment.

    b. Assess the corneal topographic change and rule out post-LASIK ectasia.

    c. Perform surface ablation to treat the refractive error.

    d. Rule out cataract formation, as nuclear cataracts can result in a myopic shift.

36. What is an appropriate initial management option to improve vision for myopic astigmatism induced by corneal ectasia after LASIK?

    a. wavefront-guided enhancement

    b. refractive lens exchange

    c. radial and astigmatic keratotomy

    d. rigid gas-permeable contact lens

37. What is the primary difference between femtosecond lenticule extraction (FLEx) and small-incision lenticule extraction (SMILE)?

    a. flap creation

    b. use of the femtosecond laser

    c. stromal lenticule creation

    d. use for myopia correction

Answer Sheet for Section 13 Study Questions

Question	Answer	Question	Answer
1	a b c d	20	a b c d
2	a b c d	21	a b c d
3	a b c d	22	a b c d
4	a b c d	23	a b c d
5	a b c d	24	a b c d
6	a b c d	25	a b c d
7	a b c d	26	a b c d
8	a b c d	27	a b c d
9	a b c d	28	a b c d
10	a b c d	29	a b c d
11	a b c d	30	a b c d
12	a b c d	31	a b c d
13	a b c d	32	a b c d
14	a b c d	33	a b c d
15	a b c d	34	a b c d
16	a b c d	35	a b c d
17	a b c d	36	a b c d
18	a b c d	37	a b c d
19	a b c d		

Answers

1. **c.** A Placido disk–based topographer captures and analyzes an image of a series of concentric rings reflected off the corneal surface. The computer measures the distance from the edge of each ring to the next ring along multiple semi-meridians and generates a map of the corneal surface that would be required to produce the captured image. These data are frequently expressed in color maps. The system can present the color maps in several ways, including axial curvature, tangential curvature, best-fit sphere, and an image of the rings themselves as seen by the computer.

2. **a.** Placido disk topography uses the image of a series of concentric rings reflected from the corneal surface, and the resulting information depends on several variables. One of the most important is the quality of the air/tear film interface, the interface that gives rise to most of the eye's focusing power. If the tear film is irregular or the eye is dry, the Placido imaging device can generate abnormal reflections that result in unreliable data about corneal curvature. In addition, if the topographer is misaligned to the optical axis, the data is less than optimal. Peripheral corneal findings or refractive error due to latent hyperopia would not be expected to affect central corneal topography measurements.

3. **c.** The amount of tissue removed centrally for myopic treatments using a broad beam laser is estimated by the Munnerlyn formula: Ablation Depth (μm) ≈ Degree of Myopia (D) × (Optical Zone diameter)^2 (mm)/3. This formula shows that for a specific degree of myopia, ablation depth increases by the square of the treated optical zone. The effective change is independent of the initial corneal curvature. The density of the cornea may change the amount of tissue ablated per unit of laser energy, but it will not change the depth of ablation required to correct a specific degree of myopia. Because excimer laser irradiation is absorbed by hydrocarbons, increasing humidity in the laser suite may require increasing power delivered to the cornea to get the same effect at the corneal surface; however, this will not affect the depth of the laser ablation required to treat a specific degree of myopia.

4. **a.** Leaving a residual stromal bed of less than 250 μm may place the patient at higher risk of developing corneal ectasia after laser in situ keratomileusis (LASIK) surgery.

5. **a.** Pregnancy and breastfeeding can cause a temporary change in refraction, which makes refractive surgery potentially less accurate. Many surgeons recommend waiting at least 3 months after delivery and cessation of breastfeeding before performing the refractive surgery evaluation and procedure.

6. **b.** Younger patients may be accommodating during the dry refraction, thereby resulting in an overminused refraction. In a myopic eye, using an inaccurate dry refraction would result in overcorrection; in a hyperopic eye, an overminused refraction would result in an undercorrection. By performing a wet, or cycloplegic, refraction, the true refractive error can be unmasked. Many surgeons perform manifest and cycloplegic refractions close together. If they are not performed close together, a post-cycloplegic dry refraction should be performed later to obtain the correct refraction for use in refractive surgery.

7. **b.** Contact lens wear may result in corneal warpage. Many surgeons recommend that patients discontinue use of soft contact lenses for 3 days to 2 weeks, soft toric contact lenses for 2 weeks or longer, and rigid contact lenses for 2–3 weeks before the refractive surgery evaluation. This allows the cornea to resume its normal, baseline characteristics, which

can then use used to plan refractive surgery. In some long-term hard contact lens wearers, the cornea may require months to return to a stable curvature, and sequential corneal mapping is recommended to document stability.

8. **a.** For an arcuate keratotomy procedure, cylindrical correction can be increased by increasing the length or depth of the incision, using multiple incisions or reducing the optical zone.

9. **c.** Progressive hyperopia is a common long-term finding due to progressive central corneal flattening after RK due to peripheral corneal instability. The Prospective Evaluation of Radial Keratotomy (PERK) study found that 43% of eyes undergoing RK developed progressive hyperopia and were overcorrected by more than 1.00 diopters at 10 years postoperatively. Loss of best-corrected visual acuity (BCVA; also called *corrected distance visual acuity*, CDVA) secondary to nuclear sclerotic cataract can occur after RK surgery; however, this usually occurs secondary to aging and is not related to the procedure itself. Increased intraocular pressure is a rare complication that can occur secondary to treatment with topical corticosteroids in the early postoperative period. Globe perforation is a rare complication that can occur during the RK procedure.

10. **b.** Intrastromal corneal ring segments may be implanted to improve vision in patients with keratoconus and post-LASIK ectasia. These segments were originally used for the refractive correction of mild myopia (−1 to 3D). They are typically contraindicated in patients with collagen vascular, autoimmune, or immunodeficiency diseases; patients who may be predisposed to future complications because of the presence of ocular conditions, such as herpetic keratitis, recurrent corneal erosion syndrome, and corneal dystrophy; and in pregnant or breastfeeding women.

11. **c.** Intrastromal corneal ring segments are made of polymethyl methacrylate (PMMA).

12. **b.** Alloplastic corneal inlays can be used to treat presbyopic patients. These inlays have several potential advantages over homoplastic inlays, such as the ability to be accurately mass-produced in a wide range of sizes and powers. Four different presbyopic inlays have been developed and are currently in investigational studies. In 2015, the United States Food and Drug Administration approved the small-aperture KAMRA corneal inlay (Acu-Focus Inc, Irvine, CA) for the improvement of near vision in presbyopic patients who require near correction.

13. **b.** Presbyopic inlays correct presbyopia via several methods: the pinhole effect, change of (increased) anterior corneal curvature, and addition of corneal convergent power. Currently, there are no presbyopic inlays based on the multifocality or corneal thickness change.

14. **c.** Several studies have compared the benefits of the mechanical microkeratome with those of femtosecond lasers for creating flaps. Minimal differences between the techniques have been found for most patients. However, the flap thickness achieved with the femtosecond laser seems to be more predictable, with less variability than flaps created with a mechanical microkeratome. Please see Table 5-2 for a summary of the advantages and disadvantages of the femtosecond laser.

15. **b.** Many surgeons make asymmetric (not symmetric) sterile ink marks on the cornea prior to laser ablation in the LASIK procedure. Because of their asymmetry, these marks can aid in alignment of the flap at the end of surgery and in proper orientation in the rare event of a free flap. It is helpful to avoid heavy ink marks that might cause epithelial toxicity. Topi-

cal anesthetics should be applied immediately before the procedure, as excess anesthetic may cause the epithelium to slough. It is important to cover the eye not being treated to prevent cross-fixation by the patient on the laser fixation target.

16. **c.** Commercially prepared preserved topical anesthetics can severely inhibit the healing process and may lead to persistent epithelial defects that can lead to corneal haze and scarring. Topical NSAIDs may be used sparingly, but they can have an anesthetic effect and may inhibit healing. If the reepithelialization of the cornea appears to be impaired, then any agent that may impair healing should be stopped to reduce the risk of haze. Mitomycin C does not help with pain and has significant toxicity.

17. **a.** Wavefront-guided and wavefront-optimized ablations offer better contrast sensitivity than conventional excimer laser ablations, because they limit the amount of induced higher-order aberrations.

18. **c.** Animal studies demonstrate an increase in keratocyte activity, which results in deposition of extracellular matrix in the anterior stroma. Corneal haze after photorefractive keratectomy (PRK) typically presents several weeks after surface ablation, not days, and peaks over several months. The haze will improve or resolve typically over 6–12 months. Risk factors for haze include larger corrections, small optical zones, and ultraviolet exposure.

19. **c.** Excimer laser vision overcorrection is more common with older individuals, with higher corrections, and can also result from dehydration of the stromal bed during the procedure. Typically, treatments are reduced by 30%–35% when performing laser vision correction enhancements in a patient who was originally hyperopic and is now myopic.

20. **c.** Vitamin B_2 (riboflavin) serves as a source for the generation of singlet oxygen and superoxide anion free radicals, which are split from its ring structure after excitation by ultraviolet A (UVA) irradiation.

21. **b.** The UVA light used to activate riboflavin in crosslinking is toxic to corneal endothelial cells. In the presence of riboflavin, approximately 95% of the UVA light is absorbed in the anterior 300 μm of the corneal stroma. A minimum corneal thickness of 400 μm is recommended in order to prevent corneal edema from endothelial toxicity, but thinner corneas may be thickened temporarily with application of a hypotonic riboflavin formulation prior to UVA treatment.

22. **b.** While Schirmer testing may be helpful for ruling out comorbid dry eye disease in both and LASIK phakic IOL (PIOL) candidates, anterior chamber depth measurements are needed for PIOL candidates to ensure that adequate room is available for the PIOL to reduce the risk of angle crowding and damage to the endothelial cells. Specular microscopy is also routinely performed for patients before PIOL implantation. All currently FDA-approved PIOLs suggest the preoperative measurement of endothelial cell counts and are contraindicated in patients with inadequate preexisting endothelial health. All PIOLs are associated with some degree of endothelial cell loss during the implantation procedure. Ongoing assessment of anterior chamber depth and endothelial cell health is typically performed after PIOL implantation.

23. **c.** Manual keratometry and simulated keratometry values can both provide information on the amount of regular corneal astigmatism present. However, preoperative corneal topography is essential to detect irregular astigmatism and to identify patients with corneal ectatic disorders, such as keratoconus and pellucid marginal degeneration. Such disorders must be recognized preoperatively in order to determine treatment options for any residual

astigmatism. Patients with regular astigmatism are potential candidates for various treatment strategies, including toric IOLs or multifocal IOLs with bioptics, using LASIK or PRK postoperatively. However, patients with significant irregular astigmatism are not candidates for bioptics and may not be suitable for toric IOLs if the irregularity is too great.

24. **b.** Monovision can be attempted with contact lenses, LASIK, PRK, or cataract surgery. It is typically done by correcting the dominant eye for a distance focus, while the nondominant eye is the near eye with a refractive error of –1.50 to –2.50 D. Before performing a monovision refractive treatment in a patient who has never experienced monovision, the surgeon should try a trial of contact lenses with the planned monofocal correction to ensure the patient can tolerate monovision. Some patients may prefer their nondominant eye for distance, and others prefer their dominant eye. Many patients do not tolerate adequate anisometropia to allow for adequate near vision, and therefore would typically not undergo refractive surgery.

25. **c.** Patients with suboptimal results or who are dissatisfied with the quality of vision after multifocal lens implantation should first undergo a comprehensive evaluation, from the ocular surface to the macula, to rule out dry eyes, residual refractive error, irregular astigmatism, cystoid macular edema, and epiretinal membrane. Decentration of the IOL, unless significant and obvious, should not be addressed as the first-line treatment, as the intervention is invasive and may be avoidable. Nd:YAG laser capsulotomy should be considered only if other causes have been ruled out, as the opening of the capsule will then cause a significant challenge if IOL exchange becomes necessary.

26. **a.** Corneal inlays improve near vision by changing corneal curvature, increasing depth of field via a small central aperture, or changing the refractive index of the cornea.

27. **c.** To create monovision in a myopic patient, it is necessary to undercorrect 1 eye (usually the nondominant eye). The amount of desired undercorrection is determined by a combination of the patient's requirements for near vision and the amount of anisometropia that is tolerable. In a 45-year-old patient, 1.50 D is generally the appropriate amount of undercorrection for providing functional near vision without generating significant problems with anisometropia, if the nondominant eye requires correction with glasses for activities such as driving at night. This refraction allows good uncorrected distance vision in the dominant eye and good near vision in the nondominant eye. If a postoperative refraction of –1.50 D is desired in a patient who has a preoperative refraction of –5.0 D, then a correction of –3.50 D needs to be programmed into the laser. All patients being evaluated for a surgical monovision correction should initially try monovision contact lenses to ensure they can tolerate the anisometropia and visual quality of monovision and to confirm the preferred distance and near eye.

28. **d.** Dry-eye symptoms are the most common adverse effects of refractive surgery, and occasionally may persist for months or years; they have been reported in 60%–70% of all patients, to varying degrees. Corneal sensitivity decreases after LASIK because of the surgical amputation of nerves during flap formation and the destruction of superficial nerve fibers during the laser ablation. This may result in corneal anesthesia lasting 3–6 months. As a result, most patients experience a decrease in tear production. Patients who had dry eyes before surgery or whose eyes were marginally compensated before surgery more have more severe symptoms. In addition, patients with dry eyes following LASIK or surface ablation have an abnormal tear film and a poor ocular surface, and they will often note fluctuating vision between blinks and at different times of the day.

29. **d.** Although the "safe" minimum residual corneal stromal bed thickness has not been definitively established, it should not be thinner than 250 μm, as this increases the risk of corneal ectasia, unstable corneal curvature, and poor visual results. In certain cases, connective tissue and autoimmune disease are relative contraindications to refractive surgery, because these conditions can adversely affect healing. However, good results can be achieved in some patients with stable, inactive, well-controlled connective tissue and autoimmune diseases. A LASIK procedure in such patients may be considered "off-label." The potential increased risk and possible "off-label" status should be discussed with the patient and documented in the medical record.

30. **c.** Active connective tissue and autoimmune diseases are absolute contraindications to refractive surgery, because these conditions can adversely affect healing. However, good results can be achieved in some patients with stable, inactive, well-controlled connective tissue and autoimmune diseases. Surgery in such patients may be considered "off-label." The potential increased risk and possible "off-label" status should be discussed with the patient and documented in the medical record. Keratometry readings lower than approximately 34.00 D and higher than approximately 50.00 D increase the risk of poor-quality vision after refractive surgery. A patient with low myopia who has a preoperative keratometry reading of 39.00 D would probably have a postoperative keratometry reading above 34.00 D. A hyperopic patient with a preoperative keratometry reading of 46.00 D would very likely have a postoperative keratometry reading below 50.00 D. Although the "safe" minimum residual corneal stromal bed thickness has not been definitively established, it should not be thinner than 250 μm, as this increases the risk of corneal ectasia, unstable corneal curvature, and poor visual results.

31. **a.** PRK is an effective means of treating hyperopia. In patients with a history of strabismus, especially esotropia, reducing or eliminating the hyperopia should reduce accommodative convergence and decrease the tendency for esotropia. Prism correction may still be necessary following PRK in patients with strabismus. PRK will usually not significantly improve dense amblyopia. Persistent diplopia has been reported after bilateral LASIK in a patient with anisometropic amblyopia and a history of intermittent diplopia in childhood. Preoperatively, this type of patient can adjust to the disparity of the retinal image sizes with spectacle correction. Refractive surgery, however, can result in a dissimilar retinal image size that the patient cannot fuse, resulting in diplopia. Strabismus surgery may not always be indicated or possible after PRK surgery, despite the persistence or worsening of diplopia. Patients need to be warned about this possible postoperative complication.

32. **c.** The blood sugar of a diabetic patient must be well controlled at the time of examination to ensure an accurate refraction, as the refractive error may fluctuate with changes in the blood glucose level. For this reason, it is not advised to prescribe eyeglasses or contact lenses in a diabetic patient with labile blood glucose control. Elective ocular surgery should not be performed in a diabetic patient with poor or erratic blood glucose control.

33. **b.** Keratoconus is considered a contraindication to LASIK and surface ablation. Creating a LASIK flap and removing stromal tissue results in a loss of structural integrity of the cornea and increases the risk of ectasia, even if keratoconus was stable prior to treatment. It is important to diagnose forme fruste keratoconus during the screening examination for refractive surgery. Although keratoconus can be diagnosed by slit-lamp examination and manual keratometry, more sensitive analyses using corneal topography and corneal

pachymetry can reveal findings consistent with early keratoconus. No specific agreed-upon test or measurement is diagnostic of a corneal ectatic disorder, but both of these diagnostic tests should be part of the evaluation, because subtle corneal thinning or curvature changes can be overlooked on slit-lamp evaluation. The existing literature on ectasia and longitudinal studies of the fellow eye of unilateral keratoconus patients indicate that asymmetric inferior corneal steepening or asymmetric bow-tie topographic patterns with skewed steep radial axes above and below the horizontal meridian are risk factors for progression to keratoconus and post-LASIK ectasia. LASIK should not be considered in such patients, using current technology.

34. **d.** Cataract surgery performed on eyes with a history of RK frequently causes short-term flattering of the cornea and hyperopic shift due to the corneal edema common after surgery. For this reason, in the event of a refractive "surprise," an IOL exchange should not be performed in post-RK eyes until the cornea and refraction stabilize, which may take several weeks to months.

35. **b.** A post-LASIK myopic shift, especially with onset of with-the-rule astigmatism, can be a sign of post-LASIK ectasia. This patient's corneas should be evaluated for ectatic changes using topographic imaging. If ectasia is noted, further ablative treatments should be avoided, as they could lead to further decompensation of the corneal integrity. The patient should then be evaluated on an ongoing basis and considered for treatment and management of the ectasia.

36. **d.** Rigid gas-permeable (RGP) contact lenses are the gold standard for the correction of reduced vision due to ectasia. Surgical procedures that thin or destabilize the cornea (eg, LASIK, PRK, incisional procedures) are inappropriate. As ectasia may be a progressive condition, refractive lens exchange is also contraindicated. Because the contact lens fit and power can be modified as the ectasia progresses, RGP contact lenses are the most appropriate treatment. In the future, corneal crosslinking may become the treatment of choice to prevent further ectasia, but it does not improve vision as much as RGP contact lenses.

37. **a.** The SMILE method is performed entirely within a pocket, thereby avoiding the need for a flap.

Index

(*f* = figure; *t* = table)

Neodymium-doped yttrium aluminum garnet laser (Nd:YAG laser) capsulotomy, for capsule opacification with multifocal IOLs, 156, 167
Night myopia, spherical aberrations and, 12, 102
Night-vision abnormalities
    after refractive/keratorefractive surgery
        contact lens use for, 199
        phakic IOLs
            angle-supported lenses, 146
            iris-fixated lenses, 145
            multifocal lenses, 156
            posterior chamber lenses, 146
        photoablation, 102
        radial keratotomy, 51
    spherical aberrations and, 12, 102
Nocardia/Nocardia asteroides, keratitis caused by, after photoablation, 106
Nonlaser lamellar keratorefractive surgery, 8t
Nonsteroidal anti-inflammatory drugs (NSAIDs)
    after LASIK, 93
        for diffuse lamellar keratitis, 117
    after surface ablation, 92, 93–94, 108
        delayed re-epithelialization and, 93–94, 108
        sterile infiltrates and, 108
NSAIDs. *See* Nonsteroidal anti-inflammatory drugs
Nuclear cataracts, after posterior chamber phakic IOL insertion, 146
Nuclear sclerosis, refractive surgery and, 44
NuLens accommodating intraocular lens, 170

OBL. *See* Opaque bubble layer
Oblate cornea, 14, 26
    Q value and, 14
    after radial keratotomy, 50
Occupation, refractive surgery selection and, 36–37
OCT. *See* Optical coherence tomography
Ocular alignment, refractive surgery and, 41
Ocular dominance, determining, 39
Ocular history, refractive surgery evaluation and, 36t, 37–38
Ocular hypertension. *See also* Elevated intraocular pressure
    refractive surgery and, 104–105, 180–183, 182f, 200–201
Ocular motility
    assessment of, before refractive surgery, 41
    contact lens trial before refractive surgery and, 199
Ocular surface disorders, refractive surgery and, 172–173
Ocular surgery. *See* Intraocular (ocular) surgery
Off-label uses
    for conductive keratoplasty, 129
    refractive surgery in ocular and systemic disease and, 171
Onlays, corneal, 59–71. *See also* Inlays, corneal
Online post-refractive intraocular lens power calculator (ASCRS), 52, 195–197, 196f
Opaque bubble layer (OBL), femtosecond laser flap creation and, 88, 122–123
Open-angle glaucoma, primary (POAG), refractive surgery and, 180–183, 182f, 200–201
Open-loop trackers, 91
Optic nerve, evaluation of, before refractive surgery, 44
Optical aberrations. *See* Aberrations

Optical coherence tomography (OCT), 20f
    before refractive lens exchange, 149–150
Optical zone, corneal
    arcuate keratotomy and, 54–55, 56
    in photoablation, 74f
        preoperative laser programming and, 81
    pupil size and, 40
    radial keratotomy and, 50, 50f, 51
        IOL power calculations affected by, 193
Optics, of human eye
    refractive states and, 7–9
    wavefront analysis and, 9–13, 10f, 11f, 12f, 13f
Orbit, assessment of before refractive surgery, 41
Orthokeratology, 70–71
Overcorrection, with photoablation, 101–102, 108–109

Pacemakers, laser surgery in patient with, 37
Pachymetry/pachymeter, 21f, 45–46
    forme fruste keratoconus and, 176, 177f
    intraoperative, 79
    for intrastromal corneal ring segment placement, 64
    before LASIK, 79, 125, 176, 177f
        corneal perforation and, 111
    before refractive surgery, 45–46, 78, 79, 125, 176, 177f
Patient selection/preparation. *See also* Preoperative assessment/preparation for ocular surgery
    for corneal crosslinking, 131–132
    expectations/motivations and, 35–36, 36t, 47
    for LASIK, 78–80
    for monovision, 39, 165
    for multifocal IOLs, 155, 166–167
    for phakic IOLs, 140–141
    for photoablation, 77–80, 78t
    for refractive lens exchange, 147–149
    for surface ablation, 77–78
    for toric IOLs, 151
PCO. *See* Posterior capsule opacification
Pellucid marginal degeneration (PMD)
    refractive lens exchange and, 149
    refractive surgery contraindicated in, 24, 44, 79, 176, 176f
        corneal topography and, 24, 44, 45f, 79, 176, 176f
"Pellucid suspect" pattern, LASIK contraindicated in, 176, 176f
Penetrating keratoplasty (PKP). *See* Keratoplasty, penetrating
Peribulbar anesthesia, for phakic IOL insertion, 141
PERK (Prospective Evaluation of Radial Keratotomy) study, 50
Persistent corneal epithelial defects
    after LASIK, 112
    after surface ablation, 107–108
Phakic intraocular lenses (PIOLs), 8t, 137, 138–147, 139t, 142f, 143f
    advantages of, 138
    for amblyopia/anisometropic amblyopia/strabismus, 185–186, 187
    ancillary preoperative tests for, 141
    angle-supported, 137, 138, 139t, 144
        complications of, 146–147
    anterior chamber, 8t
    background of, 138
    in children, 187